D1265808

Nutrition, Diet Therapy, and the Liver

Nutrition, Diet Therapy, and the Liver

Edited by

Victor R. Preedy

Raj Lakshman

Rajaventhan Srirajaskanthan

Ronald Ross Watson

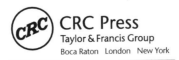

CRC Press
Taylor & Francis Group
Boca Raton   London   New York

CRC Press is an imprint of the
Taylor & Francis Group, an **informa** business

CRC Press
Taylor & Francis Group
6000 Broken Sound Parkway NW, Suite 300
Boca Raton, FL 33487-2742

© 2010 by Taylor & Francis Group, LLC
CRC Press is an imprint of Taylor & Francis Group, an Informa business

No claim to original U.S. Government works
Printed in the United States of America on acid-free paper
10 9 8 7 6 5 4 3 2 1

International Standard Book Number-13: 978-1-4200-8549-5 (Hardcover)

Library of Congress Cataloging-in-Publication Data

Nutrition, diet therapy, and the liver / edited by Victor R. Preedy ... [et al.].
    p. ; cm.
    Includes bibliographical references and index.
    ISBN-13: 978-1-4200-8549-5 (hardcover : alk. paper)
    ISBN-10: 1-4200-8549-2 (hardcover : alk. paper)
    1. Liver--Diseases--Nutritional aspects. 2. Liver--Diseases--Complications. 3. Malnutrition. I. Preedy, Victor R. II. Title.
    [DNLM: 1. Liver Diseases--therapy. 2. Diet Therapy. 3. Nutrition Therapy. WI 700 N976 2010]

RC846.N88 2010
616.3'620654--dc22
                                        2009008697

Visit the Taylor & Francis Web site at
http://www.taylorandfrancis.com

and the CRC Press Web site at
http://www.crcpress.com

Contents

SECTION I Overviews, General Nutritional Support, and Nonspecific Conditions

SECTION II Steatosis and Metabolic Liver Disease

SECTION III   Cancer, Viral, and Immune Diseases

Preface

The liver has a vital role in intermediary and whole-body metabolism. Thus, it is the major organ responsible for a whole spectrum of body functions ranging from glucose provision via the breakdown of glycogen and gluconeogenesis to the storage of vitamins; the secretion of bile; lipogenesis; lipid catabolism; the synthesis and secretion of a number of export proteins such as albumin, prothrombin, and various secretory proteins; amino acid deamination; the production of urea; the detoxification of toxins; and steroid hormone metabolism. As a consequence, any adverse effect on the liver will have devastating consequences not only on its functions but also on the functions of other tissues such as the brain and the heart. However, there are many different types of liver diseases, each with distinct etiologies and nutritional treatment regimens. Each of the facets mentioned above must be placed within the context of the particular disease under scrutiny. Nevertheless, some of the elements in a particular disease entity can be cross-transferable to some other types of liver diseases.

The understanding of liver disease and nutrition requires a holistic understanding not only of the causative elements that precipitate the disease but also the nutritional factors and regimens that reverse the deteriorating hepatic function. By implication, holistic knowledge is also gained via a broad understanding of the nutritional elements in a wide range of liver diseases. Finding this knowledge in a single coherent volume of treatise would be very vital in the treatment of liver diseases. It is precisely in this context that *Nutrition, Diet Therapy, and the Liver* addresses these aspects in a comprehensive yet succinct way.

Nutrition, Diet Therapy, and the Liver is composed of the following four sections: Overviews, General Nutritional Support, and Nonspecific Conditions; Steatosis and Metabolic Liver Disease; Cancer, Viral, and Immune Diseases; and The Young and Aging Liver, End-Stage, and Transplantation.

Contributors in the first section emphasize the fact that nutrition has an important role to play not only in the development of liver disease but also in the reversal of liver dysfunction. It is well known that mortality is significantly increased in a malnourished compared with a nourished or even an overnourished population. For example, vitamin A deficiency will lead to an exacerbation of alcoholic liver disease. Moreover, the general nutritional status of a patient with liver disease will also have a bearing on the outcome. Artificial nutritional support is also important in the treatment of patients, such as those with hepatitis, whose survival is markedly improved by enteral or parenteral feeding.

In the second section, the contributors cover various aspects of alcoholic liver disease (ALD) and nonalcoholic fatty liver disease (NAFLD) and the consequent steatohepatitis that encompasses the whole spectrum of triglyceride accumulation, inflammation, fibrosis, and, eventually, end-stage cirrhosis of the liver, which accounts for 14–20% of liver transplants worldwide. The initial stage of triglyceride accumulation leads to insulin resistance and accompanying metabolic syndrome. This leads to mitochondrial dysfunction resulting in the generation of reactive oxygen species (ROS). ROS is further increased in iron overload. ROS, in turn, causes more peroxidation of polyunsaturated fatty acids, generating more ROS, which down-regulates apolipoprotein B synthesis, which is in turn essential for exporting hepatic triglycerides in the form of very low density lipoproteins. ROS also depletes hepatic antioxidant glutathione; increases proinflammatory cytokines such as tumor necrosis factor α; suppresses adiponectin and proteasome activity; down-regulates asialoglycoprotein receptors resulting in apoptosis; leads to chemoattraction inflammatory cells to invade the liver; and activates stellate cells that produce and deposit more collagen, the hallmark of liver fibrosis. On the other hand, S-adenosylmethionine (SAMe), zinc, low levels of omega-3 fatty acids, and low-protein diets may be beneficial in the treatment of ALD and NAFLD in clinical practice, presumably by counteracting ROS and proinflammatory cytokines.

The authors of the third section focus on the mounting evidence in support of alcohol abuse, hepatitis viruses, and immune diseases as important predisposing factors in the incidence of hepatocellular carcinomas. Obviously, oxidative stress leading to ROS may be one of the major mechanisms involved in the pathogenesis of liver cancer. Therefore, dietary supplementation with antioxidants such as vitamins E and C as well as with methyl donors such as SAMe or betaine to restore liver glutathione, the natural antioxidant, may protect against alcohol-, autoimmune-, or viral-induced hepatocellular carcinomas. In addition, branched-chain amino acids and vitamins A, D, and K may also protect against hepatocarcinomas.

Finally, in the fourth section, the contributors evaluate the importance of nutrition in the treatment of liver diseases in infants versus adults, including recovery after liver transplantation. Thus, compared with the young, ROS generation within mitochondria seems to be increased with aging and may cause severe injury to mitochondrial DNA. There is also a progressive decline in the hepatic cytochrome P450 system with aging, resulting in impaired xenobiotic metabolism in the aged liver. Shortening of telomeric ends of chromosomes also correlates with aging and decline in the replicative potential of liver cell replicative senescence. Treatments with potential antioxidant cocktails including SAMe and betaine seem to show promise in recovery, even in patients with end-stage liver transplants.

The contributors to this volume are authors of international and national repute and leading experts in their respective fields. Emerging fields of science and important discoveries are also incorporated in this book and represent a one-stop shopping of material related to nutrition and the liver. *Nutrition, Diet Therapy, and the Liver* will be an essential reference book for nutritionists, dieticians, hepatologists, clinicians, health care professionals, research scientists, pathologists, molecular biologists, biochemists or cellular biochemists, and general practitioners, as well as those interested in nutrition or hepatology in general.

Editors

Victor R. Preedy is currently a professor in the Department of Nutrition and Dietetics, King's College, London. He directs studies regarding nutrition and the biochemical aspects of food health and toxicity. Dr. Preedy graduated in 1974 from the University of Aston with a combined honors degree in biology and physiology with pharmacology. He gained his PhD in nutrition and metabolism, specializing in protein turnover, in 1981. In 1992 he became a member of the Royal College of Pathologists, and in 1993 he gained a DSc degree for his outstanding contributions to protein metabolism. At the time, he was one of the university's youngest recipients of this distinguished award. Prof. Preedy was elected as a fellow to the Royal College of Pathologists in 2000. Since then he has been elected as a fellow to the Royal Society for the Promotion of Health (2004) and the Royal Institute of Public Health (2004). Prof. Preedy specializes in the field of alcohol studies within the confines of a nutrition and food environment as a senior academic member of the Department of Nutrition and Dietetics. He has published more than 550 articles, which include more than 150 peer-reviewed manuscripts based on original research and 75 reviews as well as 12 books.

Raj Lakshman is currently the deputy associate chief of staff for research and development and the chief of lipid research at the Veterans' Administration Medical Center, Washington, D.C. He also has joint appointments as a professor in the Departments of Biochemistry and Molecular Biology and in the Department of Medicine at George Washington University, Washington, D.C. He directs studies in the areas of alcoholism, alcoholic liver disease, coronary artery disease, lipids and lipoproteins, metabolic and genetic obesity, hepatotoxins, and gene regulation and expression. Dr. Lakshman earned his PhD in biochemistry from the prestigious Indian Institute of Science in 1966. He was awarded a National Research Council postdoctoral fellowship in Canada, specializing in vitamin A nutrition. He then served for 4 years as a senior research adviser at the Rockefeller Foundation, Bangkok, Thailand, after which he moved back to the United States in 1971 and worked at the Department of Physiological Chemistry, under the tutelage of Prof. John Porter and Prof. Henry Lardy, at the University of Wisconsin, making major contributions in the fields of fatty acid and cholesterol metabolism. In 1974, he joined the National Institutes of Health (NIH), where he made significant contributions in the fields of lipids and lipoproteins in relation to alcoholic hyperlipidemia under the able guidance of Prof. Richard Veech and Prof. Hans Krebs. In 1979, he received the prestigious Veterans' Administration Research Career Scientist Award while working in the field of alcohol and alcoholism at the Veterans' Administration Medical Center, Washington, D.C. He was honored with the "Washington Heart Ball" research award in 1990 in the field of hyperlipidemia. Prof. Lakshman has chaired and has been an invited speaker in several symposia in international and national meetings all over the world. He is a member of several professional societies, such as the American Society of Biochemistry and Molecular Biology, and the American Institute of Nutrition. Prof. Lakshman serves as a member of the initial review group for the evaluation of grant applications at NIH, as well as other granting agencies. He has also served as an associate editor for *Alcoholism: Clinical & Experimental Research*. He has produced more than 136 publications in peer-reviewed journals and authored several book chapters in the fields of alcohol in relation to cardioprotection, alcoholic hyperlipidemia, posttranslational modifications of proteins, alcohol biomarkers, and oxidative stress and liver injury.

Rajaventhan Srirajaskanthan trained at the prestigious Guy's, King's, and St. Thomas' School of Medicine, where he obtained his MD (MBBS) and BSc (Hons) in neuroscience with a special focus in pain pathways. His postgraduate training was undertaken at a variety of university teaching hospitals, including the John Radcliffe Hospital, Oxford, and King's College Hospital, London. During this time, he was elected as a member to the Royal College of Physicians. His specialist training has included hepatology, gastroenterology, and internal medicine. He has recently completed a two-year research fellowship in neuroendocrine tumors at the Royal Free Hospital, London. He is currently working at St. Thomas' Hospital, London, as a specialist registrar in gastroenterology and hepatology.

His academic and practical fields of interests include alcoholic liver disease, nonalcoholic steatohepatitis, metabolic syndrome, nutrition, and neuroendocrine tumors. He has been awarded numerous research prizes and presented at national and international meetings. He has published 15 peer-reviewed papers and 6 book chapters.

Ronald Ross Watson has edited 80 biomedical books, particularly in nutrition and food sciences. He presently directs or has directed several NIH-funded biomedical grants relating to dietary supplementation to modify immune function and thus cardiovascular actions in people and animal models. Prof. Watson was director of the NIH-funded Alcohol Research Center for 5 years. The main goal of the center was to understand the role of ethanol-induced immunosuppression on immune function and disease resistance in animals. He is an internationally recognized researcher, nutritionist, and immunologist. He initiated and directed other NIH-associated work at the University of Arizona College of Medicine. He is also a professor at the College of Public Health. Prof. Watson attended the University of Idaho but graduated from Brigham Young University in Provo, Utah, with a degree in chemistry in 1966. He completed his PhD in biochemistry in 1971 from Michigan State University. His postdoctoral schooling was completed at the Harvard School of Public Health in nutrition and microbiology, including a two-year postdoctoral research experience in immunology. Prof. Watson is a distinguished member of several national and international nutrition, immunology, and cancer societies and has published 450 research papers and reviews. He has a patent pending for a dietary supplement and has worked extensively for decades on the role of nutrient supplements in immune regulation; he has recently been studying Pycnogenol in heart disease therapy. He was the panel manager of the research team reviewing grants in bioactive foods for the United States Department of Agriculture.

Contributors

Mariangela Allocca
Division of Internal Medicine and Liver Unit
San Paolo Hospital School of Medicine
University of Milan
Milan, Italy

Alastair Baker
The Paediatric Liver Centre
King's College Hospital
London, United Kingdom

Bernard Campillo
Digestive Rehabilitation Service
Albert Chenevier-Henri Mondor Hospital
Creteil, France

Phunchai Charatcharoenwitthaya
Department of Medicine
Mahidol University
Bangkok, Thailand

Alan D. Cherrington
Department of Molecular Physiology and Biophysics
Vanderbilt School of Medicine
Nashville, Tennessee

Luciano D'Agostino
Department of Clinical and Experimental Medicine
"Federico II" University of Naples
Naples, Italy

Ana R. Dâmaso
Department of Biosciences
Paulista Medicine School
Federal University of São Paulo
São Paulo, Brazil

Vincent E. De Meijer
Department of Surgery and Vascular Biology
Children's Hospital Boston
Boston, Massachusetts

Aline de Piano
Multidisciplinary Obesity Research Group
Paulista Medicine School
Federal University of São Paulo
São Paulo, Brazil

Simon M. Gabe
Lennard-Jones Intestinal Failure Unit
St. Mark's Hospital
Harrow, United Kingdom
and
Division of Surgery, Oncology, Reproductive Biology and Anaesthetics
Imperial College
London, United Kingdom

Teodoro Grau
Department of Intensive Care
Hospital Universitario Doce de Octubre
Madrid, Spain

Kathleen M. Gura
Department of Pharmacy
Children's Hospital Boston
and
Harvard Medical School
Boston, Massachusetts

Daniel Gyamfi
Department of Biomedical Sciences
University of Westminster
London, United Kingdom

Mazen Issa
Division of Gastroenterology and
    Hepatology
Medical College of Wisconsin
Milwaukee, Wisconsin

Binita M. Kamath
University of Pennsylvania School of
    Medicine
and
Division of Gastroenterology,
    Hepatology, and Nutrition
The Children's Hospital of
    Philadelphia
Philadelphia, Pennsylvania

Yasunori Kawaguchi
Department of Internal Medicine
Saga University
Saga, Japan

Ralph E. Kirsch
Department of Medicine
University of Cape Town
Cape Town, South Africa

Richard Kirsch
Department of Pathology and
    Laboratory Medicine
Mount Sinai Hospital, University of
    Toronto
Toronto, Ontario, Canada

Jens Kondrup
Department of Human Nutrition
University of Copenhagen
Copenhagen, Denmark

Robin H. Lachmann
Charles Dent Metabolic Unit
National Hospital for Neurology and
    Neurosurgery
London, United Kingdom

W. Wayne Lautt
Department of Pharmacology and
    Therapeutics
University of Manitoba
Winnipeg, Manitoba, Canada

Hau D. Le
Department of Surgery and Vascular
    Biology
Children's Hospital Boston
Boston, Massachusetts

Keith D. Lindor
Division of Gastroenterology and
    Hepatology
Mayo Clinic and Foundation
Rochester, Minnesota

David A. J. Lloyd
Lennard-Jones Intestinal Failure Unit
St. Mark's Hospital
Harrow, United Kingdom

Francesco Manguso
Gastroenterology Unit
A. Cardarelli Hospital
Naples, Italy

Luis S. Marsano
Department of Medicine
University of Louisville
and
Department of Medicine
Louisville Veterans' Administration
    Medical Center
Louisville, Kentucky

Craig J. McClain
Departments of Medicine and
    Pharmacology & Toxicology
University of Louisville
Louisville, Kentucky

Marion McClain
Departments of Medicine and
  Pharmacology & Toxicology
University of Louisville
Louisville, Kentucky

Jonathan A. Meisel
Department of Surgery and Vascular
  Biology
Children's Hospital Boston
Boston, Massachusetts

Charles L. Mendenhall
Department of Medicine
Veterans Administration Medical
  Center
and
University of Cincinnati Medical Center
Cincinnati, Ohio

Zhi Ming
Department of Pharmacology and
  Therapeutics
University of Manitoba
Winnipeg, Manitoba, Canada

Toshihiko Mizuta
Department of Internal Medicine
Saga University
Saga, Japan

Juan Carlos Montejo
Department of Intensive Care
Hospital Universitario Doce de Octubre
Madrid, Spain

Mary Courtney Moore
Department of Molecular Physiology
  and Biophysics
Vanderbilt School of Medicine
Nashville, Tennessee

Amanda Muir
Department of Pediatrics
Children's Hospital of Philadelphia
Philadelphia, Pennsylvania

Helen Mundy
Department of Inherited Metabolic
  Disease
Evelina Children's Hospital
London, United Kingdom

Amin A. Nanji
Department of Pathology and
  Laboratory Medicine
Dalhousie University School of
  Medicine
Halifax, Nova Scotia, Canada

Kristina Norman
Department of Gastroenterology,
  Hepatology, and Endocrinology
Charite–University Medicine Berlin
Berlin, Germany

Vinood Patel
Department of Biomedical Sciences
University of Westminster
London, United Kingdom

Danielle Pigneri
Department of Medicine
University of Louisville
Louisville, Kentucky

Matthias Pirlich
Department of Gastroenterology,
  Hepatology, and Endocrinology
Charite–University Medicine Berlin
Berlin, Germany

Mark Puder
Department of Surgery and Vascular
  Biology
Children's Hospital Boston
Boston, Massachusetts

Elizabeth B. Rand
University of Pennsylvania School of
    Medicine
and
Division of Gastroenterology,
    Hepatology, and Nutrition
Children's Hospital of Philadelphia
Philadelphia, Pennsylvania

Kia Saeian
Division of Gastroenterology and
    Hepatology
Medical College of Wisconsin
Milwaukee, Wisconsin

Carlo Selmi
Department of Internal Medicine
Humanitas Clinical Institute
University of Milan
Milan, Italy
and
Division of Rheumatology, Allergy, and
    Clinical Immunology
University of California, Davis
Davis, California

Susumu Shiomi
Department of Nuclear Medicine
Graduate School of Medicine
Osaka City University
Osaka, Japan

Zhenyuan Song
Department of Kinesiology and
    Nutrition
College of Applied Health Sciences
University of Illinois at Chicago
Chicago, Illinois

Rajaventhan Srirajaskanthan
Department of Nutrition and Dietetics
King's College London
London, United Kingdom

Kazuyuki Suzuki
Department of Gastroenterology and
    Hepatology
Iwate Medical University
Morioka, Japan

Yasuhiro Takikawa
Department of Gastroenterology and
    Hepatology
Iwate Medical University
Morioka, Japan

Akihiro Tamori
Department of Hepatology
Graduate School of Medicine
Osaka City University
Osaka, Japan

Lian Tock
Multidisciplinary Obesity Research
    Group
Paulista Medicine School
Federal University of São Paulo
São Paulo, Brazil

Zhanxiang Zhou
Division of Gastroenterology/
    Hepatology
University of Louisville
Louisville, Kentucky

Section I

Overviews, General
Nutritional Support, and
Nonspecific Conditions

1 Liver Metabolism: Biochemical and Molecular Regulations

Daniel Gyamfi and Vinood Patel

CONTENTS

1.1 INTRODUCTION

The liver is the largest organ in the body and is involved in numerous metabolic pathways, such as the regulation of carbohydrate, lipids, and proteins. The specific functions of the liver also include steroid hormone synthesis, drug detoxification, and bilirubin conjugation (Figure 1.1). More recently, investigations have been focusing on how components of the diet, in particular fatty acids, may regulate lipogenic pathways. As a consequence, current and future research is now heavily targeting transcriptional factors that are possibly involved in these pathways. This may lead to newer drug interventions for disorders such as obesity and fatty liver disease (alcoholic and nonalcoholic).

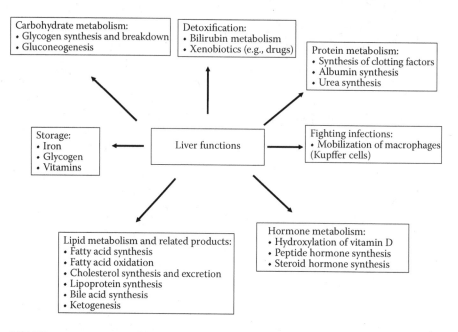

FIGURE 1.1   Main liver functions are indicated together with examples in each category.

1.2   ROLE OF THE LIVER IN CARBOHYDRATE METABOLISM

1.2.1   GLYCOGEN SYNTHESIS AND BREAKDOWN

The liver plays an important role in carbohydrate metabolism under two main conditions: absorptive (feeding) state and postabsorptive (fasting) state.

1.2.1.1   Feeding Conditions

During feeding, the absorbed intestinal glucose is transported to the liver via the hepatic portal vein. In the liver, glucose is carried across the hepatocyte membrane through glucose transporters known as glucose transporter 2. They are irresponsive to insulin and also have a very high Michaelis constant (K_m), ranging from 15 to 20 mmol/L. Thus, the rate of glucose uptake by the hepatocytes is proportional to the plasma glucose concentration. In the hepatocyte, glucose is phosphorylated to form glucose-6-phosphate (G6P) by the enzyme glucokinase. Glucokinase is a distinctive enzyme in the family of hexokinases with a high K_m for glucose and, under physiological conditions, is unaffected by its product, G6P (Figure 1.2). These characteristic features of the liver make it capable of rapidly taking up and phosphorylating glucose when the plasma glucose concentration is high and also its ability to release glucose when the need arises (as outlined below).

The synthesized G6P may be used in glycolysis, which is activated under fed conditions or fed into the pathway of glycogen synthesis. Glycogen formation in the liver is activated by insulin and glucose, which are of easy proximity to the liver

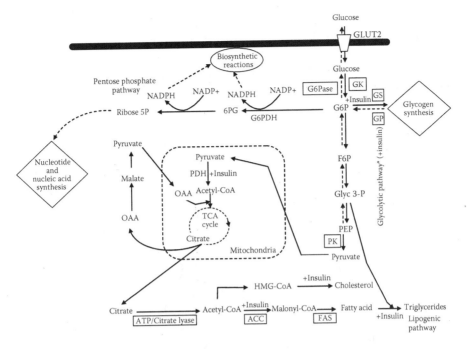

FIGURE 1.2 Glucose enters hepatocytes mainly through the glucose transporter 2 and undergoes glycolysis in the cytosol to form pyruvate. Stored liver glycogen is also broken down by the enzyme glycogen phosphorylase (GP) to glucose 6-phosphate (G6P), which can join the glycolytic and pentose phosphate pathways or be converted by the enzyme glucose 6-phosphatase (G6Pase) to produce glucose when the need arises (e.g., during fasting). Pyruvate can enter the Krebs cycle in the mitochondria via acetyl-CoA to form citrate. Citrate also enters the lipogenesis pathway via acetyl-CoA to produce triglycerides and cholesterol in the cytosol. Hormonal regulation by insulin is shown throughout. Furthermore, enzymes involved in the lipogenic pathway are induced by insulin. FAS, fatty acid synthase; F6P, fructose 6-phosphate; GK, glucokinase; Glyc 3-P, glyceraldehydes 3-phosphate; G6PD, glucose 6-phosphate dehydrogenase; GS, glycogen synthase; OAA, oxaloacetate; PK, pyruvate kinase; PEP, phosphoenol pyruvate; 6PG, 6-phosphogluconate.

due to direct secretion of insulin by the pancreas and quick delivery of intestinal glucose via the hepatic portal vein. Insulin and glucose stimulate glycogen synthesis by activating the main regulatory enzyme glycogen synthase and suppress glycogen breakdown by inhibiting the enzyme glycogen phosphorylase (GP), resulting in the final glycogen storage. On the other hand, under fed conditions, glycolysis is activated and G6P can also be used by hepatocytes to produce pyruvate, which can then enter the tricarboxylic acid (TCA) cycle or be transformed into lactate. However, evidence shows that glycogen synthesis after meals is derived from both the contribution of the pathway that directly produces glycogen from glucose, and also the indirect route, whereby glycogen is synthesized from three-carbon gluconeogenic substrates such as lactate (Nuttall, Ngo, and Gannon, 2008).

1.2.1.2 Fasting Conditions

When the concentration of glucose in the blood drops (e.g., during starvation/fasting), glycogen stored in the liver is then broken down to release glucose into the bloodstream. This process is the reverse of glycogen formation; thus, GP is activated whereas glycogen synthase is inhibited. Hormones such as glucagon, and the catecholamines adrenaline and noradrenaline, under stressful situation effect the phosphorylation of GP to cause its activation, leading to glycogenolysis. The resultant product of glycogen breakdown is glucose-1-phosphate, which is reversibly converted to G6P by the enzyme phosphoglucomutase. G6P is finally acted upon by the enzyme glucose-6-phosphatase to produce glucose (Figure 1.2) and released into the circulation.

1.2.2 GLUCONEOGENESIS

Gluconeogenesis is the synthesis of glucose from noncarbohydrate sources, and the liver is the main organ that plays an important role in this process. Gluconeogenesis resembles the direct reciprocal of glycolysis but with some significant differences at strategic points in the pathway where regulation occurs. The main substrates involved in gluconeogenesis are lactate, pyruvate, glycerol, amino acids (e.g., alanine), and intermediate metabolites of the TCA cycle.

The regulation of gluconeogenesis is under the control of two main factors: (1) regulation of the enzymes involved in the pathway by hormones and (2) rate of substrate supply (Jahoor, Peters, and Wolfe, 1990; Frayn, 2003). The hormone glucagon activates gluconeogenesis, whereas insulin inhibits it. Whenever glucagon predominates, the resultant effect is the production of G6P in the liver with the subsequent release of glucose into the bloodstream. This pattern of glucagon dominance is in resemblance of glycogenolysis. This means that the two processes happen almost at the same time but for a short term. For instance, during an overnight fast, the contribution of gluconeogenesis and glycogenolysis to overall glucose production is roughly equal (Rothman et al., 1991). However, in prolonged fasting/starvation, gluconeogenesis predominates (Landau et al., 1996).

In the case of substrate supply, postulated in the past to be a major mechanism for regulating the rate of gluconeogenesis, this pathway is enhanced when substrates are increased. One good example is after physical exercise, when lactate concentration rises in the blood, and the liver is the main organ in the body that mobilizes and converts lactate into glucose, increasing gluconeogenesis. However, several current studies performed using different gluconeogenic substrates such as amino acids, lactate, glycerol, and the monosaccharides fructose and galactose have revealed that only a small variation in glucose production occurred postabsorptively despite the increased availability of substrates (Nuttall, Ngo, and Gannon, 2008).

1.2.3 REGULATION OF BLOOD GLUCOSE LEVELS

Stable maintenance of blood glucose levels is under carefully regulated homeostatic mechanisms in the body because serious metabolic consequences will arise if this process is not tightly controlled. This is so for two main reasons: (1) the utilization of glucose by the brain as a primary fuel is imperative and (2) the toxicity of high concentrations of glucose in causing protein modification and oxidative damage (Nuttall, Ngo, and Gannon, 2008). Insulin, which plays a central role in the regulation of blood glucose, is secreted by the β cells of the Islets of Langerhans in the pancreas. Increasing levels of blood glucose stimulates insulin secretion. Also, amino acids, free fatty acids (FFAs), and ketone bodies will cause a similar effect. Insulin decreases blood glucose levels by enhancing its entrance into insulin-sensitive tissues. It also promotes glucose metabolism via glycolysis and glucose storage via glycogenesis. Under low blood glucose conditions (hypoglycemia), the hormone glucagon (secreted by the α cells of the Islets of Langerhans) is released into circulation to promote the release of glucose by stimulating glycogenolysis and gluconeogenesis (Figures 1.2 and 1.3). Other hormones with similar effects such as glucagon include adrenaline, thyroid hormones, glucocorticoids, and growth hormones.

In the longer-term regulation, insulin has been identified to have long-term effects on glucose (and lipid) metabolism through its control on the expression of specific genes involved in the metabolic pathways of glucose. In insulin-sensitive tissues, particularly in the liver, the transcription factor sterol regulatory element–binding protein 1c (SREBP-1c) mediates the insulin signal. Thus, insulin activates the transcription and proteolytic maturation of SREBP-1c, which in turn induces the expression of a family of genes involved in glucose utilization (and also fatty acid synthesis as explained in section 1.3.2.1) and as such can be considered a thrifty gene (Foufelle and Ferré, 2002; Denechaud et al., 2008). Besides the transcription factor SREBP-1c, glucose also causes the activation of the carbohydrate responsive element–binding protein (ChREBP), which stimulates the gene expression of most enzymes involved in glucose metabolism and lipogenesis (as explained in section 1.3.2.1).

1.3 ROLE OF THE LIVER IN FAT METABOLISM

The liver has both synthetic and catabolic functions in terms of fat metabolism. Its synthetic role is of more importance when fatty acids are synthesized from nonfat sources such as glucose, which, in humans, contributes a small amount to the body fatty acid pool. Mostly, dietary fatty acids are the main source of fatty acids in the body. After a meal, more than 95% of dietary fat (85–90% in infants) is absorbed by the small intestine and fed into the portal (fatty acids with fewer than 10 carbon units) or lymphatic systems to form chylomicrons (CMs), the largest group of the circulating lipoproteins (Sampath and Ntambi, 2005). Besides these CMs, very low density lipoproteins (VLDLs), packaged by the liver, and adipose tissue lipolysis, also contribute to the plasma fatty acid pool. Principally, fatty acids entering the liver either undergo oxidation or are involved in triacylglycerol (TAG) formation (Figure 1.3).

1.3.1 Fatty Acid Oxidation

In humans, the breakdown of fatty acids in the liver (also known as β oxidation) occurs in the mitochondria. It can also occur in other intracellular sites, particularly in peroxisomes, which are involved in the metabolism of a variety of fatty acids, especially very long chain fatty acids and branched-chain fatty acids (Reddy and

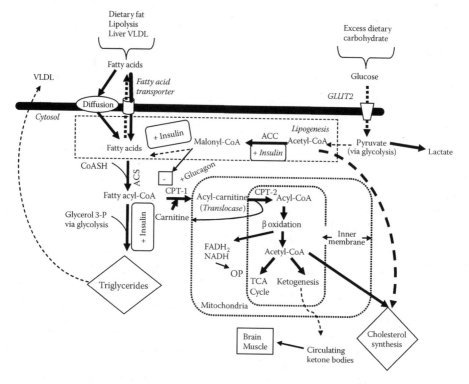

FIGURE 1.3 Fatty acid transporters carry fatty acids across the membrane into the cytosol. They can also enter via diffusion or with the assistance of specific binding proteins. Fatty acids become activated by forming a thioester bond with coenzyme A (CoASH) catalyzed by the enzyme acyl-CoA synthase (ACS) to produce fatty acyl-CoA. In conditions of excess and/or under the influence of insulin, fatty acyl-CoA will lead to triglyceride formation by the enzyme fatty acid synthase. Small- to medium-sized acyl-CoAs enter the mitochondrion for oxidation by simple diffusion, but longer ones are aided by forming acyl-carnitine derivatives by the enzyme carnitine-palmitoyl transferase 1 (CPT-1) with the subsequent formation of acyl-CoA by the inner mitochondrial membrane enzyme carnitine palmitoyl transferase 2 (CPT-2). The function of CPT-1 is inhibited by malonyl-CoA. Acyl-CoA derivatives undergo β oxidation leading to acetyl-CoA production. The fate of acetyl-CoA depends on the energy status of the cell and can (1) enter the Krebs cycle and (2) lead to the formation of ketone bodies (e.g., under conditions of starvation), which are subsequently released into the circulation and metabolized by the muscle, heart, and brain. Fatty acid oxidation also produces flavin adenine dinucleotide (reduced form) ($FADH_2$) and nicotinamide adenine dinucleotide (reduced form) (NADH), which can enter the oxidation phosphorylation (OP) pathway to produce ATP. Hormonal regulation occurs by insulin inhibiting fatty acid oxidation by activating acetyl-CoA carboxylase (ACC) to increase the production of malonyl-CoA and fatty acid esterification, whereas glucagon increases fatty acid oxidation through its action on CPT-1.

Hashimoto, 2001). There are other types of fatty acid oxidation, including α oxidation and ω oxidation by members of the cytochrome P450 4A family in the endoplasmic reticulum (microsomes). Cytochrome P450s belong to a superfamily of hemoproteins that catalyze the oxidation of endogenous and exogenous compounds, including fatty acids. These extramitochondrial fatty acid oxidation systems are essential during periods of increased influx of fatty acids into the liver. Thus, a variety of agents (known as peroxisome proliferators) such as fatty acids and fatty acid–derived molecules can stimulate peroxisome proliferation, which is associated with increased expression of genes involved in peroxisomal β oxidation. Other essential enzymes involved in fatty acid oxidation are long-chain acyl-coenzyme A (CoA) dehydrogenase, which converts long-chain fatty acids (LCFAs) to medium-chain fatty acids (MCFAs; C12–C14); medium-chain acyl-CoA dehydrogenase, which make short-chain fatty acids (SCFAs), and short-chain acyl-CoA dehydrogenase (Reddy and Hashimoto, 2001).

When the circulatory fatty acids reach the liver, they are transported across the membrane of hepatocytes by transporters (e.g., CD36 fatty acid transporters, fatty acid transport proteins) into the cytosol (Kalant and Cianflone, 2004). Within the cytosol, they bind to specific fatty acid binding proteins to effect their movements and then become activated by forming thioester link with CoA (i.e., esterification), catalyzed by the enzyme acyl-CoA synthase present in the outer mitochondrial membrane, to produce acyl-CoA derivatives of the fatty acids in question. Small- and medium-chain fatty acyl-CoA molecules (usually up to 10 carbon atoms) have the ability to cross the inner mitochondrial membrane into the matrix by diffusion, whereas longer fatty acyl-CoAs require a specialized transport mechanism as they cannot readily cross the inner mitochondrial membrane. To accomplish this, the longer fatty acyl-CoAs form a link with a polar molecule carnitine catalyzed by the enzyme carnitine palmitoyl transferase 1 (CPT-1) (located on the outer face of the inner mitochondrial membrane) resulting in the substitution of the CoA group with carnitine molecule to form acylcarnitine (Figure 1.3). With the help of the enzyme acylcarnitine translocase, the acylcarnitine is transported across the inner mitochondrial membrane into the mitochondrial matrix, where it is converted back to fatty acyl-CoA by the enzyme carnitine acyltransferase-2 (located on the matrix side of the inner mitochondrial membrane) with the release of carnitine. The fatty acyl-CoA is then degraded by the sequential removal of two-carbon units in the form of acetyl CoA from the end of the fatty acid. The acetyl CoA produced enters the TCA cycle. This pathway also results in the production of flavin adenine dinucleotide (reduced form) ($FADH_2$) and nicotinamide adenine dinucleotide (reduced form) (NADH), which feed directly into mitochondrial oxidative phosphorylation to yield energy in the form of adenosine 5′-triphosphate (ATP).

In excess, the acetyl CoA is converted into acetoacetate and 3-hydroxybutyrate via a process called ketogenesis. Acetoacetate can undergo decarboxylation to form acetone. These products, 3-hydroxybutyrate, acetoacetate, and acetone, are known as ketone bodies. They are mainly produced by the liver but cannot be reused by the liver; rather, they are released into circulation. Ketone bodies play an important physiological role as a source of energy for certain tissues such as heart muscle and kidney cortex. Also, during starvation and in diabetes, the brain can use 3-hydroxybutyrate as its main energy source (Cahill and Veech, 2003).

1.3.1.1 Regulation of Fatty Acid Oxidation

The major regulatory point of β oxidation of fatty acids is fatty acid availability. One of the main sources of FFAs in the blood is from the degradation of stored TAG in adipose tissue, which is regulated by the action of hormone-sensitive triacylglycerol lipase. Another point of regulation is the inhibition of the enzyme CPT-1 by malonyl-CoA, an intermediate of *de novo* lipogenesis. Insulin inhibits fatty acids β oxidation by first increasing the concentration of malonyl-CoA through the activation of acetyl-CoA carboxylase (ACC), and then by stimulating fatty acid esterification to form TAG. Another hormone, glucagon, is known to increase fatty acid oxidation, probably by its direct effect on CPT-1.

In longer-term regulation, peroxisomal proliferator–activated receptors (PPARs) (nuclear receptors activated by peroxisome proliferators; e.g., fatty acids, fatty acid–derived molecules) have been identified to play an important regulatory role. (For a comprehensive review, see Reddy and Hashimoto, 2001.) Members of this family include PPARα, PPARγ, and PPARδ. PPARα is mainly expressed in tissues involved in fatty acid metabolism, including the liver. Recently, it has been discovered that PPARα tightly regulates the expression of genes involved in mitochondrial and extramitochondrial fatty acid oxidation in the liver, and as such, any defect in the expression of these genes can affect the degree of hepatic fatty acid oxidation. Thus, elevated levels of plasma fatty acids lead to the activation of PPARα, which results in peroxisomal proliferation and increased expression of genes encoding for enzymes involved in fatty acid oxidation, ultimately leading to increased fatty acid oxidation (Jump et al., 1993, 1994; Reddy and Hashimoto, 2001). However, in humans, PPARα is weakly expressed and its role is not fully understood, although a number of splice variants of the isoform have been characterized (Jump and Clarke, 1999; Palmer et al., 1998).

1.3.1.1.1   *Dietary Regulation of Fatty Acid Oxidation*

Currently, for health interest, structure-dependent stimulation of fatty acid oxidation has become a point of attraction. Thus, choice of food may greatly impact the separation of dietary fat for oxidation versus retention for storage and structural utilization in humans. This is so for mainly two reasons (Jones and Kubow, 2006): (1) eating of fats associated with greater retention may increase the possibility of developing obesity; (2) the more one accumulates less oxidized fatty acids in cells, the greater the chance of occurrence of structural and functional alterations resulting from changes in membrane phospholipids fatty acid patterns or in the prostaglandin/thromboxane ratio. The effect of tissue fatty acid composition on functional capability, for instance, insulin sensitivity, is well known (Clandinin et al., 1993).

Clinically, consumption of SCFAs and MCFAs leads to increase in energy production, likely due to the direct movement of SCFAs and MCFAs from the intestine to the liver via the hepatic portal vein. Moreover, SCFAs are rapidly oxidized because of their transport by diffusion into the mitochondria. For LCFAs, polyunsaturated FAs (PUFAs), especially n-6 and n-3, are preferentially oxidized for energy than saturated FAs (Jones and Kubow, 2006).

1.3.2   LIPID SYNTHESIS

Depending on the energy status, another fate of fatty acids upon arrival in the liver is their esterification to form TAG, stored within the hepatocytes as a reserved energy for the liver but also subsequently secreted into the circulation as VLDLs, which contributes to the body fatty acid pool.

The liver can synthesize lipids from nonlipid precursors such as glucose (pathway commonly known as *de novo* lipogenesis) in the cytosol through acetyl-CoA (Figure 1.2). Acetyl-CoA, a product of pyruvate (e.g., from glycolysis or amino acid catabolism), is synthesized in the mitochondria. Since the inner mitochondrial membrane is impermeable to acetyl-CoA transport into the cytosol, entry is achieved by its conversion into citrate via the enzyme citrate synthase. In the cytosol, the citrate is broken down by ATP/citrate lyase to regenerate the acetyl-CoA, where it is carboxylated by the enzyme ACC to form malonyl CoA. Fatty acid synthesis proceeds from the intermediates of acetyl-CoA and malonyl CoA by successive addition of two-carbon units facilitated by the enzyme fatty acid synthase. The synthesized fatty acids may combine with glyceraldehyde 3-phosphate (an intermediate of glycolysis) to form TAG and phospholipids.

1.3.2.1 Regulation of Lipid Synthesis

Fatty acid synthesis occurs in the fed state, when carbohydrate and energy sources are in abundance. The main enzyme involved in the regulation of fatty acid synthesis is ACC, which synthesizes malonyl CoA, the committed step in the metabolic pathway. ACC is inactivated by phosphorylation via the enzyme adenosine 5′-monophosphate (AMP)–activated protein kinase (which is activated by AMP and inhibited by ATP). However, ACC is activated via dephosphorylation by the enzyme protein phosphatase 2A (PP2A). At low cellular energy (i.e., when the AMP/ATP ratio is high), the kinase is activated, which then inactivates ACC, and fatty acid synthesis is switched off.

ACC is also under hormonal regulation. In a well-fed state, insulin levels become elevated and stimulate ACC, leading to high levels of malonyl CoA (which, in turn, inhibits fatty acids oxidation) (Figure 1.3), which finally promotes fatty acid synthesis and storage. In situations where energy is required, glucagon and epinephrine inhibit the activity of PP2A, leading to prevention of ACC activation and blocking of fatty acid synthesis.

In longer-term regulation, *de novo* lipogenesis is nutritionally regulated, and recently it has been discovered that both glucose and insulin signaling pathways are involved, in response to dietary carbohydrates, to synergistically induce glycolytic and lipogenic gene expression (Figure 1.4) and not insulin alone (Denechaud et al., 2008). Insulin acts by activating SREBP-1c, an important transcription factor that regulates a number of genes promoting lipogenesis. SREBP-1c is synthesized as a precursor in the membranes of the endoplasmic reticulum and requires posttranslational modification to produce a transcriptionally active nuclear form. Thus, insulin promotes the synthesis and posttranslational modification/maturation of SREBP-1c, which subsequently enhances the expression of lipogenic genes, such as acetyl CoA carboxylase, fatty acid synthase, and stearoyl-CoA desaturase-1 (Foufelle and Ferré, 2002). It has been identified that SREBP-1c alone cannot cause the activation of glycolytic and lipogenic gene expression in response to dietary carbohydrate because studies in SREBP-1c gene deletion mice only led to a 50% reduction in fatty acid synthesis (Liang et al., 2002; Denechaud et al., 2008). Also, it has been

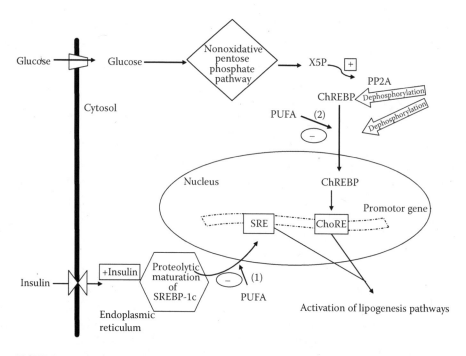

FIGURE 1.4 Under high glucose concentration, xylulose 5-phosphate, an intermediate of the nonoxidative branch of the pentose phosphate pathway, stimulates the enzyme protein phosphatase 2A to cause the activation of ChREBP via double dephosphorylation (i.e., before and after entry into the nucleus). Activated ChREBP then binds to the ChoRE binding site of its promoter gene, in the nucleus leading to transcriptional activation of lipogenic genes. Insulin also activates the proteolytic maturation of SREBP-1c in the endoplasmic reticulum and its attachment to the sterol regulatory element (SRE) binding site of its promoter gene, causing an increase in lipogenic gene expression. Polyunsaturated fatty acids inhibit lipogenesis by (1) reducing SRE gene transcription and increasing the proteolytic degradation of mRNA SREBP-1C (Jump et al., 2005) and (2) inhibiting ChREBP nuclear translocation (Dentin et al., 2006). ChREBP, carbohydrate responsive element-binding protein; ChoRE, carbohydrate responsive element; SREBP-1c, sterol regulatory element–binding protein 1c.

shown that the activity of L-pyruvate kinase, one of the rate-limiting enzymes of glycolysis, is entirely under the control of glucose (Decaux et al., 1989) and not under SREBP-1c regulation (Stoeckman and Towle, 2002). The nature of the glucose-signaling compound was not known until recently and has been identified to be a glucose-responsive transcription factor named ChREBP (Yamashita et al., 2001; Uyeda and Repa, 2006). ChREBP is a large protein of nearly 100 kDa (864 amino acids) having several domains such as a nuclear localization signal near the N terminus, polyproline domains, a basic loop-helix-leucine zipper, and a leucine-zipper-like domain (Postic et al., 2007; Denechaud et al., 2008). Thus, glucose acts through its intermediate, xylulose 5-phosphate (X5P) (from the nonoxidative branch of the pentose phosphate pathway), to cause the activation of the enzyme PP2A, which subsequently activates ChREBP via dephosphorylation where it now moves from the cytosol into the nucleus, where through another dephosphorylation cycle by PP2A it allows ChREBP to bind to the carbohydrate responsive element (ChoRE) present in the promoter regions of glycolytic and lipogenic genes (Ishii et al., 2004; Postic et al., 2007) (Figure 1.4). Therefore, in excess carbohydrate (i.e., when liver glycogen storage is full to capacity), the liver converts glucose to fat to control blood glucose and prevent hyperglycemia.

1.4 SUMMARY POINTS

The liver plays a central role in many metabolic processes to address the energy needs of the body (Figure 1.5).

Liver glucose is stored as glycogen (via glycogenesis) from high dietary carbohydrate under the influence of insulin; glucose release from glycogen (via glycogenolysis) occurs via glucagon stimulation when the blood glucose concentration falls, whereas insulin inhibits this process.

When glycogen stores are exhausted (e.g., during starvation), the liver synthesizes glucose from other carbohydrate sources such as lactate and glycerol through the pathway gluconeogenesis. This is under the control of hormones, such as glucagons, and substrate availability.

Fatty acids are either oxidized via β oxidation to generate energy or stored as triglycerides by the liver. Fatty acid oxidation is enhanced by fatty acid availability, which triggers PPARα to increase expression of the enzymes involved in this pathway and possibly also by glucagon, but oxidation is inhibited by insulin.

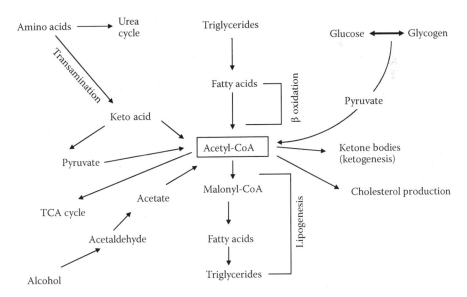

FIGURE 1.5 Summary of the main metabolic pathways leading to acetyl-CoA formation and possible metabolic products.

Fatty acids can also be synthesized in the cytosol by the liver from nonlipids such as glucose via *de novo* lipogenesis. Besides hormonal regulation (e.g., by insulin), this pathway is also activated by glucose via ChREBP and insulin via SREBP-1c.

REFERENCES

Cahill, G. F., and R. L. Veech. 2003. Ketoacids? Good medicine? *Trans Am Clin Climatol Assoc* 114:149–163.

Clandinin, M. T., S. Cheema, C. J. Field, and V. E. Baracos. 1993. Dietary lipids influence insulin action. *Ann N Y Acad Sci* 683:151–163.

Decaux, J. F., B. Antoine, and A. Kahn. 1989. Regulation of the expression of the L-type pyruvate kinase gene in adult rat hepatocytes in primary culture. *J Biol Chem* 264: 11584–11590.

Denechaud, P.-D., R. Dentin, J. Girard, and C. Postic. 2008. Role of ChREBP in hepatic steatosis, and insulin resistance. *FEBS Lett* 582:68–73.

Dentin, R., P.-D. Denechaud, F. Benhamed, J. Girard, and C. Postic. 2006. Hepatic gene regulation by glucose and polyunsaturated fatty acids: A role for ChREBP. *J Nutr* 136:1145–1149.

Foufelle, F., and P. Ferré. 2002. New perspectives in the regulation of hepatic glycolytic and lipogenic genes by insulin and glucose: A role for the transcription factor sterol regulatory element binding protein–1c. *Biochem J* 366:377–391.

Frayn, K. N. 2003. *Metabolic regulation: A human perspective.* Oxford: Blackwell Science Limited.

Ishii, S., K. Iizuka, B. C. Miller, and K. Uyeda. 2004. Carbohydrate response element binding protein directly promotes lipogenic enzyme gene transcription. *Proc Natl Acad Sci U S A* 101:15597–15602.

Jahoor, F., E. J. Peters, and R. R. Wolfe. 1990. The relationship between gluconeogenic substrate supply and glucose production in humans. *Am J Physiol* 258:E288–E296.

Jones, P. J. H., and S. Kubow. 2006. Lipids, sterols and their metabolites. In: *Modern nutrition in health and disease*, ed. M. E. Shils, M. Shike, A. C. Ross, B. Caballero, and R. J. Cousins. Philadelphia: Lippincott Williams and Wilkins.

Jump, D. B., D. Botolin, Y. Wang, J. Xu, B. Christian, and O. Demeure. 2005. Fatty acid regulation of hepatic gene transcription. *J Nutr* 135:2503–2506.

Jump, D. B., and S. D. Clarke. 1999. Regulation of gene expression by dietary fat. *Annu Rev Nutr* 19:63–90.

Jump, D. B., S. D. Clarke, O. A. MacDougald, and A. T. Thelen. 1993. Polyunsaturated fatty acids inhibit S14 gene transcription in rat liver and cultured hepatocytes. *Proc Natl Acad Sci U S A* 90:8454–8458.

Jump, D. B., S. D. Clarke, A. T. Thelen, and M. Liimata. 1994. Coordinate regulation of glycolytic and lipogenic gene expression by polyunsaturated fatty acids. *J Lipid Res* 35:1076–1084.

Kalant, D., and K. Cianflone. 2004. Regulation of fatty acid transport. *Curr Opin Lipidol* 15:309–314.

Landau, B. R., R. Wahren, V. Chandramouli, W. C. Schumann, and K. Ekberg. 1996. Contributions of gluconeogenesis to glucose production in the fasted state. *J Clin Invest* 98:378–385.

Liang, G., J. Yang, J. D. Horton, R. E. Hammer, J. L. Goldstein, and M. S. Brown. 2002. Diminished hepatic response to fasting/refeeding and liver X receptor agonists in mice with selective deficiency of sterol regulatory element–binding protein–1c. *J Biol Chem* 277:9520–9258.

Nuttall, F. Q., A. Ngo, and M. C. Gannon. 2008. Regulation of hepatic glucose production and the role of gluconeogenesis in humans: Is the rate of gluconeogenesis constant? *Diabetes Metab Res Rev* 24:438–458.

Palmer, C. N., M. H. Hsu, K. J. Griffin, J. L. Rauchy, and E. F. Johnson. 1998. Peroxisome proliferators activated receptor–alpha expression in human liver. *Mol Pharmacol* 53:14–22.

Postic, C., R. Dentin, P. Denechaud, and J. Girard. 2007. ChREBP, a transcriptional regulator of glucose and lipid metabolism. *Annu Rev Nutr* 27:179–192.

Reddy, J. K., and T. Hashimoto. 2001. Peroxisomal β-oxidation and peroxisome proliferator–activated receptor α: An adaptive metabolic system. *Annu Rev Nutr* 21:193–230.

Rothman, D. L., I. Magnusson, L. D. Katz, R. G. Shulman, and G. I. Shulman. 1991. Quantitation of hepatic glycogenolysis and gluconeogenesis in fasting humans with ^{13}C NMR. *Science* 254:573–576.

Sampath, H., and J. M. Ntambi. 2005. Polyunsaturated fatty acid regulation of genes of lipid metabolism. *Annu Rev Nutr* 25:317–340.

Stoeckman, A. K., and H. C. Towle. 2002. The role of SREBP-1c in nutritional regulation of lipogenic enzyme gene expression. *J Biol Chem* 277:27029–27035.

Uyeda, K., and J. J. Repa. 2006. Carbohydrate response element binding protein, ChREBP, a transcription factor coupling hepatic glucose utilization and lipid synthesis. *Cell Metab* 4:107–110.

Yamashita, H., M. Takenoshita, M. Sakurai, R. K. Bruick, W. J. Henzel, W. Shillinglaw, D. Arnot, and K. Uyeda. 2001. A glucose-responsive transcription factor that regulates carbohydrate metabolism in the liver. *Proc Natl Acad Sci U S A* 98:9116–9121.

2 Regulation of Hepatic Metabolism by Enteral Delivery of Nutrients

Mary Courtney Moore and Alan D. Cherrington

CONTENTS

2.1 RESPONSE OF THE LIVER TO A GLUCOSE LOAD

The liver is known to play an important role in the disposal of a glucose load, but exact measurements of the liver's contribution in humans is hampered by methodological and ethical concerns regarding portal vein blood sampling under most conditions. Human studies using splanchnic balance measurements and tracer techniques indicate that the liver disposes approximately 25–35% of an oral glucose load (Ferrannini et al., 1985; Mari et al., 1994). Direct assessment of net hepatic glucose uptake (NHGU) during oral or enteral delivery of glucose in the dog has yielded data remarkably consistent with estimates from the human (Ishida et al., 1983; Moore et al., 1991). The canine liver accounted for the disposition of 25–40% of the administered glucose, with the exact percentage being largely determined by the load of glucose and insulin reaching the liver.

2.1.1   ENTERAL OR INTRAPORTAL GLUCOSE DELIVERY: THE PORTAL SIGNAL

Peripheral venous glucose infusion, even in the presence of marked hyperinsuline-mia and hyperglycemia, does not result in as high a rate of NHGU as the infusion of a similar amount of glucose via the hepatic portal vein (Moore et al., 2000). The ability of combined changes in insulin and glucose to cause greater hepatic glucose uptake when they are associated with oral glucose delivery led DeFronzo et al. (1978) to propose the existence of a gut factor that augments NHGU after administration of an oral glucose load. However, several independent investigations in dogs produced hyperglycemia via an intraportal glucose infusion that mimicked the absorption of oral glucose. In these studies, NHGU was not different after intraportal and oral glucose entry, ruling out a gut factor and strongly suggesting that the liver responds differently to portally delivered glucose than it does to peripherally delivered glu-cose. Studies in which pancreatic hormone concentrations and the load of glucose reaching the liver were maintained equivalent with the two delivery routes conclu-sively demonstrated that entry of glucose into the portal vein significantly stimu-lated NHGU and hepatic glycogen synthesis, in comparison to glucose delivery via a peripheral vein (Figure 2.1A and B) (Myers et al., 1991b; Pagliassotti et al., 1996). The rate of NHGU during portal glucose infusion was determined to be inversely related to the magnitude of the arterial-portal (A-P) vein glucose gradient (Figure 2.1C). Thus, a "portal signal," rather than a gut factor, is responsible for enhancement of NHGU during oral, enteral, or portal venous glucose delivery.

The effects of the portal signal are not limited to the liver. One study conducted in the mouse indicated that portal glucose delivery at a rate similar to that of basal endogenous hepatic glucose output stimulated whole body glucose disposal suffi-ciently to induce hypoglycemia (Burcelin et al., 2000). Portal glucose delivery in this model increased glucose uptake by the heart, brown adipose tissue, and soleus muscle, but not the liver. However, these data could not be replicated in the mouse by other investigators (Chueh et al., 2006), and virtually all data demonstrate that the portal signal does not enhance whole body glucose clearance (e.g., Pagliassotti et al., 1996; Vella et al., 2002). Instead, nonhepatic glucose uptake, especially that in skeletal muscle glucose, is suppressed in the presence of the portal signal (Galassetti et al., 1998). As a result of its reciprocal actions, the portal signal ensures that a glu-cose load is appropriately distributed between the skeletal muscle, the liver, and the other tissues of the body.

Although the portal signal has been demonstrated to operate in species other than the dog, the importance of the route of glucose delivery in humans has been more difficult to evaluate because of the inability to catheterize the portal vein and the dif-ficulty in controlling the insulin and glucagon levels reaching the liver. Intraduodenal glucose enhanced hepatic glucose extraction by 40–125% over that evident during peripheral intravenous (IV) glucose infusion in a human study in which a pancreatic clamp was used to fix the insulin and glucagon concentrations (Vella et al., 2002). Whole body glucose kinetics in humans did not differ between IV and intraduodenal glucose delivery (Fery et al., 2001), consistent with findings in the mouse and dog (Chueh et al., 2006; Pagliassotti et al., 1996). In summary, evidence strongly sug-gests that the portal signal functions in humans, but definitive data are unavailable.

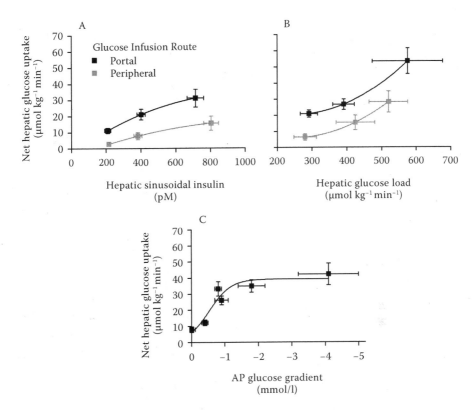

FIGURE 2.1 Net hepatic glucose uptake (NHGU) during portal or peripheral glucose delivery in the presence of a range of physiological plasma insulin concentrations and hepatic glucose loads, and the effect of a negative arterial-portal (A-P) glucose gradient on NHGU. In the presence of physiological (A) plasma insulin concentrations and (B) hepatic glucose loads, NHGU is approximately twofold to threefold greater with portal versus peripheral glucose infusion. (C) NHGU during portal glucose delivery is linearly associated with the magnitude of the negative A-P gradient (the amount that the portal vein concentration exceeds that in the artery), up to ≈1 mmol/l. Data are mean ± SEM, $n = 6$–7/group. The line of best fit for the data in each plot is shown. (Panels A and B are from Myers, S. R., Biggers, D. W., Neal, D. W., et al., *J Clin Invest*, 88, 158–167, 1991; Myers, S. R., McGuinness, O. P., Neal, D. W., et al., *J Clin Invest*, 87, 930–939, 1991. With permission. Data from panel C is derived from Pagliassotti, M. J., Myers, S. R., Moore, M. C., et al., *Diabetes*, 40, 1659–1668, 1991.)

2.1.2 MEDIATORS OF THE PORTAL GLUCOSE SIGNAL

2.1.2.1 Humoral Mediators

The mediator or mediators of the portal signal are unclear as yet, but possible candidates are humoral agents and/or neural networks. Lautt (2004) hypothesized that whole body insulin sensitivity, particularly that of the skeletal muscle, is modulated by the hepatic insulin sensitizing substance (HISS), a humoral factor released by the liver after the generation of nitric oxide (NO) in response to parasympathetic signaling in the presence of hyperinsulinemia. Most studies on HISS actions have been carried out in the euglycemic state, when the liver plays little role in glucose disposal. However, NHGU in dogs during a hyperinsulinemic hyperglycemic clamp in the presence of the portal signal was significantly reduced by intraportal infusion of the NO donor 3-morpholinosydnonimine (SIN-1) (An et al., 2008). Conversely, NHGU was stimulated by intraportal infusion of the NO synthase inhibitor N_ω-nitro-L-arginine methyl ester under hyperinsulinemic hyperglycemic conditions during peripheral glucose delivery (Moore et al., 2008). Murine studies suggested that glucagon-like peptide 1 (GLP-1) might mediate the portal signal (Burcelin et al., 2001), but this is unlikely, given that portal glucose infusion does not stimulate the release of GLP-1 (Johnson et al., 2007).

2.1.2.2   Neural Mediators

Both the sympathetic and parasympathetic nervous systems are involved in regulation of hepatic glucose metabolism (Shimazu, 1987). Complete surgical denervation of the liver blocked the enhancement of NHGU during portal glucose infusion in the dog (Adkins-Marshall et al., 1992), and hepatic vagotomy in the rat reduced hepatic glucose uptake and glycogen accumulation during portal glucose infusion by 40% and 55%, respectively (Matsuhisa et al., 2000). Afferent signals from the hepatoportal region are conducted to the hypothalamus by the vagus nerve, with the afferent firing rate in the hepatic branch of the vagus being inversely proportional to the D-glucose concentration in the portal vein (Niijima, 1982). Whether the vagus nerve carries the afferent limb of the portal signal, however, is as yet unclear. Cooling the vagus nerves to halt neural firing did not inhibit the response to the portal signal in dogs (Cardin et al., 2004), and bilateral cervical vagotomy in rats did not prevent changes in firing in lateral hypothalamic neurons in response to portal glucose injection (Schmitt, 1973). Other pathways could be responsible for communicating data regarding hepatoportal glucose levels to the brain, including splanchnic (Schmitt, 1973) or spinal (Berthoud, 2004) afferents. Alternative possibilities for the mediation of the portal signal include an intrahepatic reflex, as suggested by studies in the neurally isolated liver (Niijima, 1984; Stumpel and Jungermann, 1997), and/or a spinal reflex, analogous to that reported to stimulate hepatic glucose output in hypoglycemia (Fujita et al., 2007).

An efferent neural pathway for the actions of the portal signal also remains undefined. Atropine blocked the effect of the portal glucose signal in the perfused rat liver (Stumpel and Jungermann, 1997), although results from cultured hepatocytes indicate that acetylcholine is permissive of insulin action but is unlikely to bring about the marked, rapid effects of the portal signal (Hampson and Agius, 2007). Thus, the parasympathetic nervous system, or at least acetylcholine, seems unlikely to be involved in the enhancement of NHGU by the portal glucose signal. Selective hepatic sympathectomy enhanced NHGU approximately 70% during IV glucose infusion but did not affect NHGU during portal glucose infusion, suggesting that the sympathetic innervation might exert a tonic inhibition of glucose uptake that is relieved by portal glucose delivery (Dicostanzo et al., 2006). The liver contains nitrergic nerves, and modulation of hepatic NO levels alters NHGU, as discussed above. Thus, the release of NO by these nerves might also be involved in the regulation of NHGU.

The pathway or pathways bringing about the nonhepatic response to the portal signal also remain undefined. Electrical stimulation of the ventromedial hypothalamus enhances muscle glucose uptake, an effect that can be prevented with sympathetic blockade (Minokoshi et al., 1994). In addition to receiving neural signals from the periphery, the hypothalamus is sensitive to circulating hormones and substrates, including insulin and glucose (Perrin et al., 2004; Schmitt, 1973). Both insulin and glucose modulate the phosphorylation of cerebral AMP-activated protein kinase (AMPK), which can play a role in the regulation of muscle glucose disposal (Perrin et al., 2004). Thus, although numerous possibilities exist in regard to the identities of the afferent and efferent limbs associated with the portal glucose signal, it is unclear at present which are key to the response.

2.2   HEPATIC PROTEIN METABOLISM: EFFECT OF DIETARY AMINO ACIDS

The splanchnic bed (liver and gastrointestinal tract) accounts for 25% of whole body protein synthesis (Barle et al., 1997). Dietary amino acids (AAs) are the preferential source of substrate for small intestine and hepatic protein synthesis, and AA uptake by the liver is tightly coupled to the gastrointestinal release of AAs. The dietary requirements for lysine, methionine, leucine, valine, isoleucine, and threonine in piglets (based on the indicator AA oxidation technique) are lower with total parenteral nutrition than with enteral nutrition (Burrin and Davis, 2004), demonstrating the increased demand for AAs by the digestive tract, pancreas, and liver in orally or enterally fed animals.

2.2.1   AA AVAILABILITY AND AA SIGNALING

A number of studies in healthy humans indicate that increasing AA levels result in an increase in albumin and/or splanchnic protein synthesis and a decrease in hepatic protein breakdown (e.g., Nygren and Nair, 2003). However, in other human (Ballmer et al., 1995) and animal (e.g., Mosoni et al., 1993) investigations, no effect of AA delivery on hepatic protein synthesis has been observed, leading to the suggestion that most of the AAs extracted by the liver undergo catabolism or are involved in suppressing tissue catabolism (Mosoni et al., 1993). The discrepant results likely reflect the differences in experimental design, as the studies varied in numerous respects, including the route of AA delivery (oral/enteral vs. IV), circulating AA concentrations, postprandial versus postabsorptive conditions, and insulin concentrations. Few of the reports included glucagon concentrations; when glucagon was reported, it differed among treatments (Nygren and Nair, 2003). Despite the conflicting results *in vivo*, AA levels comparable to postprandial portal blood concentrations stimulated synthesis of 16 specific liver proteins, including albumin, in isolated hepatocytes (Jaleel and Nair, 2004).

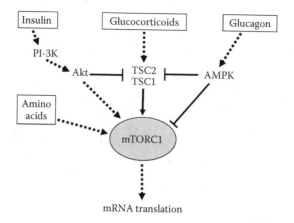

FIGURE 2.2 Signaling through the mammalian target of rapamycin complex 1 (mTORC1). mTORC1 is involved in the regulation of anabolic processes such as mRNA translation and cell growth. In turn, the activity of mTORC1 is impacted by a number of factors, including nutrient availability [i.e., amino acids (AAs), particularly leucine], pancreatic hormones, and glucocorticoids. Dotted lines indicate multistep processes with intermediate steps omitted. Akt is also known as protein kinase B (PKB). TSC, tuberous sclerosis complex (or tuberin-hamartin). AMPK, AMP-activated protein kinase.

Protein synthesis, or mRNA translation, is a highly complex process requiring a number of initiation and elongation factors extrinsic to the ribosome. The mammalian target of rapamycin complex 1 (mTORC1) is a protein kinase that directly or indirectly controls the activity of several of the initiation and elongation factors (Kimball and Jefferson, 2006). mTORC1, in turn, is regulated by multiple inputs, including hormonal changes and nutrient (amino acids) availability (Figure 2.2). Branched-chain AAs, particularly leucine, are especially important regulators of mTORC1.

2.2.1.1 Protein Synthesis and the Route of AA Delivery

Concomitant intraportal glucose and AA infusions resulted in a blunting of NHGU, in comparison to glucose delivered without AAs (Moore et al., 1998). The data further suggested that AA utilization for protein synthesis might be increased by portal AA delivery. This raised the question of whether intraportally delivered AAs might generate a signal, similar to the portal glucose signal, that would stimulate their uptake and utilization by the liver.

The rate of hepatic protein synthesis was quantified in the conscious dog during portal or peripheral delivery of an AA mixture that reproduced the normal elevation of AAs in the portal vein in the postprandial state (Dardevet et al., 2008). Insulin and glucagon were clamped at normal physiological postprandial levels, that is, fourfold and threefold basal, respectively, and glucose was infused via peripheral vein to maintain the hepatic glucose load 50% above the fasting level. In one group, a mixture of 20 AAs was infused intravenously to maintain postabsorptive plasma AA levels, since hyperinsulinemia normally brings about a drop in AA concentrations, and in two other groups, the mixture was infused either intravenously or intraportally to increase the hepatic load of each AA approximately twofold basal, mimicking postprandial concentrations. Although the hepatic AA loads were well matched in the latter two groups, the net hepatic uptakes of most AAs were significantly greater during portal AA infusion (Figure 2.3). Synthesis of both albumin and resident hepatic proteins was enhanced by portal AA delivery. A negative A-P AA gradient (portal vein concentration greater than that in the artery) was most closely associated with enhancement of protein synthesis (Figure 2.4).

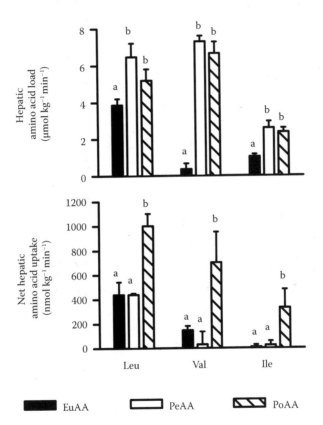

FIGURE 2.3 Net hepatic uptake of AAs is increased by intraportal AA delivery. Conscious dogs were studied during a pancreatic clamp, with insulin and glucagon infused at fourfold and threefold basal rates, respectively, and the hepatic glucose load increased to 1.5-fold basal by peripheral glucose infusion. A mixture of 20 AAs was delivered via a peripheral vein or the hepatic portal vein to maintain euaminoacidemia (EuAA) or to increase the hepatic load of each AA twofold basal via peripheral (PeAA) or portal vein (PoAA) infusion (top panel). Net hepatic uptakes of most AAs, including leucine, valine, and isoleucine, were enhanced during portal AA infusion (bottom panel). Bars with the same letters are not significantly different from each other. Data are mean ± SEM, n = 9/group. (From Dardevet et al., *Am J Clin Nutr*, 88, 986–996, 2008. With permission.)

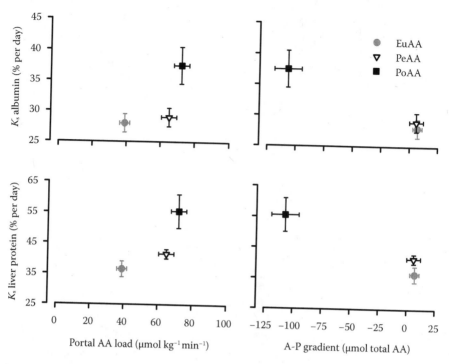

FIGURE 2.4 Hepatic protein synthesis is stimulated by portal AA delivery. The fractional synthetic rates (K_s) of albumin (top panels) and resident liver proteins (bottom panels) were significantly increased by portal AA delivery. This was not due to differences in the total hepatic AA load (not shown) or portal AA load (left panels). K_s increased significantly in the presence of a negative A-P AA gradient (right panels). Data are mean ± SEM, n = 9/group. EuAA, AA infused via peripheral vein to maintain euaminoacidemia; PeAA and PoAA, AAs infused via peripheral and portal vein, respectively, to increase the hepatic load of each AA twofold. (Data derived from Dardevet et al., *Am J Clin Nutr*, 88, 986–996, 2008.)

2.2.1.1.1 *Portal AA Signal: Potential Neural Involvement*

An "amino acid signal" resulting from dietary or portal delivery of AAs and impacting hepatic protein metabolism could be neurally mediated. Hepatoportal sensors for at least 15 different AAs modulate the afferent firing rate of the hepatic branch of the vagus nerve (Niijima and Meguid, 1995). Moreover, the syntheses of transferrin (Watanabe et al., 1990) and tyrosine transferase (Black and Reis, 1971a, 1971b) by the liver are neurally regulated. Either hepatic branch vagotomy or selective hepatic sympathetic denervation retards liver regeneration after partial hepatectomy in the rat (Sakaguchi and Liu, 2002; Xia et al., 2006). Regulation of protein synthesis in liver and muscle is similar in many respects, and neural stimuli in muscle can modulate signaling through mTORC1 (e.g., Thomson et al., 2008). Thus, there is evidence for neural control of protein synthesis, but the role of the autonomic nervous system remains incompletely defined.

2.3   PORTAL VEIN LIPIDS: IMPACT ON HEPATIC
AND WHOLE BODY METABOLISM

The liver is the site of formation of very low density lipoproteins (VLDLs), the synthesis of which is determined in part by the supply of substrates—triglycerides, free fatty acids (FFAs), and cholesterol ester. FFA concentrations normally fall during the postprandial period, and splanchnic and net hepatic FFA uptakes decline correspondingly. However, FFA concentrations in individuals with type 2 diabetes remain higher than in nondiabetic controls (Reaven, 2005).

Elevated circulating FFA impair insulin-mediated suppression of endogenous glucose production under euglycemic conditions (Homko et al., 2003). Interestingly, the reduction in net splanchnic glucose uptake after glucose or meal ingestion observed in patients with type 2 diabetes is primarily due to an increase in splanchnic glucose output, relative to that in normal volunteers, rather than to an impairment of splanchnic glucose uptake (Ludvik et al., 1997; Woerle et al., 2006). Therefore, the effect of preventing the normal postprandial decline in FFAs on hepatic glucose disposal was examined (Moore et al., 2004). When dogs were studied during a hyperinsulinemic hyperglycemic clamp in the presence of the portal signal, infusion of a lipid emulsion to prevent the normal fall in FFAs reduced NHGU by more than 50% (Figure 2.5), and this was due almost entirely to impaired suppression of endogenous glucose R_a, and not a defect in hepatic glucose uptake. Both hepatic glucose oxidation and hepatic glycolysis were reduced during lipid infusion (Figure 2.5), however, and as a consequence, glycogen synthesis was not suppressed in the presence of elevated FFAs.

2.3.1   VISCERAL AND INTRAPORTAL LIPID AND THE LIVER

Visceral adipose tissue releases FFAs into the portal vein, and suppression of lipolysis in the visceral adipose is poorly responsive to insulin. Visceral adiposity has been implicated in the development of inflammation and steatohepatitis (reviewed by Schäffler et al., 2005). Omentectomy at the time of adjustable gastric banding in humans was associated with improved insulin sensitivity 2 years later, compared with gastric banding alone (Thorne et al., 2002). In Zucker fatty rats, omentectomy at the time of gastric banding did not reduce body weight, insulin resistance, or plasma glucose or triglyceride concentrations 8 weeks later, in comparison to gastric banding alone; however, it significantly decreased plasma FFA levels and increased adiponectin mRNA expression in visceral adipose tissue, suggesting that lipolysis was reduced (Endo et al., 2008).

Chronic intraportal infusion of a lipid emulsion (3 hours a day for 15 days) during the early postprandial period induced insulin resistance both at the liver and in the adipose tissue in dogs but did not increase liver triglyceride content (Everett et al., 2005). Findings in the dog are in general agreement with those from individuals with type 2 diabetes and normal volunteers receiving a mixed meal (Woerle et al., 2006). Neither the basal nor the postprandial FFA concentrations differed between the two groups in that investigation. However, over the first 90 min of the postprandial period, FFAs declined significantly more slowly in the diabetic group.

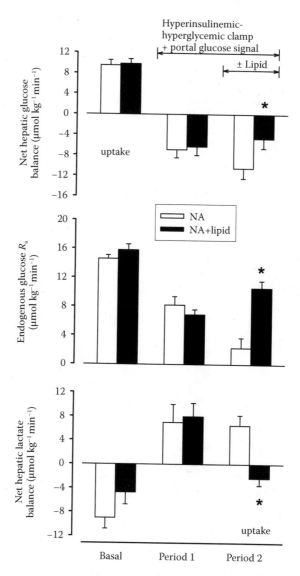

FIGURE 2.5   Elevated free fatty acid (FFA) concentrations alter NHGU and hepatic glucose disposition under postprandial conditions. Dogs were studied under basal conditions and in the presence of hyperinsulinemia, hyperglycemia, and the portal glucose signal. All animals received a peripheral infusion of nicotinic acid (NA) during periods 1 and 2 to suppress lipolysis. During period 2, one group (NA) served as the control, another group (NA + lipid) received a long-chain lipid emulsion infusion, and a third group (NA + glycerol; data not shown) received a glycerol infusion at the rate that glycerol was supplied by the lipid emulsion. Glucose metabolism in the NA and NA + glycerol groups did not differ significantly. Maintaining FFA concentrations at postabsorptive levels by lipid infusion reduced NHGU (top panel), impaired suppression of endogenous glucose R_a (middle panel), and reduced net hepatic lactate output (bottom panel). Data are mean ± SEM, $n = 7$–8/group. *$p < .05$ for NA + lipid versus NA. (Derived from data of Moore et al., *Diabetes*, 53, 32–40, 2004.)

Tracer-determined splanchnic glucose uptake did not differ between the groups, but endogenous glucose R_a was significantly less suppressed in the diabetic group, and therefore, net splanchnic glucose uptake was impaired.

The splanchnic tissues apparently play an important role in the postprandial regulation of plasma lipid concentrations. Insulin-resistant men had greater postprandial lipemia than age- and BMI-matched insulin-sensitive men, due to increased VLDL, rather than chylomicron, triglyceride (Hodson et al., 2007). In addition, the splanchnic tissues were the largest source of substrate for VLDLs in insulin-resistant men. Only ≈4% of the fatty acids incorporated into VLDLs were derived from dietary fat in either group. Rapid flux of fatty acids into and out of the liver occurs in the postprandial period, and the liver may buffer the remainder of the body from acute changes in FFA concentrations (Ravikumar et al., 2005).

2.4 PRACTICAL APPLICATIONS

Under normal conditions, the liver plays a significant role in disposing of orally or enterally delivered carbohydrate and, therefore, in limiting postprandial hyperglycemia. Hepatic glucose uptake is reduced in impaired glucose tolerance or diabetes (Basu et al., 2000), however, and postprandial hyperglycemia contributes to the development and progression of cardiovascular disease. The relative insulin resistance of lipolysis, particularly that of the visceral adipose tissue, in individuals with prediabetes and diabetes likely explains at least part of the impairment in liver glucose uptake. Not only carbohydrate metabolism, but also protein synthesis, is altered in type 2 diabetes and obesity (Pereira et al., 2008). Thus, it is important to understand the factors that promote hepatic glucose uptake, glycogen storage, and protein anabolism under normal conditions in order to design appropriate interventions for those with alterations in metabolism. Recognition of the importance of the route of nutrient delivery for normal hepatic metabolism is also of key importance in designing nutrition support regimens for those individuals with impaired ability to ingest, digest, or assimilate feedings.

2.5 SUMMARY POINTS

The unique position of the liver gives it early exposure to absorbed nutrients, as well as to lipids released from visceral adipose tissue. This allows various substrates to modulate hepatic nutrient metabolism in a number of important ways.

Hepatic glucose extraction is enhanced by enteral or intraportal glucose delivery, which reduces the glucose that must be disposed of in the peripheral tissues and enhances hepatic glycogen synthesis.

AAs reaching the liver via the portal vein stimulate hepatic protein synthesis, in comparison to AAs administered intravenously.

Elevated lipid concentrations in the portal circulation may impair both hepatic and peripheral insulin sensitivity.

The route of delivery—portal versus peripheral vein—is an important determinant of nutrient disposition in both hepatic and extrahepatic tissues.

REFERENCES

Adkins-Marshall, B., M. J. Pagliassotti, J. R. Asher, et al. 1992. Role of hepatic nerves in response of liver to intraportal glucose delivery in dogs. *Am J Physiol* 262:E679–E686.

An, Z., C. A. DiCostanzo, M. C. Moore, et al. 2008. Effects of the nitric oxide donor SIN-1 on net hepatic glucose uptake in the conscious dog. *Am J Physiol Endocrinol Metab* 294:E300–E306.

Ballmer, P. E., M. A. McNurlan, P. Essen, et al. 1995. Albumin synthesis rates measured with [2H5ring]phenylalanine are not responsive to short-term intravenous nutrients in healthy humans. *J Nutr* 125:512–519.

Barle, H., B. Nyberg, P. Essen, et al. 1997. The synthesis rates of total liver protein and plasma albumin determined simultaneously in vivo in humans. *Hepatology* 25:154–158.

Basu, A., R. Basu, P. Shah, et al. 2000. Effects of type 2 diabetes on the ability of insulin and glucose to regulate splanchnic and muscle glucose metabolism: Evidence for a defect in hepatic glucokinase activity. *Diabetes* 49:272–283.

Berthoud, H. R. 2004. Anatomy and function of sensory hepatic nerves. *Anat Rec A Discov Mol Cell Evol Biol* 280:827–835.

Black, I. B., and D. J. Reis. 1971a. Central neural regulation by adrenergic nerves of the daily rhythm in hepatic tyrosine transaminase activity. *J Physiol* 219:267–280.

Black, I. B., and D. J. Reis. 1971b. Cholinergic regulation of hepatic tyrosine transaminase activity. *J Physiol* 213:421–433.

Burcelin, R., A. Da Costa, D. Drucker, et al. 2001. Glucose competence of the hepatoportal vein sensor requires the presence of an activated glucagon-like peptide–1 receptor. *Diabetes* 50:1720–1728.

Burcelin, R., W. Dolci, and B. Thorens. 2000. Portal glucose infusion in the mouse induces hypoglycemia: Evidence that the hepatoportal glucose sensor stimulates glucose utilization. *Diabetes* 49:1635–1642.

Burrin, D. G., and T. A. Davis. 2004. Proteins and amino acids in enteral nutrition. *Curr Opin Clin Nutr Metab Care* 7:79–87.

Cardin, S., M. J. Pagliassotti, M. C. Moore, et al. 2004. Vagal cooling and concomitant portal norepinephrine infusion do not reduce net hepatic glucose uptake in the conscious dog. *Am J Physiol Regul Integr Comp Physiol* 287:R742–R748.

Chueh, F. Y., C. Malabanan, and O. P. McGuinness. 2006. Impact of portal glucose delivery on glucose metabolism in conscious, unrestrained mice. *Am J Physiol Endocrinol Metab* 291:E1206–E1211.

Dardevet, D., S. R. Kimball, L. S. Jefferson, et al. 2008. Portal infusion of amino acids is more efficient than peripheral infusion in stimulating liver protein synthesis at the same amino acid load in dogs. *Am J Clin Nutr* 88:986–996.

DeFronzo, R. A., E. Ferrannini, R. Hendler, et al. 1978. Influence of hyperinsulinemia, hyperglycemia and the route of glucose administration on splanchnic glucose exchange. *Proc Natl Acad Sci U S A* 75:5173–5177.

Dicostanzo, C. A., D. P. Dardevet, D. W. Neal, et al. 2006. Role of the hepatic sympathetic nerves in the regulation of net hepatic glucose uptake and the mediation of the portal glucose signal. *Am J Physiol Endocrinol Metab* 290:E9–E16.

Endo, Y., M. Ohta, T. Hirashita, et al. 2008. Additional effect of visceral fat resection in an obese rat model of gastric banding. *Obes Surg*, epub ahead of print.

Everett, C. A., N. Rivera, T. Rodewald, et al. 2005. Chronic postprandial intraportal infusion of FFA results in hepatic and adipose tissue insulin resistance. *Diabetes* 54:A329.

Ferrannini, E., O. Bjorkman, G. A. Reichard Jr., et al. 1985. The disposal of an oral glucose load in healthy subjects. A quantitative study. *Diabetes* 34:580–588.

Fery, F., J. Deviere, and E. O. Balasse. 2001. Metabolic handling of intraduodenal vs. intravenous glucose in humans. *Am J Physiol Endocrinol Metab* 281:E261–E268.

Fujita, S., M. Bohland, G. Sanchez-Watts, et al. 2007. Hypoglycemic detection at the portal vein is mediated by capsaicin-sensitive primary sensory neurons. *Am J Physiol Endocrinol Metab* 293:E96–E101.

Galassetti, P., M. Shiota, B. A. Zinker, et al. 1998. A negative arterial-portal venous glucose gradient decreases skeletal muscle glucose uptake. *Am J Physiol* 275:E101–E111.

Hampson, L. J., and L. Agius. 2007. Acetylcholine exerts additive and permissive but not synergistic effects with insulin on glycogen synthesis in hepatocytes. *FEBS Lett* 581: 3955–3960.

Hodson, L., A. S. Bickerton, S. E. McQuaid, et al. 2007. The contribution of splanchnic fat to VLDL triglyceride is greater in insulin-resistant than insulin-sensitive men and women: Studies in the postprandial state. *Diabetes* 56:2433–2441.

Homko, C. J., P. Cheung, and G. Boden. 2003. Effects of free fatty acids on glucose uptake and utilization in healthy women. *Diabetes* 52:487–491.

Ishida, T., Z. Chap, J. Chou, et al. 1983. Differential effects of oral, peripheral intravenous, and intraportal glucose on hepatic glucose uptake and insulin and glucagon extraction in conscious dogs. *J Clin Invest* 72:590–601.

Jaleel, A., and K. S. Nair. 2004. Identification of multiple proteins whose synthetic rates are enhanced by high amino acid levels in rat hepatocytes. *Am J Physiol Endocrinol Metab* 286:E950–E957.

Johnson, K. M., D. S. Edgerton, T. Rodewald, et al. 2007. Intraportal GLP-1 infusion increases nonhepatic glucose utilization without changing pancreatic hormone levels. *Am J Physiol Endocrinol Metab* 293:E1085–E1091.

Kimball, S. R., and L. S. Jefferson. 2006. Signaling pathways and molecular mechanisms through which branched-chain amino acids mediate translational control of protein synthesis. *J Nutr* 136:227S–2231S.

Lautt, W. W. 2004. A new paradigm for diabetes and obesity: The hepatic insulin sensitizing substance (HISS) hypothesis. *J Pharmacol Sci* 95:9–17.

Ludvik, B., J. J. Nolan, A. Roberts, et al. 1997. Evidence for decreased splanchnic glucose uptake after oral glucose administration in non-insulin-dependent diabetes mellitus. *J Clin Invest* 100:2354–2361.

Mari, A., J. Wahren, R. A. DeFronzo, et al. 1994. Glucose absorption and production following oral glucose: Comparison of compartmental and arteriovenous-difference methods. *Metabolism* 43:1419–1425.

Matsuhisa, M., Y. Yamasaki, Y. Shiba, et al. 2000. Important role of the hepatic vagus nerve in glucose uptake and production by the liver. *Metabolism* 49:11–16.

Minokoshi, Y., Y. Okano, and T. Shimazu. 1994. Regulatory mechanism of the ventromedial hypothalamus in enhancing glucose uptake in skeletal muscles. *Brain Res* 649:343–347.

Moore, M. C., A. D. Cherrington, G. Cline, et al. 1991. Sources of carbon for hepatic glycogen synthesis in the conscious dog. *J Clin Invest* 88:578–587.

Moore, M. C., C. A. Dicostanzo, M. S. Smith, et al. 2008. Hepatic portal venous delivery of a nitric oxide synthase inhibitor enhances net hepatic glucose uptake. *Am J Physiol Endocrinol Metab* 294:E768–E777.

Moore, M. C., P. J. Flakoll, P. S. Hsieh, et al. 1998. Hepatic glucose disposition during concomitant portal glucose and amino acid infusions in the dog. *Am J Physiol* 274:E893–E902.

Moore, M. C., P. S. Hsieh, D. W. Neal, et al. 2000. Nonhepatic response to portal glucose delivery in conscious dogs. *Am J Physiol Endocrinol Metab* 279:E1271–E1277.

Moore, M. C., S. Satake, M. Lautz, et al. 2004. Nonesterified fatty acids and hepatic glucose metabolism in the conscious dog. *Diabetes* 53:32–40.

Mosoni, L., M. L. Houlier, P. P. Mirand, et al. 1993. Effect of amino acids alone or with insulin on muscle and liver protein synthesis in adult and old rats. *Am J Physiol* 264:E614–E620.

Myers, S. R., D. W. Biggers, D. W. Neal, et al. 1991a. Intraportal glucose delivery enhances the effects of hepatic glucose load on net hepatic glucose uptake in vivo. *J Clin Invest* 88:158–167.

Myers, S. R., O. P. McGuinness, D. W. Neal, et al. 1991b. Intraportal glucose delivery alters the relationship between net hepatic glucose uptake and the insulin concentration. *J Clin Invest* 87:930–939.

Niijima, A. 1982. Glucose-sensitive afferent nerve fibres in the hepatic branch of the vagus nerve in the guinea-pig. *J Physiol* 332:315–323.

Niijima, A. 1984. Reflex control of the autonomic nervous system activity from the glucose sensors in the liver in normal and midpontine-transected animals. *J Auton Nerv Syst* 10:279–285.

Niijima, A., and M. M. Meguid. 1995. An electrophysiological study on amino acid sensors in the hepato-portal system in the rat. *Obes Res* 3 Suppl 5:741S–745S.

Nygren, J., and K. S. Nair. 2003. Differential regulation of protein dynamics in splanchnic and skeletal muscle beds by insulin and amino acids in healthy human subjects. *Diabetes* 52:1377–1385.

Pagliassotti, M. J., L. C. Holste, M. C. Moore, et al. 1996. Comparison of the time courses of insulin and the portal signal on hepatic glucose and glycogen metabolism in the conscious dog. *J Clin Invest* 97:81–91.

Pagliassotti, M. J., S. R. Myers, M. C. Moore, et al. 1991. Magnitude of negative arterial-portal glucose gradient alters net hepatic glucose balance in conscious dogs. *Diabetes* 40:1659–1668.

Pereira, S., E. B. Marliss, J. A. Morais, et al. 2008. Insulin resistance of protein metabolism in type 2 diabetes. *Diabetes* 57:56–63.

Perrin, C., C. Knauf, and R. Burcelin. 2004. Intracerebroventricular infusion of glucose, insulin, and the adenosine monophosphate–activated kinase activator, 5-aminoimi-dazole-4-carboxamide-1-beta-D-ribofuranoside, controls muscle glycogen synthesis. *Endocrinology* 145:4025–4033.

Ravikumar, B., P. E. Carey, J. E. Snaar, et al. 2005. Real-time assessment of postprandial fat storage in liver and skeletal muscle in health and type 2 diabetes. *Am J Physiol Endocrinol Metab* 288:E789–E797.

Reaven, G. M. 2005. Compensatory hyperinsulinemia and the development of an atherogenic lipoprotein profile: The price paid to maintain glucose homeostasis in insulin-resistant individuals. *Endocrinol Metab Clin North Am* 34:49–62.

Sakaguchi, T., and L. Liu. 2002. Hepatic branch vagotomy can block liver regeneration enhanced by ursodesoxycholic acid in 66% hepatectomized rats. *Auton Neurosci* 99:54–57.

Schäffler, A., J. Schölmerich, and C. Büchler. 2005. Mechanisms of disease: Adipocytokines and visceral adipose tissue—Emerging role in nonalcoholic fatty liver disease. *Nat Clin Pract Gastroenterol Hepatol* 2:273–280.

Schmitt, M. 1973. Influences of hepatic portal receptors on hypothalamic feeding and satiety centers. *Am J Physiol* 225:1089–1095.

Shimazu, T. 1987. Neuronal regulation of hepatic glucose metabolism in mammals. *Diabetes Metab Rev* 3:185–206.

Stumpel, F., and K. Jungermann. 1997. Sensing by intrahepatic muscarinic nerves of a portal-arterial glucose concentration gradient as a signal for insulin-dependent glucose uptake in the perfused rat liver. *FEBS Lett* 406:119–122.

Thomson, D. M., C. A. Fick, and S. E. Gordon. 2008. AMPK activation attenuates S6K1, 4E-BP1, and eEF2 signaling responses to high-frequency electrically stimulated skeletal muscle contractions. *J Appl Physiol* 104:625–632.

Thorne, A., F. Lonnqvist, J. Apelman, et al. 2002. A pilot study of long-term effects of a novel obesity treatment: Omentectomy in connection with adjustable gastric banding. *Int J Obes Relat Metab Disord* 26:193–199.

Vella, A., P. Shah, R. Basu, et al. 2002. Effect of enteral vs. parenteral glucose delivery on initial splanchnic glucose uptake in nondiabetic humans. *Am J Physiol Endocrinol Metab* 283:E259–E266.

Watanabe, Y., A. Takahashi, and T. Shimazu. 1990. Neural control of biosynthesis and secretion of serum transferrin in perfused rat liver. *Biochem J* 267:545–548.

Woerle, H. J., E. Szoke, C. Meyer, et al. 2006. Mechanisms for abnormal postprandial glucose metabolism in type 2 diabetes. *Am J Physiol Endocrinol Metab* 290:E67–E77.

Xia, F., Z. He, K. Li, et al. 2006. Evaluation of the role of sympathetic denervation on hepatic function. *Hepatol Res* 36:259–264.

3 Assessment of Nutritional Status and Diagnosis of Malnutrition in Patients with Liver Disease

Bernard Campillo

CONTENTS

Malnutrition is a common finding in liver cirrhosis, and protein energy malnutrition may be present in 20% of patients with well-compensated disease and in more than 60% of patients with severe liver insufficiency.[1] See Table 3.1 for general facts regarding malnutrition in liver cirrhosis. Many mechanisms are involved in the pathogenesis of malnutrition, and the two main factors are insufficient dietary intake and anorexia.[2] In patients with end-stage liver disease, protein-calorie malnutrition

TABLE 3.1

Key Facts of Malnutrition in Liver Cirrhosis

1. Malnutrition is a common finding in liver cirrhosis and may be present in 20% of patients with well-compensated disease and in more than 60% of patients with severe liver insufficiency.
2. Many mechanisms are involved in the pathogenesis of malnutrition: The main factor is insufficient dietary intake.
3. Malnutrition has a prognostic value and is associated with adverse outcomes in patient and graft survival after liver transplantation.
4. The assessment of nutritional status is difficult in cirrhotic patients owing to confounding factors related with liver failure.
5. Anthropometry, measurement of muscle strength, and composite score are simple, inexpensive, and reliable methods in assessing nutritional status.
6. Nutritional status should be assessed in every patient with chronic liver disease to recognize malnutrition and prevent nutritional depletion in hospital.
7. Assessment of dietary intake has a considerable importance in management of nutritional support.
8. Nutritional support is achievable using oral route with supplements or artificial feeding, mainly enteral feeding.

Note: This table lists the key features of malnutrition in liver cirrhosis including the prevalence of malnutrition, the consequences of malnutrition, the most suitable methods for assessing nutritional status, and the management of malnutrition.

is almost universal. The presence of protein-calorie malnutrition has been associated with adverse outcomes in patient and graft survival after liver transplantation.[1] The association of protein-calorie malnutrition with adverse outcomes has increased the importance of identifying reliable and cost-effective methods for assessing the nutritional status of patients with end-stage liver disease. Unfortunately, traditional methods of measuring nutritional status (including plasma levels of hepatically synthesized plasma proteins, total lymphocyte count, delayed type hypersensitivity, and anthropometrics) are confounded by the changes in metabolism, body composition, and immune function that occur in liver disease independent of nutritional status.

In this chapter, we shall describe the changes in body composition occurring in liver cirrhosis, the results of the different methods for assessing these changes, and the impairment in nutritional status with the purpose of showing the most suitable methods for detecting malnutrition in clinical practice.

3.1 CHANGES IN BODY COMPOSITION IN LIVER CIRRHOSIS

The two most important metabolic and nutritional body compartments are the body cell mass and body fat stores. Bone mineral is considered as a third compartment. The body cell mass represents the oxygen-exchanging, glucose-oxidizing, and work-performing tissue and is the best reference for expressing rates of metabolic processes. It is principally composed of muscle and viscera and is therefore an excellent nutritional parameter because these tissues are affected by periods of nutritional deprivation. Body fat has several minor functions including insulation and mechanical padding. However, its principal function is to provide a reservoir of energy. Some studies using reference methods such as total body and extracellular water measurements by deuterium oxide and bromide dilution techniques, neutron activation analysis, and total body potassium index have shown increased total body and extracellular water, decreased total body protein, body cell mass, and fat mass in cirrhotic patients. Impairment in body composition parallels the severity of liver failure, but increased total body and extracellular water as well as depletion in protein stores are found in nonascitic patients with a preserved liver function.[3–5] Although these methods give an accurate analysis of body composition, they are not available for routine assessment of nutritional status. Therefore, use of more simple and less expensive tools is required for detection of malnutrition in clinical practice.

3.2 ASSESSMENT OF NUTRITION STATUS IN CLINICAL PRACTICE

3.2.1 ANTHROPOMETRY

3.2.1.1 Mid-Arm Circumference and Triceps Skinfold Thickness

The two measurements are easy to make. The first reflects muscle mass and the second body fat. Mid-arm muscle circumference (MAMC) is derived from mid-arm circumference (MAC) and triceps skinfold thickness (TST) = MAMC (cm) = MAC (cm) − $\pi \times$ TST (cm).

MAC is usually measured with a spring tape at a point between the tip of acromion and the ulnar process with the arm hanging vertically and the forearm supinated. TST can be measured with a skinfold caliper (the Harpenden or the Holtrain caliper is recommended). Skinfold thickness can be measured at three other sites: subscapular, biceps, and suprailiac. The relations between the sum of the four skinfold thicknesses and the percentage of body fat derived from density can be calculated from regression equations according to Durnin and Womersley.[6] However, these equations are not validated in cirrhotic patients. Local standards are recommended for interpretation of measurements. Because they are not available everywhere, measurements made on large numbers of U.S. citizens 30 years ago are usually used.[7,8] Sex and age of the patients must be taken into account for interpretation of measurements. Values of MAMC or TST below the fifth percentile of a reference population are considered as severely altered and those below the 10th percentile as moderately altered.

A number of studies have assessed nutritional status in cirrhotic patients using MAMC and TST or upper mid-arm muscle area and upper mid-arm fat area measurements.[9–11] Impairment of nutritional status parallels the severity of liver failure. Male subjects are characterized by a depleted muscle mass, whereas fat mass is reduced to a greater extent in female patients. The study including the largest number of patients has shown that about 50% of male Child C cirrhotic patients have a severely reduced muscle mass, whereas 40% of female Child C patients have a severely reduced fat mass (Figure 3.1). Prevalence of malnutrition may be higher in hospitalized patients.[11] Furthermore, altered nutritional status assessed by reduced MAMC and TST have a prognostic value: patients with reduced MAMC and TST measurements have a lower survival rate when compared to normal and overnourished patients. The prognostic power of MAMC is higher than that of TST.[9]

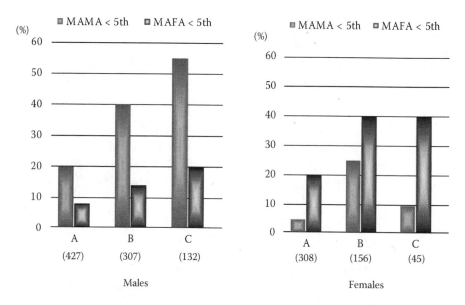

FIGURE 3.1 Prevalence of malnutrition in cirrhotic patients. Percentage of male and female patients with cirrhosis with a reduction in mid-arm muscle area (MAMA) and mid-arm fat area (MAFA) below the fifth percentile of standard for an age- and sex-matched healthy population.[10] (From Italian Multicentre Cooperative Project on nutrition in liver cirrhosis. *J Hepatol*, 21, 317–325, 1994. With permission.)

The limitations of anthropometric measurements are the presence of edema at the upper extremities, which is seldom observed, and the intraobserver and inter-observer variability. Thus, measurements by a trained observer are recommended, and if measurements are made by several observers, reproducibility of measurements must be tested among them. When these conditions are respected, anthropometry based on the measurement of MAMC and TST is a reliable bedside method to assess nutritional status in patients with liver cirrhosis, especially in epidemiological studies including a large number of patients.

3.2.1.2   Body Mass Index

Body weight, change in body weight, and body mass index (BMI) are the most simple parameters to assess nutritional status; however, it is admitted that fluid retention and ascites preclude their interpretation in cirrhotic patients. Campillo et al.[12] have shown in a large series of cirrhotic patients that BMI was dependent on nutritional status and ascites. BMI decreased with impairment in nutritional status, whereas the prevalence of tense ascites increased. Therefore, BMI could have acceptable value in the diagnosis of malnutrition provided that adequate cutoff values are defined according to the presence of ascites: optimal cutoff values were 22 in nonascitic patients, 23 in patients with mild ascites, and 25 in patients with tense ascites with sensitivities and specificities ranging from 86% to 90% and areas under the ROC curves (AUROC) ranging from 0.783 to 0.863 (Figure 3.2).

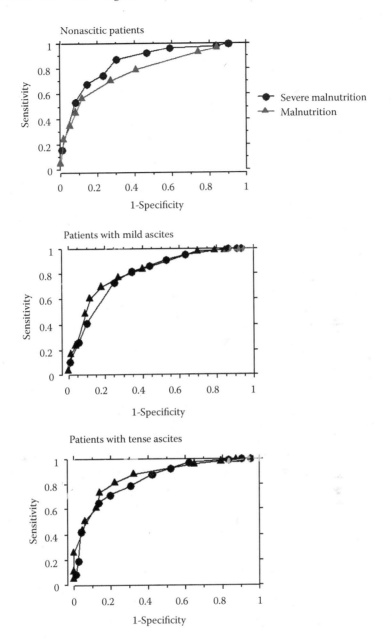

FIGURE 3.2 Receiver operator characteristics (ROC) curves for the diagnosis of malnutrition and severe malnutrition according to the presence of ascites. Areas under the ROC curves (AUROC) (95% confidence interval) for the diagnosis of severe malnutrition and malnutrition were 0.854 (0.801–0.907) and 0.783 (0.732–0.834) in nonascitic patients, 0.806 (0.749–0.862) and 0.822 (0.767–0.877) in patients with mild ascites, and 0.843 (0.796–0.890) and 0.863 (0.804–0.922) in patients with tense ascites, respectively. Comparisons of AUROC in each group showed that there was a significant difference for the diagnosis of malnutrition and severe malnutrition in nonascitic patients ($p = .016$), but not in the other two groups.

3.2.2   THE 24-HOUR URINARY CREATININE APPROACH

The 24-hour urinary creatinine approach is the most common chemical method of estimating whole body muscle mass in humans. It is based on the assumptions that creatine is almost totally within the skeletal and smooth muscle and in a constant concentration per kilogram of muscle, creatine is converted irreversibly to creatinine at a constant daily rate and creatinine undergoes renal excretion at a constant rate. In healthy subjects, the rate of limiting step of creatine biosynthesis, the synthesis of guanidinoacetic acid from glycine and arginine, is predominantly located in the kidney. The next step of creatine biosynthesis, which is located in the liver (the trans-methylation from S-adenosylmethionine to guanidinoacetate), could become rate limiting when reduced liver function of liver cell mass is present. Pirlich et al.[13] have shown that renal dysfunction, but not reduced liver function, systematically affects the urinary creatinine method for the estimation of skeletal muscle mass in cirrhosis.

3.2.3   ASSESSMENT OF MUSCLE STRENGTH

Muscle wasting in liver cirrhosis is related to reduced protein intake, decreased muscle protein synthesis, increased myofibrillar degradation, and physical inactivity associated with severe liver disease. Muscle strength has been studied in patients with alcoholic liver cirrhosis, and it has been shown that muscle weakness is related to the severity of malnutrition but not to the severity of liver disease, duration of alcohol abstinence, or neuropathy.[14] Measurement of handgrip strength has the advantage of being simple, quick to perform, inexpensive, and noninvasive. In patients with end-stage liver disease, handgrip strength is a sensitive marker of body cell mass depletion, and a correlation of grip strength with morbidity and mortality in alcoholic hepatitis and postoperative morbidity has previously been reported. Serial measurements of muscle function might be useful in assessing the nutritional status of these patients, both as a screening tool and for measuring response to therapy, because muscle function indices have been shown to improve with refeeding.[15]

3.2.4   BIOELECTRICAL IMPEDANCE ANALYSIS

This is an indirect method of assessing body composition based on the resistance and reactance of the body to a small electrical current. Regression equations are devised, using the subject's height, weight, age, and resistance and reactance to a known current, which are then used to calculate the subject's total body water, fat free mass, and, by derivation, fat mass and percentage body fat. The technique is easy to perform and reproducible and provides valid assessments of body composition in healthy individuals and in disease states when hydration is constant. However, it is of little value for assessing body composition in patients whose state of hydration is variable, and the validity of bioelectrical impedance analysis (BIA) in patients with cirrhosis has been questioned because of erroneous estimates of body fluid compartments. Pirlich et al.[16] have shown that BIA is a valid tool for the assessment of protein malnutrition by the detection of reduced body cell mass in cirrhotic patients, especially in nonascitic patients. There was an excellent and highly significant correlation between body cell mass estimated by BIA and body cell mass estimated by total body potassium in controls as well as in patients without ascites; the correlation was lower in patients with ascites. In comparison with controls and nonascitic patients, the agreement was somewhat less strong in patients with ascites.[16] Madden and Morgan[17] have shown that BIA could not be used interchangeably with skinfold anthropometry for assessment of body fat percentage in patients with cirrhosis, regardless of their state of hydration, since there was considerable variation in individual values such that measurements made using BIA could be from 9% less to 8% more than the corresponding anthropometric values. Another study[18] has shown that bifrequency BIA (5 and 100 kHz) agrees with anthropometry to a greater extent than monofrequency (50 kHz) and may be useful for assessing change in nutritional status of cirrhotic patients.

3.2.5 DUAL-ENERGY X-RAY ABSORPTIOMETRY

Dual-energy x-ray absorptiometry (DXA) is a precise, safe, and relatively inexpensive tool of measuring body composition in humans. DXA is associated with a low radiation exposure and provides bone mineral as well as fat and lean tissue mass, and thus, body composition may be estimated according to the three-compartment model. Analysis of body composition by DXA has shown a significant reduction in percentage of body fat in cirrhotic patients. The reduction in percentage body fat is evident in female cirrhotic patients only, particularly in the trunk. In male cirrhotic patients, fat-free mineral-free mass is reduced in the whole body and the limbs. For both sexes and in each body segment bone mineral content and density are reduced. Percentage body fat can be evaluated by skinfold anthropometry or DXA with a difference of less than 5% in the majority of cirrhotic patients without overt fluid retention.[19] The validity of DXA may be questionable in ascitic patients. However, it has been shown that paracentesis of ascites does not significantly change total and regional fat mass assessment by DXA.[20]

3.2.6 BIOLOGICAL PARAMETERS

All biological parameters used as nutritional assessment indices are influenced by numerous interacting factors. Circulating concentrations of many visceral proteins (albumin, transthyretin, retinol binding protein) are highly affected by the presence of liver disease, excessive alcohol, and inflammatory state. Immune status, which is often considered a functional test of malnutrition, may be affected by hypersplenism, abnormal immunologic reactivity, and alcohol abuse. Therefore, none of these parameters can be used as a reliable index of nutritional status in clinical practice in patients with liver cirrhosis.

3.2.7 SUBJECTIVE GLOBAL ASSESSMENT

The technique of subjective global assessment (SGA) uses clinical information collected during history taking and physical examination to determine nutritional status without recourse to objective measurements. This method of assessment, which has

TABLE 3.2
Baylor University Medical Center Revised Subjective Nutrition Assessment Criteria for Adult Liver Transplant Candidates

I.   History
A.   Weight
    Height
    Current weight   ___
    Pre-illness weight   ___
    IBW   ___
    Weight in past 6 months: High ___   Low ___
    Overall change in past 6 months: ___
B.   Appetite
    1.   Dietary intake change—relative to normal. Appetite in past 2 wk
          Good ☐   Fair ☐   Poor ☐
    2.   Early satiety
          None ☐   1–2 wk ☐   >2 wk ☐
    3.   Taste changes
          None ☐   1–2 wk ☐   >2 wk ☐
C.   Current intake per recall
          Calories   ___   Protein   ___
          Calorie needs ___   Protein needs ___
D.   Persistent gastrointestinal symptoms
    1.   Nausea
          None ☐   1–2 wk ☐   >2 wk ☐
    2.   Vomiting
          None ☐   1 wk ☐   >1 wk ☐
    3.   Diarrhea (loose stools, > 3/day)
          Number of stools per day ___
          Consistency   ___
          None ☐   1 wk ☐   >1 wk ☐
    4.   Constipation
          None ☐   1–2 wk ☐   >2 wk ☐
    5.   Difficulty chewing
          None ☐   1–2 wk ☐   >2 wk ☐
    6.   Difficulty swallowing
          None ☐   1–2 wk ☐   >2 wk ☐
E.   Functional capacity
        ___ No dysfunction
        ___ Dysfunction
        ___ Weeks
        ___ Working suboptimally
        ___ Ambulatory
        ___ Bedridden

TABLE 3.2 (CONTINUED)
Baylor University Medical Center Revised Subjective Nutrition Assessment Criteria for Adult Liver Transplant Candidates

II. Physical

A. Status of subcutaneous fat (triceps, chest)

      Good stores ☐   Fair stores ☐   Poor stores ☐

B. Muscle wasting (quadriceps, deltoids, shoulders)

      None ☐   Mild to moderate ☐   Severe ☐

C. Edema and ascites

      None ☐   Mild to moderate ☐   Severe ☐

III. Existing conditions

A. Encephalopathy

      None ☐   Stage I–II ☐   Stage III ☐   Stage IV ☐

B. Chronic or recurrent infection

      None ☐   1 wk ☐   > 1 wk ☐

C. Kidney function

      ___ Good

      ___ Decreased (no dialysis)

      ___ Decreased (with dialysis)

D. Varices

      ___ None

      ___ Varices (no bleeds)

      ___ Varices (with bleeds)

IV. Subjective nutrition-assessment rating

      A. ___ Well nourished

      B. ___ Moderately (or suspected of being malnourished)

      C. ___ Severely malnourished

V. Additional information

      A. History of diabetes mellitus _____

      B. Vitamin/mineral supplements _____

      C. Other dietary supplements _____

      D. Alcohol _____

      E. Current diet _____

      F. Compliance to diet based on history _____

      G. Food intolerances/allergies _____

      H. Drugs _____

Source: From Hasse J., Strong, S., Gorman, M. A., and Liepa, G., *Nutrition*, 9, 339–343, 1993. With permission.

Note: Subjective global assessment is an alternative test for assessing the nutrition status of adult liver transplant candidates with an overall fair to good interobserver reproducibility rate. Muscle wasting and fat depletion were determined to be the strongest predictors of the final SGA rating.

been successfully used to assess nutritional status in general medical and surgical patients, shows good to excellent interobserver reproducibility and good convergent validity when compared with measured anthropometric variables. In patients with liver cirrhosis, Hasse et al.[21] have shown that SGA has an overall fair to good inter-observer reproducibility rate for assessing the nutrition status of adult liver transplant candidates, whereas Naveau et al.[22] have cautioned against the use of SGA because the results do not accord with those obtained using anthropometry. SGA adapted for assessment of adult liver transplant candidate according to Hasse et al.[21] is shown in Table 3.2.

3.2.8   ENERGY BALANCE

Energy requirements can be calculated from resting energy expenditure (REE). Prediction formulae can be used to estimate REE. Individual predicted values in cirrhotic patients vary widely from measured values, therefore measurement of REE rather than prediction has been recommended in these patients.[23] Hypermetabolism is found in 20–30% of cirrhotic patients and has a negative effect on prognosis.[24] Energy expenditure and energy requirements are usually expressed per kilogram of body weight. It remains controversial whether actual body weight, "dry" weight, or ideal body weight should be used for calculation. Actual body weight in case of severe fluid retention as well as errors in estimates of "dry" weight may lead to erro-neous values; therefore, ideal body weight may be accepted as a safe approach.[1]

Assessment of dietary intake has a great importance because low intake is associ-ated with a poor outcome.[11] Inadequacy of spontaneous dietary intake is obvious in hospitalized cirrhotic patients, mainly Child C patients, since it has been shown that 80% and 65% have caloric and protein intakes, respectively, which are below the usual recommendations.[11] In clinical practice, a systematic dietary recall obtained by a skilled dietician will provide adequate information in most cases.

3.2.9   COMPOSITE SCORES

The composite score used by the Veterans Administration Study Group investigator includes mid-arm muscle area, skinfold thickness, creatinine excretion, lymphocyte count, recall antigen testing, and circulating levels of visceral proteins that are of questionable value in chronic liver disease.[25] All composite scores including serum protein levels are dependent on liver function and have limited value in cirrhotic patients.

Morgan et al.[26] have validated a global nutritional assessment scheme called Royal Free Hospital–Subjective Global Assessment (RFH-SGA), including measures of BMI calculated from estimated dry weight, MAMC, and details of dietary intake. Intakes were categorized as adequate if they met estimated requirements, inadequate if they failed to meet estimated requirements but exceeded 500 kcal/day, or negli-gible if they provided fewer than 500 kcal/day. The three variables were incorporated into a semistructured, algorithmic construct, which allocates patients to one of three nutritional categories as shown in Figure 3.3.[26] RFH-SGA has a prognosis value since patients categorized as severely malnourished have shorter subsequent survival;

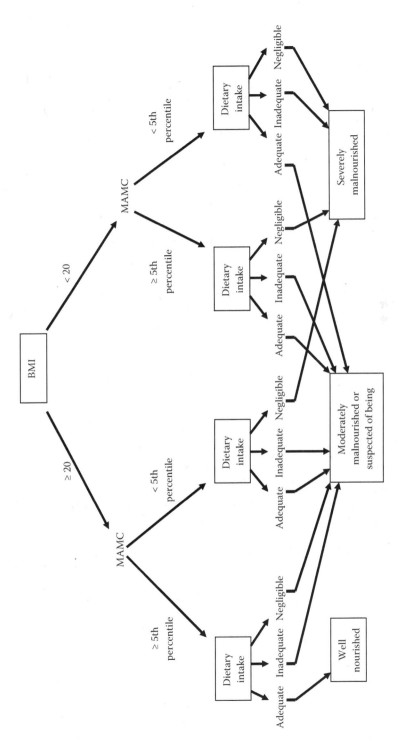

FIGURE 3.3 Royal Free Hospital–Subjective Global Assessment scheme for determining nutritional status in patients with cirrhosis. Patients are categorized in relation to their body mass index (BMI), mid-arm muscle circumference (MAMC), and dietary intake into one of three categories: adequately nourished, moderately (or suspected to be) malnourished, and severely malnourished. A subjective override based on such factors as profound recent weight loss or recent significant improvements in appetite and dietary intake can be used to modify the classification by one category only.[26] (From Morgan M. Y., Madden, A. M., Soulsby, C. T., and Morris, R. W., *Hepatology*, 44, 823–835, 2006. With permission.)

moreover, this nutritional index adds significantly to Child-Pugh grade and model for end-stage liver diseases when assessing the patient prognosis (Figure 3.4).[27]

3.3   CONCLUSION

Many methods can be used for assessment of nutritional status in patients with liver cirrhosis. Regarding both the high prevalence of malnutrition and the consequences on outcome, assessment of nutritional status should be performed in every patient, especially at admission in hospital. Anthropometry, including measurements of EMI, MAMC, and TST, is a reliable and inexpensive method and seems sufficiently robust for detection of malnutrition in clinical practice. Measurement of dietary intake should be added, although this may be a limiting factor because a dietician is required for this purpose. Combination of anthropometric parameters and dietary intake in a composite score, such as RFH-SGA scheme, provides an interesting and valid tool to assess both nutritional status and prognosis in patients with liver cirrhosis.

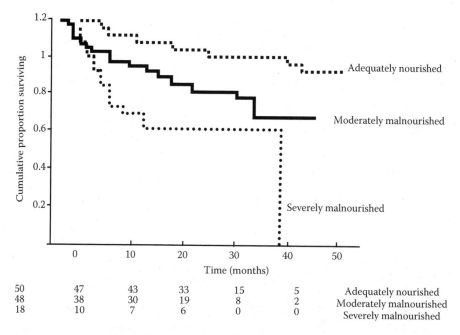

FIGURE 3.4   Cumulative survival in 116 patients with cirrhosis by a category of nutritional status determined using the Royal Free Hospital–Subjective Global Assessment scheme. Numbers of patients at risk at each time point are tabulated below the figure by nutritional category. Significance of the difference between the groups (χ^2 = 15.04; df = 2; p = .0005).[26] (From Morgan M. Y., Madden, A. M., Soulsby, C. T., and Morris, R. W., *Hepatology*, 44, 823–835, 2006. With permission.)

3.4 SUMMARY POINTS

- Total body protein, body cell mass, and fat mass decrease early in the course of liver cirrhosis.
- Malnutrition parallels the severity of liver failure.
- BMI may be incorporated to a reliable index with the use of dry weight or the definition of threshold values according to the importance of ascites.
- Measurement of MAMC and TST is a simple method that can be used at bedside.
- Measurement of handgrip strength is simple, quick, inexpensive, and a sensitive marker of body cell mass depletion.
- Ascites limit the value of BIA and DXA.
- Confounding factors induced by liver failure preclude the use of visceral proteins and markers of immune status.
- SGA and composite scores including anthropometric parameters and dietary intake are reliable indexes for diagnosis of malnutrition.

REFERENCES

1. Plauth, M., M. Merli, J. Kondrup, A. Weiman, P. Ferenci, and M. J. Müller. 1997. ESPEN guidelines for nutrition in liver disease and transplantation. *Clin Nutr* 16:43–55.
2. Campillo, B. 2006. Nutritional aspects of liver and biliary disease. In *Texbook of Hepatology. From Basic Science to Clinical Practice*, Third Edition, ed. J. Rodes, J. P. Benhamou, A. T. Blei, J. Reichen, and M. Rizzetto. 1905–1911. Oxford: Blackwell Publishing Ltd. UK.
3. McCullough, A. J., K. D. Mullen, and S. C. Kalhan. 1991. Measurements of total body and extracellular water in cirrhotic patients with and without ascites. *Hepatology* 14:1102–1111.
4. Prijatmoko, D., B. J. G. Strauss, J. R. Lambert, et al. 1993. Early detection of protein depletion in alcoholic cirrhosis: Role of body composition analysis. *Gastroenterology* 105:1839–1845.
5. Peng, S., L. D. Plank, J. L. McCall, L. K. Gillanders, K. McIlroy, and E. J. Gane. 2007. Body composition, muscle function, and energy expenditure in patients with liver cirrhosis: A comprehensive study. *Am J Clin Nutr* 85:1257–1266.
6. Durnin, J. V. G. A., and J. Wormersley. 1974. Body fat assessed from total body density and its estimation from skinfold thickness: Measurements on 481 men and women aged from 16 to 72 years. *Br J Nutr* 32:77–97.
7. Bishop, C. W., P. E. Bowen, and S. J. Ritchey. 1981. Norms for nutritional assessment of American adults by upper arm anthropometry. *Am J Clin Nutr* 34:2530–2539.
8. Frisancho, A. R. 1981. New norms of upper limb fat and muscle area for assessment of nutritional status. *Am J Clin Nutr* 31:2540–2545.
9. Caregaro, L., F. Alberberino, P. Amodio, et al. 1996. Malnutrition in alcoholic and virus-related cirrhosis. *Am J Clin Nutr* 63:602–609.
10. Italian Multicentre Cooperative Project on nutrition in liver cirrhosis. 1994. Nutritional status in cirrhosis. *J Hepatol* 21:317–325.
11. Campillo, B., J. P. Richardet, E. Scherman, and P. N. Bories. 2003. Evaluation of nutritional practice in hospitalized cirrhotic patients; results of a prospective study. *Nutrition* 19:515–521.

12. Campillo, B., J. P. Richardet, and P. N. Bories. 2006. Validation of body mass index for the diagnosis of malnutrition in patients with liver cirrhosis. *Gastroenterol Clin Biol* 30:1137–1143.

13. Pirlich, M., O. Selberg, K. Böker, M. Schwarze, and M. J. Müller. 1996. The creatinine approach to estimate skeletal muscle mass in patients with cirrhosis. *Hepatology* 24: 1422–1427.

14. Andersen, H., M. Borre, J. Jakobsen, P. H. Andersen, and H. Vilstrup. 1998. Decreased muscle strength in patients with alcoholic liver cirrhosis in relation to nutritional status, alcohol abstinence, liver function and neuropathy. *Hepatology* 27:1200–1206.

15. Figueiredo, F. A., E. R. Dickson, T. M. Pasha, et al. 2000. Utility of standard nutritional parameters in detecting body cell mass depletion in patients with end-stage liver disease. *Liver Transpl* 6:575–581.

16. Pirlich, M., T. Schütz, T. Spachos, et al. 2000. Bioelectrical impedance analysis is a useful bedside technique to assess malnutrition in cirrhotic patients with and without ascites. *Hepatology* 32:1208–1215.

17. Madden, A. M., and M. Y. Morgan. 1994. A comparison of skinfold anthropometry and bioelectrical impedance analysis for measuring percentage body fat in patients with cirrhosis. *J Hepatol* 21:878–883.

18. Campillo, B., P. N. Bories, and B. Pornin. 1997. Assessment of body composition by skinfold anthropometry and mono-frequency and bi-frequency bio-electrical impedance technique: A comparative study. *Nutr Clin Metab* 11:81–89.

19. Fiore, P., M. Merli, A. Andreoli, et al. 1999. A comparison of skinfold anthropometry and dual-energy X-ray absorptiometry for the evaluation of body fat in cirrhotic patients. *Clin Nutr* 18:349–351.

20. Haderslev, K. V., O. L. Svendsen, and M. Staun. 1999. Does paracentesis of ascites influence measurements of bone mineral, or body composition by dual-energy x-ray absorptiometry? *Metabolism* 48:373–377.

21. Hasse, J., S. Strong, M. A. Gorman, and G. Liepa. 1993. Subjective global assessment: Alternative nutrition-assessment technique for liver transplant candidates. *Nutrition* 9:339–343.

22. Naveau, S., E. Belda, E. Borotto, F. Genuist, and J. C. Chaput. 1995. Comparison of clinical judgment and anthropometric parameters for evaluating nutritional status in patients with alcoholic liver disease. *J Hepatol* 23:234–235.

23. Madden, A. M., and M. Y. Morgan. 1999. Resting energy expenditure should be measured in patients with cirrhosis, not predicted. *Hepatology* 30:655–664.

24. Müller, M. J., J. Böttcher, O. Selberg, et al. 1999. Hypermetabolism in clinically stable patients with liver cirrhosis. *Am J Clin Nutr* 69:1194–1201.

25. Mendenhall, C. L., T. Tosch, R. E. Weesner, et al. 1986. VA Cooperative study on alcoholic hepatitis II: Prognostic significance of protein calorie malnutrition. *Am J Clin Nutr* 43:213–218.

26. Morgan, M. Y., A. M. Madden, C. T. Soulsby, and R. W. Morris. 2006. Derivation and validation of a new global method for assessing nutritional status in patients with cirrhosis. *Hepatology* 44:823–835.

27. Gunsar, F., M. L. Raimondo, S. Jones, et al. 2006. Nutritional status and prognosis in cirrhotic patients. *Aliment Pharmacol Ther* 24:563–572.

4 Managing Liver Dysfunction in Parenteral Nutrition

Simon M. Gabe and David A. J. Lloyd

CONTENTS

4.1 INTRODUCTION

Since it was developed in the second half of the twentieth century, parenteral nutrition has become established as a life-saving treatment for patients with intestinal failure. However, patients receiving parenteral nutrition are at risk of developing hepatic complications. Parenteral nutrition–associated liver disease (PNALD) was first described in the early 1970s (Peden et al., 1971). Hepatic complications are observed in both adults and children, although the patterns of liver disease differ between these two groups. The incidence of hepatic dysfunction, possible etiologies, and strategies to avoid and manage these complications will be discussed.

4.2 INCIDENCE OF LIVER DYSFUNCTION IN PATIENTS RECEIVING PARENTERAL NUTRITION

4.2.1 SHORT-TERM HOME PARENTERAL NUTRITION AND PNALD

Abnormalities of liver function tests (LFTs) are common in adults with acute intestinal failure receiving short-term parenteral nutrition. Early reports (Lindor et al., 1979) describe the development of abnormal LFTs occurring after only 2 weeks of a lipid-free parenteral nutrition with a high glucose content (elevated aspartate aminotransferase, alkaline phosphatase, and bilirubin concentrations in 68%, 54%, and 21% of patients, respectively). More recent reports in which more balanced parenteral regimens are used (Clarke et al., 1991) describe less frequently abnormal LFTs, although this is still clearly a common phenomenon (after 4 weeks of parenteral nutrition, aspartate aminotransferase, alkaline phosphatase, and bilirubin concentrations were elevated in 27%, 32%, and 31% of patients, respectively). In general, these elevations are mild, and they often normalize even if parenteral nutrition is continued and usually resolve fully once it is discontinued (Quigley et al., 1993). A more recent audit of patients revealed that 34% of patients had abnormal LFTs before the parenteral nutrition was started (Baker and Nightingale, 2004). In those patients, the LFTs worsened in 60% and resolved in 30% while receiving parenteral nutrition. Only 9% of patients developed abnormal LFTs during parenteral nutrition. For patients who developed abnormal LFTs or worsening LFTs on parenteral nutrition, the underlying cause was thought to be sepsis in 46% and the underlying liver disease in 24%.

The abnormalities of LFT observed in patients receiving acute parenteral nutrition are influenced by factors relating to underlying disease, especially ongoing sepsis and preexisting liver disease.

4.2.2 LONG-TERM PARENTERAL NUTRITION

The incidence of abnormal LFTs, abnormal liver histology, and more advanced liver disease in adults receiving long-term home parenteral nutrition varies between studies. Deranged LFTs have been reported in 48% of patients receiving home parenteral nutrition, with an elevated alkaline phosphatase level being the commonest abnormality (Luman and Shaffer, 2002). However, in this study none of the patients developed decompensated or end-stage liver disease. Similarly, abnormal LFTs have been reported in 95% of patients who had received parenteral nutrition for an average of 2 years, but severe liver disease was observed in only 4% of patients (Salvino et al., 2006). Chronic biochemical cholestasis is defined as the persistent elevation to > 1.5 times the upper limit of the normal range for more than 6 months of two of three biochemical variables (alkaline phosphatase, γ-glutamyl transferase, and conjugated bilirubin). Using this definition, we demonstrated a point prevalence of 24% chronic cholestasis in adult home parenteral nutrition patients at our institution (Lloyd et al., 2008) and a prospective cohort study by Cavicchi et al. (2000) noted that 65% of patients on home parenteral nutrition developed chronic cholestasis after 6 months. The wide range in the reported prevalence of chronic cholestasis reflects other factors such as the amount of lipid in the parenteral nutrition. The study by Cavicchi et al. also demonstrated that the development of chronic cholestasis was predictive of the development of complicated liver disease (defined according to liver histology), which was seen in 26% and 50% of all patients at 2 and 6 years, respectively. Six patients died of PNALD during the course of the study. The most common histological finding in this cohort of patients was intrahepatic cholestasis with varying degrees of fibrosis progressing to cirrhosis. In addition, macrovesicular steatosis, microvesicular steatosis, and phospholipidosis were commonly observed. These findings are consistent with other reports, suggesting that although steatosis is the most common initial finding in adults with PNALD, intrahepatic cholestasis develops later and is persistent (Quigley et al., 1993). A lower incidence of advanced liver disease of 14–19% has been described in other studies (Chan et al. 1999; Ito and Shils, 1991).

PNALD is common in neonates and infants. Unlike in adults, intrahepatic cholestasis rather than steatosis is the most common finding, perhaps reflecting the immaturity of the biliary excretion system in neonates and its susceptibility to hypoxia. The exact incidence varies between studies, reflecting the patient-group studies and the exact definitions used. Neonatal cholestasis relates closely to birth weight, prematurity, and duration of parenteral nutrition. Infants with a very low birth weight have a high incidence of cholestasis (Beale et al., 1979, 1996), whereas in those treated for more than 3 months a 90% incidence of cholestasis has been reported (Beale et al., 1979). Neonatal cholestasis is related to bacterial and fungal sepsis and, unlike adults, occurs early with rapidly progressive liver dysfunction and a reported hepatic failure rate of 17% (Sondheimer et al., 1998).

4.3 HISTOPATHOLOGY OF PNALD

The acute perturbations of LFT seen in adults receiving parenteral nutrition are characterized by hepatic steatosis, with accumulation of macrovesicular and microvesicular fat within the hepatocytes, which may be accompanied by an extent of steatohepatitis (Quigley et al., 1993). These abnormalities are strongly influenced by the underlying disease state, especially ongoing sepsis. Abnormal liver histology has been shown to correlate more closely with the presence of intra-abdominal sepsis, renal failure, and preexisting liver disease than with the use of parenteral nutrition (Wolfe et al., 1988).

For patients with abnormal LFTs receiving long-term parenteral nutrition, the most common histopathological features include intracellular and intracanalicular cholestasis, macrovesicular steatosis, microvesicular steatosis, and periportal fibrosis. Other features include hepatocellular injury, multinucleated giant cells, phospholipidosis, portal inflammation, acute cholangitis, extramedullary hematopoiesis, bile duct proliferation, varying degrees of fibrosis, and cirrhosis (Carter and Shulman, 2007; Cavicchi et al., 2000).

4.4 ETIOLOGY OF PNALD

The etiology of hepatic dysfunction in both adults and children receiving parenteral nutrition is complex and multifactorial. An understanding of the mechanisms behind the biochemical and histological changes observed in patients receiving parenteral nutrition is further complicated by differences in the patient populations studied and in the parenteral nutrition formulations used. In general, possible etiological factors can be divided into those that are patient-dependent, related to a lack of enteral intake, and those resulting from either nutrient deficiencies or nutrient toxicities in the parenteral formulations used (Figure 4.1).

4.4.1 PATIENT-DEPENDENT CAUSES

Abnormalities of LFTs may relate to underlying liver disease in patients receiving parenteral nutrition rather than the effects of the parenteral nutrition itself. Patients with inflammatory bowel disease may have occult sclerosing cholangitis with histological evidence of steatosis, or pericholangitis in the presence of normal LFT (Nightingale, 2003). Adults receiving long-term parenteral nutrition in the presence of preexisting liver disease have been shown to have a threefold increased risk of developing chronic cholestasis (Cavicchi et al., 2000).

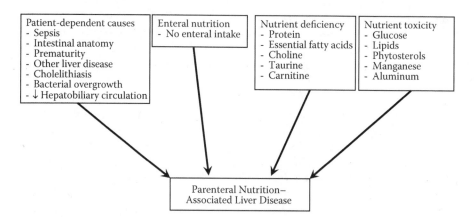

FIGURE 4.1 Factors implicated in the etiology of parenteral nutrition associated liver disease.

4.4.1.1   Sepsis

The presence of sepsis is an important precipitant of cholestasis in neonates and of abnormal LFTs in adults receiving short-term parenteral nutrition. Bacterial overgrowth is relatively common in both children and adults with intestinal failure as a result of intestinal stasis. It has been proposed that bacterial overgrowth may be causative in the development of liver dysfunction in patients receiving parenteral nutrition due to the generation of secondary bile salts such as lithocholic acid as a result of bacterial dehydroxylation of chenodeoxycholic acid (Quigley et al., 1993), endotoxin, and bacterial translocation. Recent studies on humans support the concept of bacterial translocation previously only seen in animal models (Reddy et al., 2007), and experiments performed in animals suggest that effects of bacterial endotoxins on the liver may be mediated by cytokines such as tumor necrosis alpha (Pappo et al., 1995).

4.4.1.2   Intestinal Anatomy

PNALD has been shown to be related to small intestinal length in a number of studies. One study has reported that a small intestinal length of < 1 m is associated with abnormal LFTs in adults receiving long-term parenteral nutrition (Luman and Shaffer, 2002), whereas another study has reported an increased risk of chronic cholestasis in adults with a small intestinal length of < 0.5 m (Cavicchi et al., 2000). Some authors have postulated that short bowel syndrome predisposes to liver dysfunction as a result of impairment of enterohepatic bile salt circulation and abnormal bile acid metabolism (Cavicchi et al., 2000). Other researchers have argued that bowel length may simply be a surrogate marker of parenteral energy requirement (Lloyd et al., 2008; Luman and Shaffer, 2002). In addition, it is of interest that LFTs have been noted to improve after isolated small intestinal transplantation, even in a small number of cases in which there was biopsy-proven hepatic fibrosis (Lauro et al., 2006).

The presence or absence of colon in continuity with small intestine has recently been associated with the development of PNALD in our institution (Lloyd et al., 2008). The reason for this association is not yet clear. Effects may be mediated by the metabolic and hormonal actions of products of colonic bacterial metabolism such as short chain fatty acids and phytoestrogens (van Munster et al., 1994) or may be because of release of a range of gastrointestinal hormones such as PYY (Nightingale et al., 1996).

4.4.1.3   Infant Prematurity

PNALD is common in neonates (section 4.2.2) with the smallest premature infants being the most susceptible (Beale et al., 1979, 1996). Birth weight is inversely related to PNALD (Beale et al., 1979). This association may be due to the immaturity of the hepatic transport mechanisms and metabolism of bile acids. Neonates have abnormalities in each step involved in the enterohepatic circulation of bile acids: affecting bile acid synthesis and conjugation (Balistreri et al., 1983), hepatic uptake and secretion (Suchy et al., 1986), and intestinal uptake and recirculation of bile acids (de Belle et al., 1979).

4.4.2 LACK OF ENTERAL NUTRITION

Reduced enteral nutrition is associated with an increased reliance on parenteral nutrition. It is difficult to determine if increased risk of liver dysfunction in individuals with very little oral intake is a result of the lack of enteral nutrition, or the effect of parenteral feeding.

Fasting coupled with total parenteral nutrition reduces the secretion of a number of gastrointestinal hormones, including gastrin, motilin, pancreatic polypeptide, insulinotropic polypeptide, and glucagon (Greenberg et al., 1981). This reduction may reduce intestinal motility, promoting bacterial overgrowth, and may predispose to biliary stasis.

4.4.3 NUTRIENT DEFICIENCY

Individuals with kwashiorkor, resulting from severe protein-energy malnutrition, develop hepatic steatosis because there is insufficient protein for the manufacture of very low density lipoprotein (VLDL), which is needed for hepatic triacylglycerol (TAG) export (Cook and Hutt, 1967). However, patients receiving parenteral nutrition should receive adequate amino acids for VLDL synthesis. Similarly, inadequate supply of linoleic acid may result in essential fatty acid deficiency, which is also associated with steatosis (Richardson and Sgoutas, 1975). Since the majority of parenteral lipid infusions are manufactured using soybean oil, which is rich in linoleic acid, essential fatty acid deficiency is rare, unless fat-free parenteral regimens are used in individuals with little or no enteral lipid intake.

It has been recently proposed that deficiencies of a number of methionine metabolites, such as carnitine, choline, and taurine, may be responsible for both steatosis and cholestasis in patients receiving parenteral nutrition. Orally ingested methionine can be converted to these metabolites via hepatic transulfuration pathways, although these pathways are underdeveloped in premature infants (Vina et al., 1995). Methionine administered parenterally to the systemic circulation rather than to the portal circulation is also transaminated to mercaptans, hence reducing the synthesis of carnitine, choline, and taurine (Chawla et al., 1985). Carnitine, choline, and taurine are not routinely administered as part of parenteral formulations, and there is evidence that levels are low in individuals receiving parenteral nutrition.

4.4.3.1 Carnitine

Carnitine is involved in the transport of long-chain fatty acids across the mitochondrial membrane so that they can undergo oxidation. In deficiency states in which carnitine levels are very low (< 10% normal levels), hepatic steatosis can develop (Karpati et al., 1975). Plasma carnitine is about 50% of normal levels in patients receiving parenteral nutrition, which is considerably higher than in patients with a congenital or acquired deficiency (Bowyer et al., 1986; Moukarzel et al., 1992). There is limited evidence suggesting an inverse relationship between carnitine levels and alkaline phosphatase in patients receiving parenteral nutrition (Berner et al., 1990).

However, intervention studies have failed to show any benefit of parenteral carnitine supplementation in patients receiving long-term parenteral nutrition in relation to hepatic abnormalities (Bowyer et al., 1988).

4.4.3.2 Choline

Choline, like carnitine, is normally synthesized from methionine. Levels are low in > 90% of patients receiving parenteral nutrition (Buchman et al., 1993) as a result of the abnormal metabolism described above and the lack of choline in standard parenteral formulations. Choline is required for the synthesis of VLDL and hence hepatic TAG export. Choline deficiency results in impaired hepatic TAG secretion and subsequent steatosis (Buchman et al., 1993). Choline deficiency in patients receiving parenteral nutrition has been shown to correlate with elevated transaminase levels and steatosis in both adults and children receiving parenteral nutrition (Buchman et al., 1993, 2001b). Small studies have shown that both parenteral choline supplementation and high-dose oral supplementation can reverse these abnormalities (Buchman et al., 1992, 2001a).

4.4.3.3 Taurine

Taurine is important for bile salt conjugation, particularly in preterm infants. It promotes bile flow and attenuates the cholestatic effects of secondary bile salts such as lithocholate (Belli et al., 1991). Taurine deficiency in neonates is associated with cholestatic liver disease (Cooper et al., 1984), and there is evidence that this condition can be prevented by parenteral taurine supplementation (Spencer et al., 2005). Studies in adults have shown that both plasma and biliary taurine levels are low (Schneider et al., 2006), probably as a result of a combination of reduced synthesis via hepatic transulfuration pathways coupled with an increased loss of bile acids associated with ileocolonic resection. Supplementation has been shown to improve plasma but not biliary taurine levels, this change being accompanied by an improvement in plasma transaminase concentrations (Schneider et al., 2006).

4.4.3.4 Antioxidants

Individuals receiving parenteral nutrition may be deficient in antioxidants, in particular, vitamin E and selenium (Nightingale, 2003). Increased oxidative stress might predispose to lipid peroxidation of hepatic lipid stores resulting in inflammation and steatohepatitis (Buchman et al., 2006). Experiments using animal models suggest that antioxidants such as glutathione may attenuate the hepatic dysfunction induced by parenteral feeding (Hong et al., 2007). However, although markers of oxidative stress are increased in adults receiving parenteral nutrition, there is little evidence that oxidative damage is increased despite infusion of soybean-based lipid infusions rich in polyunsaturated fatty acids (Schepens et al., 2006). Studies in children suggest that the occurrence of parenteral nutrition–associated cholestasis is independent of oxidant load (Lavoie et al., 2005). In addition, there is little evidence that antioxidant levels are depleted in patients receiving parenteral nutrition, and vitamin E is commonly added to intravenous lipid emulsions (Buchman et al., 2006).

4.4.4 NUTRIENT TOXICITY

4.4.4.1 Glucose

Early parenteral nutrition formulations contained large amounts of energy supplied as glucose, and the total glucose content often exceeded the maximum glucose oxidation rate. It is likely that this factor partly explains the high incidence of steatosis seen in these early studies (Lindor et al., 1979). Glucose infusion at rates of > 5 mg/kg body weight/min result in steatosis (Burke et al., 1979). High glucose infusion rates stimulate insulin release, which stimulates hepatic lipogenesis and the production of acylglycerol from glucose while concomitantly inhibiting mitochondrial fatty acid oxidation (Li et al., 1988). This results in a buildup of TAG within the hepatocytes. The adverse effects of insulin hypersecretion may also explain why continuous parenteral nutrition infusion is associated with a greater extent of hepatic dysfunction than cyclic infusion. Allowing ≥ 8 h each day without parenteral glucose infusion has been shown to lower insulin levels and improve LFT (Hwang et al., 2000). It was initially thought that the failure of the liver to secrete excess TAG into the circulation was the result of an inadequate amino acid content relative to carbohydrate content limiting adequate lipoprotein production (Quigley et al., 1993). However, steatosis has been shown to result from excessive glucose infusion even if amino acid intake is adequate (Guglielmi et al. 2006).

4.4.4.2 Lipid

The replacement of a proportion of glucose energy with parenteral lipid has been shown to reduce the incidence of steatosis (Meguid et al., 1984). However, excess lipid may also increase hepatic complications. Very high parenteral lipid intakes of > 4 g/kg body weight/day may result in a lipid overload syndrome due to the inability of the reticuloendothelial system to clear large amounts of polyunsaturated fatty acids and phospholipids (Bigorgne et al., 1998). An association has been found between more modest parenteral lipid intake and the incidence of both chronic cholestasis and advanced liver disease (Cavicchi et al., 2000). In multivariate analysis, parenteral intake of soybean-based lipid emulsion of > 1 g/kg body weight/day is associated with a relative risk of chronic cholestasis of 2.3 and a relative risk of advanced liver disease (fibrosis or cirrhosis on liver biopsy) of 5.5 (Cavicchi et al., 2000). The exact mechanism behind this effect is unclear. It has been postulated that lipid overloading of hepatic macrophages might impair phospholipid excretion into bile and cause intrahepatic cholestasis (Cavicchi et al., 2000). Other authors have suggested that lipid infusion may inhibit hepatic TAG release (Luman and Shaffer, 2002) or may cause accumulation of phytosterols (Clayton et al., 1998). High plasma phytosterol concentrations have been documented in children but not in adults receiving parenteral lipid emulsions (Clayton et al., 1993). There has been some suggestion that lipid infusions with a lower soybean oil content may cause fewer hepatic complications, with studies showing a lower incidence of cholestasis in patients receiving lipid emulsions in which a proportion of the soybean oil has been replaced with either medium-chain TAG (Carpentier et al., 1990) or monounsaturated fatty acids (olive oil) (Palova et al., 2008). There are also case reports of parenteral fish oil supplementation improving hepatic function in children (Gura et al., 2008), although similar studies in adults have not been published.

4.4.4.3 Other Components

A number of other components of parenteral infusions have been suggested to cause abnormal LFT in patients receiving parenteral nutrition. High amino acid content has been proposed to promote cholestasis in neonates (Vileisis et al., 1980). Studies in children have shown an association between plasma manganese concentrations and cholestasis (Fell et al., 1996). Hypermanganesemia may also be a consequence of cholestasis; however, omitting parenteral manganese in cholestatic children can still improve hepatic function (Fell et al., 1996). Also, copper is excreted via the biliary route and can accumulate in the liver if there is substantial cholestasis, exacerbating hepatic dysfunction (Blaszyk et al., 2005).

4.5 MANAGEMENT OF PNALD

The strategies used in the management of PNALD are illustrated in Figure 4.2.

4.5.1 Treatment of Nonnutritional Causes

Given the importance of sepsis as a causative factor for PNALD, it is vital that every effort is made to reduce its incidence. Intra-abdominal sepsis should be treated using a procedure that is clinically appropriate, usually with a combination of antibiotics and/or minimally invasive drainage procedures. It is also important to avoid central venous catheter–associated sepsis. To this end, studies in both adult and pediatric populations have demonstrated reduced rates of central venous catheter–associated sepsis in patients managed by specialist nutrition teams using strict aseptic techniques (Kennedy and Nightingale, 2005). Efforts to reduce bacterial overgrowth have been more successful in neonates than in adults, suggesting a greater pathophysiological role in the former. Several small studies have suggested that antibiotics such as metronidazole and gentamicin may reduce the incidence of cholestasis in neonates receiving parenteral nutrition (Kubota et al., 1990; Spurr et al., 1989). To date, other approaches that may reduce bacterial translocation, such as increased dietary fiber intake and parenteral glutamine supplementation, have not been shown to have a beneficial effect on PNALD in human subjects.

Cholelithiasis is common in both adults and children receiving parenteral nutrition due to a combination of factors including reduced oral intake, ileal resection, weight loss, and drug treatment (Nightingale, 2003). The incidence of biliary sludge in adults receiving parenteral nutrition has been estimated to approach 100% after more than 6 weeks of treatment (Messing et al., 1983), and gallstones have been demonstrated to form in 45% of patients with short bowel syndrome (Nightingale et al., 1992).

Medications, especially antibiotics, are a common cause of abnormal LFT and should always be considered in a patient receiving parenteral nutrition with abnormal LFT. All hepatotoxic medications should be minimized.

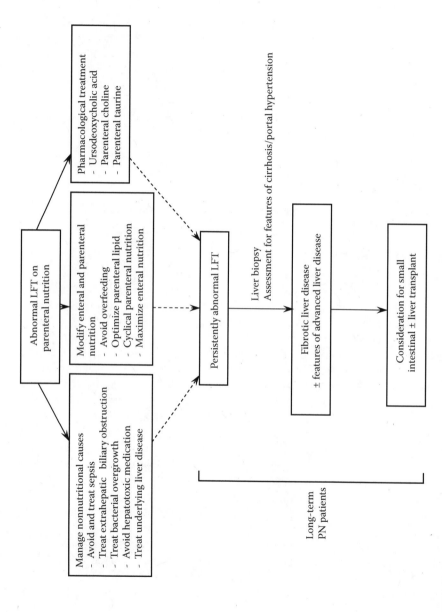

FIGURE 4.2 Management of parenteral nutrition–associated liver disease. LFT, liver function test.

4.5.2   ADJUSTMENTS TO PARENTERAL AND ENTERAL NUTRITION

It is important not to overfeed patients receiving parenteral nutrition, given the deleterious effects of infusion of excess parenteral glucose and lipid described earlier. Both U.S. and U.K. guidelines suggest a total daily energy intake of 105–146 kJ (25–35 kcal)/kg body weight and a daily protein intake of 0.8–1.5 g/kg body weight (Buchman et al., 2003; National Institute for Health and Clinical Excellence, 2006), although more accurate assessment of the basal metabolic rate and energy requirements can be made by performing indirect calorimetry. Given that the majority of patients receiving long-term parenteral nutrition will continue to eat, it is also necessary to estimate enteral energy and protein absorption and reduce parenteral provision accordingly. It is important to try to maximize enteral nutrition, although this approach may not always be possible. The oral route is preferable, although enteral tube feeding can be used and is often useful in infants. As well as countering the adverse effects of fasting described earlier and reducing parenteral requirements, enteral feeding promotes intestinal adaptation, which is of particular importance in infants for whom it may allow complete weaning from parenteral nutrition (Wallis et al., 2007).

The optimal dose and type of parenteral lipid that should be provided to minimize hepatic dysfunction remains unclear. In patients who have no enteral intake, some parenteral lipid is needed to prevent essential fatty acid deficiency (Buchman et al., 2003). A linoleic acid intake of 2–4% total energy intake is adequate for this purpose (Food and Agriculture Organization/World Health Organization/United Nations University, 1993) and, given the very high linoleic acid content of soybean-based lipid emulsions, this level of intake is easily achievable. U.S. guidelines suggest that parenteral lipid infusion should supply 20–30% total energy and daily intake should be < 2.5 g/kg body weight and ideally < 1.5 g/kg body weight (Buchman et al., 2003). However, experimental data suggest that the intake of soybean-based lipid should be < 1.0 g/kg body weight/day (Cavicchi et al., 2000). As previously discussed, there is growing evidence that lipid emulsions containing a mixture of long- and medium-chain TAG (Chan et al., 1998) (e.g., Lipofundin MCT/LCT1; B Braun, Melsungen, Germany), emulsions with a high monounsaturated fatty acids content (Palova et al., 2008) (e.g., Clinoleic1; Baxter, Maurepas, France), and emulsions containing fish oils (Gura et al., 2008) (e.g., SMOF Lipid1; Fresenius Kabi, Bad Homburg, Germany) may be preferable to soybean-based emulsions in relation to hepatic complications, but the latter remain in widespread use. Further clinical trials are necessary to explore this area further.

Finally, cyclical rather than continuous parenteral nutrition should be administered to minimize the adverse effects of prolonged insulin hypersecretion. Allowing an 8-h break from parenteral nutrition has been shown to improve LFT and reduce insulin levels (Hwang et al., 2000). Cyclical parenteral nutrition also allows greater patient freedom, which may be associated with an improved quality of life in patients receiving long-term parenteral nutrition (National Institute for Health and Clinical Excellence, 2006). At a practical level, this is achieved by slowly increasing the parenteral nutrition infusion rate and checking for hyperglycemia. In diabetic patients, it is more important to achieve tight glucose control, and this may limit or preclude cyclical parenteral nutrition.

4.5.3 Pharmacological Treatment

Ursodeoxycholic acid (UDCA) is an exogenous bile acid used in the management of a number of cholestatic conditions, including primary biliary cirrhosis and chole-lithiasis, with the aim of promoting biliary flow. There have been several small studies in neonates with parenteral nutrition associated cholestasis that have shown a beneficial effect of orally administered UDCA in doses of 10–30 mg/kg body weight/day (Chen et al., 2004; De Marco et al., 2006). In this patient group, UDCA improved LFTs and reduced the duration of cholestasis (Chen et al., 2004; De Marco et al., 2006). This outcome was achieved despite a very short residual intestine in some neonates. In addition, a rebound cholestasis occurs on withdrawal of UDCA in children (De Marco et al., 2006). Evidence of a benefit of UDCA in adults is more limited, with a single study showing that treatment with an average of 11.2 mg oral UDCA/kg body weight/day is associated with a reduction in γ-glutamyl transferase and alanine aminotransferase levels but not alkaline phosphatase, aspartate amino-transferase, or bilirubin levels (Beau et al., 1994). UDCA may also worsen diarrhea in some individuals.

As previously mentioned (section 4.4.3), there is evidence that levels of the S-containing amino acids choline and taurine are reduced in patients receiving par-enteral nutrition. Taurine is especially low in neonates and is now often added to neonatal parenteral nutrition formulations, but not to those of adults. Multivariate analysis of data collected as part of a larger multicenter trial investigating the man-agement of cholestasis in neonates receiving parenteral nutrition has suggested that parenteral taurine reduces the incidence of cholestasis in severely premature infants and those with necrotizing enterocolitis (Spencer et al., 2005). There is considerably less evidence of a benefit of taurine supplementation in adults, with a reduction in aspartate aminotransferase levels being reported in a single small study of adults receiving long-term parenteral nutrition (Schneider et al., 2006). Similarly, small-scale trials of choline supplementation in adults have demonstrated that both paren-teral choline and high-dose oral lecithin can increase plasma choline concentrations (Buchman et al., 1992, 1995, 2001a). This outcome has been shown to be associated with a reduction in hepatic steatosis, assessed by computerized tomography scan-ning, and improvements in plasma alkaline phosphatase, alanine aminotransferase, and aspartate aminotransferase concentrations (Buchman et al., 2001a).

4.5.4 Small Intestinal and Liver Transplantation

Impending or overt liver failure associated with PNALD is recognized as an indica-tion for small intestinal transplantation (Buchman et al., 2003), and PNALD is one of the most common reasons for performing intestinal transplantation (Grant et al., 2005). The definition of impending and overt liver failure includes patients with ele-vated serum bilirubin and/or liver enzymes, splenomegaly, thrombocytopenia, gas-troesophageal varices, coagulopathy, stomal bleeding, or hepatic fibrosis or cirrhosis (Buchman et al., 2003). This definition is very broad and would include patients ranging from those with relatively mild LFT abnormalities to those with end-stage liver disease. U.K. transplant units have suggested consideration of transplantation only if there is portal hypertension, cirrhosis, or bridging fibrosis (Middleton and Jamieson, 2005). Survival after intestinal transplantation is not as good as after other solid organ transplants (Grant et al., 2005). Survival is worst for individuals undergoing combined liver and small intestinal transplantation, with a 1-year survival of only 60%; 1-year survival after transplantation of small intestine alone is better at 77% (Grant et al., 2005). There is evidence to suggest that for individuals who do not have irreversible PNALD, small intestinal transplantation alone may be a viable option because of recovery of liver dysfunction after transplantation (Lauro et al., 2006). However, in adults with end-stage liver disease, a combined liver and small intestinal transplant will be required. In neonates and infants, for whom there is a possibility of an extent of intestinal adaptation and weaning from parenteral nutrition, transplantation of liver alone, which has a considerably better outcome than combined small intestinal and liver transplantation, may be possible as a bridging measure until enteral nutrition is established. In the meantime, the selection of patients for intestinal transplantation (with or without a liver transplant) presents a considerable challenge and recent consensus guidance is now published (Beath et al., 2008).

4.6   SUMMARY POINTS

- Liver dysfunction is common in individuals receiving parenteral nutrition and particularly in neonates and infants.
- Abnormalities of LFT in patients receiving short-term parenteral nutrition are usually transient.
- Individuals receiving long-term parenteral nutrition rarely develop end-stage liver disease.
- The etiology of PNALD is complex, with a large number of patient- and nutrition-related factors implicated.
- Effort should be made to prevent liver dysfunction by managing sepsis, avoiding parenteral overfeeding, using cyclical parenteral feeding, and encouraging enteral nutrition where possible.
- Intake of soybean-based parenteral lipid emulsions should be reduced in individuals with established PNALD.
- Patients with intestinal failure and PNALD who develop irreversible liver disease should be referred for a small intestinal and/or liver transplantation.

REFERENCES

Baker, M. L., and J. M. D. Nightingale. 2004. Abnormal liver function tests and parenteral nutrition. *Clin Nutr* 23:864–865.

Balistreri, W. F., J. E. Heubi, and F. J. Suchy. 1983. Immaturity of the enterohepatic circulation in early life: Factors predisposing to "physiologic" maldigestion and cholestasis. *J Pediatr Gastroenterol Nutr* 2:346–354.

Beale, E. F., R. M. Nelson, R. L. Bucciarelli, W. H. Donnelly, and D. V. Eitzman. 1979. Intrahepatic cholestasis associated with parenteral nutrition in premature infants. *Pediatrics* 64:342–347.

Beath, S. V., P. Davies, A. Papadopoulou, A. R. Khan, R. G. Buick, J. J. Corkery, P. Gornall, and I. W. Booth. 1996. Parenteral nutrition-related cholestasis in postsurgical neonates: Multivariate analysis of risk factors. *J Pediatr Surg* 31:604–606.

Beath, S., L. Pironi, S. Gabe, S. Horslen, D. Sudan, G. Mazeriegos, E. Steiger, O. Goulet, and J. Fryer. 2008. Collaborative strategies to reduce mortality and morbidity in patients with chronic intestinal failure including those who are referred for small bowel transplantation. *Transplantation* 85:1378–1384.

Beau, P., J. Labat-Labourdette, P. Ingrand, and M. Beauchant. 1994. Is ursodeoxycholic acid an effective therapy for total parenteral nutrition-related liver disease? *J Hepatol* 20:240–244.

Belli, D. C., C. C. Roy, L. A. Fournier, B. Tuchweber, R. Giguere, and I. M. Yousef. 1991. The effect of taurine on the cholestatic potential of sulfated lithocholate and its conjugates. *Liver* 11:162–169.

Berner, Y. N., W. A. Larchian, S. F. Lowry, R. R. Nicroa, M. F. Brennan, and M. Shike. 1990. Low plasma carnitine in patients on prolonged total parenteral nutrition: Association with low plasma lysine. *J Parenter Enteral Nutr* 14:255–258.

Bigorgne, C., A. Le Tourneau, K. Vahedi, B. Rio, B. Messing, T. Molina, J. Audouin, and J. Diebold. 1998. Sea-blue histiocyte syndrome in bone marrow secondary to total parenteral nutrition. *Leuk Lymphoma* 28:523–529.

Blaszyk, H., P. J. Wild, A. Oliveira, D. G. Kelly, and L. J. Burgart. 2005. Hepatic copper in patients receiving long-term total parenteral nutrition. *J Clin Gastroenterol* 39:318–320.

Bowyer, B. A., C. R. Fleming, D. Ilstrup, J. Nelson, S. Reek, and J. Burnes. 1986. Plasma carnitine levels in patients receiving home parenteral nutrition. *Am J Clin Nutr* 43:85–91.

Bowyer, B. A., J. M. Miles, M. W. Haymond, and C. R. Fleming. 1988. L-Carnitine therapy in home parenteral nutrition patients with abnormal liver tests and low plasma carnitine concentrations. *Gastroenterology* 94:434–438.

Buchman, A. L., M. E. Ament, M. Sohel, M. Dubin, D. J. Jenden, D. Roch, H. Pownall, W. Farley, M. Awal, and C. Ahn. 2001a. Choline deficiency causes reversible hepatic abnormalities in patients receiving parenteral nutrition: Proof of a human choline requirement: A placebo-controlled trial. *J Parenter Enteral Nutr* 25:260–268.

Buchman, A. L., M. Dubin, D. Jenden, A. Moukarzel, M. H. Roch, K. Rice, J. Gornbein, M. E. Ament, and C. D. Eckhert. 1992. Lecithin increases plasma free choline and decreases hepatic steatosis in long-term total parenteral nutrition patients. *Gastroenterology* 102:1363–1370.

Buchman, A. L., M. D. Dubin, A. A. Moukarzel, D. J. Jenden, M. Roch, K. M. Rice, J. Gornbein, and M. E. Ament. 1995. Choline deficiency: A cause of hepatic steatosis during parenteral nutrition that can be reversed with intravenous choline supplementation. *Hepatology* 22:1399–1403.

Buchman, A. L., K. Iyer, and J. Fryer. 2006. Parenteral nutrition-associated liver disease and the role for isolated intestine and intestine/liver transplantation. *Hepatology* 43:9–19.

Buchman, A. L., A. Moukarzel, D. J. Jenden, M. Roch, K. Rice, and M. E. Ament. 1993. Low plasma free choline is prevalent in patients receiving long term parenteral nutrition and is associated with hepatic aminotransferase abnormalities. *Clin Nutr* 12:33–37.

Buchman, A. L., J. Scolapio, and J. Fryer. 2003. AGA technical review on short bowel syndrome and intestinal transplantation. *Gastroenterology* 124:1111–1134.

Buchman, A. L., M. Sohel, A. Moukarzel, D. Bryant, R. Schanler, M. Awal, P. Burns, K. Dorman, M. Belfort, D. J. Jenden, D. Killip, and M. Roch. 2001b. Plasma choline in normal newborns, infants, toddlers, and in very-low-birth-weight neonates requiring total parenteral nutrition. *Nutrition* 17:18–21.

Burke, J. F., R. R. Wolfe, C. J. Mullany, D. E. Mathews, and D. M. Bier. 1979. Glucose requirements following burn injury. Parameters of optimal glucose infusion and possible hepatic and respiratory abnormalities following excessive glucose intake. *Ann Surg* 190:274–285.

Carpentier, Y. A., M. Richelle, D. Haumont, and R. J. Deckelbaum. 1990. New developments in fat emulsions. *Proc Nutr Soc* 49:375–380.

Carter, B. A., and R. J. Shulman. 2007. Mechanisms of disease: Update on the molecular etiology and fundamentals of parenteral nutrition associated cholestasis. *Nat Clin Pract Gastroenterol Hepatol* 4:277–287.

Cavicchi, M. P. Beau, P. Crenn, C. Degott, and B. Messing. 2000. Prevalence of liver disease and contributing factors in patients receiving home parenteral nutrition for permanent intestinal failure. *Ann Intern Med* 132:525–532.

Chan, S., K. C. McCowen, and B. Bistrian. 1998. Medium-chain triglyceride and n-3 poly-unsaturated fatty acid-containing emulsions in intravenous nutrition. *Curr Opin Clin Nutr Metab Care* 1:163–169.

Chan, S., K. C. McCowen, B. R. Bistrian, A. Thibault, M. Keane-Ellison, R. A. Forse, T. Babineau, and P. Burke. 1999. Incidence, prognosis, and etiology of end-stage liver disease in patients receiving home total parenteral nutrition. *Surgery* 126:28–34.

Chawla, R. K., C. J. Berry, M. H. Kutner, and D. Rudman. 1985. Plasma concentrations of transulfuration pathway products during nasoenteral and intravenous hyperalimentation of malnourished patients. *Am J Clin Nutr* 42:577–584.

Chen, C. Y., P. N. Tsao, H. L. Chen, H. C. Chou, W. S. Hsieh, and M. H. Chang. 2004. Ursodeoxycholic acid (UDCA) therapy in very-low-birth-weight infants with parenteral nutrition-associated cholestasis. *J Pediatr* 145:317–321.

Clarke, P. J., M. J. Ball, and M. G. Kettlewell. 1991. Liver function tests in patients receiving parenteral nutrition. *J Parenter Enteral Nutr* 15:54–59.

Clayton, P. T., A. Bowron, K. A. Mills, A. Massoud, M. Casteels, and P. J. Milla. 1993. Phytosterolemia in children with parenteral nutrition-associated cholestatic liver disease. *Gastroenterology* 105:1806–1813.

Clayton, P. T., P. Whitfield, and K. Iyer. 1998. The role of phytosterols in the pathogenesis of liver complications of pediatric parenteral nutrition. *Nutrition* 14:158–164.

Cook, G. C., and M. S. Hutt. 1967. The liver after kwashiorkor. *Br Med J* 3:454–457.

Cooper, A., J. M. Betts, G. R. Pereira, and M. M. Ziegler. 1984. Taurine deficiency in the severe hepatic dysfunction complicating total parenteral nutrition. *J Pediatr Surg* 19: 462–466.

de Belle, R. C., V. Vaupshas, B. B. Vitullo, L. R. Haber, E. Shaffer, G. G. Mackie, H. Owen, J. M. Little, and R. Lester. 1979. Intestinal absorption of bile salts: Immature development in the neonate. *J Pediatr* 94:472–476.

De Marco, G., D. Sordino, E. Bruzzese, S. Di Caro, D. Mambretti, A. Tramontano, C. Colombo, P. Simoni, and A. Guarino. 2006. Early treatment with ursodeoxycholic acid for cholestasis in children on parenteral nutrition because of primary intestinal failure. *Aliment Pharmacol Ther* 24:387–394.

Fell, J. M., A. P. Reynolds, N. Meadows, K. Khan, S. G. Long, G. Quaghebeur, W. J. Taylor, and P. J. Milla. 1996. Manganese toxicity in children receiving long-term parenteral nutrition. *Lancet* 347:1218–1221.

Food and Agriculture Organization/World Health Organization/United Nations University. 1993. *Fats and Oils in Human Nutrition*. Report of a Joint Expert Consultation. Geneva: WHO.

Grant, D., K. Abu-Elmagd, J. Reyes, A. Tzakis, A. Langnas, T. Fishbein, O. Goulet, and D. Farmer. 2005. 2003 report of the intestine transplant registry: A new era has dawned. *Ann Surg* 241:607–613.

Greenberg, G. R., S. L. Wolman, N. D. Christofides, S. R. Bloom, and K. N. Jeejeebhoy. 1981. Effect of total parenteral nutrition on gut hormone release in humans. *Gastroenterology* 80:988–993.

Guglielmi, F. W., D. Boggio-Bertinet, A. Federico, G. B. Forte, A. Guglielmi, C. Loguercio, S. Mazzuoli, M. Merli, A. Palmo, C. Panella, L. Pironi, and A. Francavilla. 2006. Total parenteral nutrition-related gastroenterological complications. *Dig Liver Dis* 38:623–642.

Gura, K. M., S. Lee, C. Valim, J. Zhou, S. Kim, B. P. Modi, D. A. Arsenault, R. A. Strijbosch, S. Lopes, C. Duggan, and M. Puder. 2008. Safety and efficacy of a fish-oil–based fat emulsion in the treatment of parenteral nutrition-associated liver disease. *Pediatrics* 121:e678–e686.

Hong, L., J. Wu, and W. Cai. 2007. Glutathione decreased parenteral nutrition-induced hepatocyte injury in infant rabbits. *J Parenter Enteral Nutr* 31:199–204.

Hwang, T. L., M. C. Lue, and L. L. Chen. 2000. Early use of cyclic TPN prevents further deterioration of liver functions for the TPN patients with impaired liver function. *Hepatogastroenterology* 47:1347–1350.

Ito, Y., and M. E. Shils. 1991. Liver dysfunction associated with long-term total parenteral nutrition in patients with massive bowel resection. *J Parenter Enteral Nutr* 15:271–276.

Karpati, G., S. Carpenter, A. G. Engel, G. Watters, J. Allen, S. Rothman, G. Klassen, and O. A. Mamer. 1975. The syndrome of systemic carnitine deficiency. Clinical, morphologic, biochemical and pathophysiologic features. *Neurology* 25:16–24.

Kennedy, J. F., and J. M. Nightingale. 2005. Cost savings of an adult hospital nutrition support team. *Nutrition* 21:1127–1133.

Kubota, A., A. Okada, K. Imura, H. Kawahara, R. Nezu, S. Kamata, and Y. Takagi. 1990. The effect of metronidazole on TPN-associated liver dysfunction in neonates. *J Pediatr Surg* 25:618–621.

Lauro, A., C. Zanfi, G. Ercolani, A. Dazzi, L. Golfieri, A. Amaduzzi, G. L. Grazi, M. Vivarelli, M. Cescon, G. Varotti, M. Del Gaudio, M. Ravaioli, L. Pironi, and A. D. Pinna. 2006. Recovery from liver dysfunction after adult isolated intestinal transplantation without liver grafting. *Transplant Proc* 38:3620–3624.

Lavoie, J. C., P. Chessex, C. Gauthier, E. Levy, F. Alvarez, P. St-Louis, and T. Rouleau. 2005. Reduced bile flow associated with parenteral nutrition is independent of oxidant load and parenteral multivitamins. *J Pediatr Gastroenterol Nutr* 41:108–114.

Li, S., M. S. Nussbaum, D. Teague, C. L. Gapen, R. Dayal, and J. E. Fischer. 1988. Increasing dextrose concentrations in total parenteral nutrition (TPN) causes alterations in hepatic morphology and plasma levels of insulin and glucagon in rats. *J Surg Res* 44:639–648.

Lindor, K. D., C. R. Fleming, A. Abrams, and M. A. Hirschkorn. 1979. Liver function values in adults receiving total parenteral nutrition. *JAMA* 241:2398–2400.

Lloyd, D. A., A. A. Zabron, and S. M. Gabe. 2008. Chronic biochemical cholestasis in patients receiving home parenteral nutrition: Prevalence and predisposing factors. *Aliment Pharmacol Ther* 27:552–560.

Luman, W., and J. Shaffer. 2002. Prevalence, outcome and associated factors of deranged liver function tests in patients on home parenteral nutrition. *Clin Nutr* 21:337–343.

Meguid, M. M., M. P. Akahoshi, S. Jeffers, R. J. Hayashi, and W. G. Hammond. 1984. Amelioration of metabolic complications of conventional total parenteral nutrition. A prospective randomized study. *Arch Surg* 119:1294–1298.

Messing, B., C. Bories, F. Kunstlinger, and J. J. Bernier. 1983. Does total parenteral nutrition induce gallbladder sludge formation and lithiasis? *Gastroenterology* 84:1012–1019.

Middleton, S. J., and N. V. Jamieson. 2005. The current status of small bowel transplantation in the UK and internationally. *Gut* 54:1650–1657.

Moukarzel, A. A., K. A. Dahlstrom, A. L. Buchman, and M. E. Ament. 1992. Carnitine status of children receiving long-term total parenteral nutrition: A longitudinal prospective study. *J Pediatr* 120:759–762.

National Institute for Health and Clinical Excellence. 2006. *Nutrition Support in Adults: Oral Nutrition Support, Enteral Tube Feeding and Parenteral Nutrition.* London, NICE.

Nightingale, J. M. 2003. Hepatobiliary, renal and bone complications of intestinal failure. *Best Pract Res Clin Gastroenterol* 17:907–929.

Nightingale, J. M., M. A. Kamm, J. R. van der Sijp, M. A. Ghatei, S. R. Bloom, and J. E. Lennard-Jones. 1996. Gastrointestinal hormones in short bowel syndrome. Peptide YY may be the "colonic brake" to gastric emptying. *Gut* 39:267–272.

Nightingale, J. M., J. E. Lennard-Jones, D. J. Gertner, S. R. Wood, and C. I. Bartram. 1992. Colonic preservation reduces need for parenteral therapy, increases incidence of renal stones, but does not change high prevalence of gall stones in patients with a short bowel. *Gut* 33:1493–1497.

Palova, S., J. Charvat, and M. Kvapil. 2008. Comparison of soybean oil- and olive oil–ased lipid emulsions on hepatobiliary function and serum triacylglycerols level during realimentation. *J Int Med Res* 36:587–593.

Pappo, I., H. Bercovier, E. Berry, R. Gallilly, E. Feigin, and H. R. Freund. 1995. Antitumor necrosis factor antibodies reduce hepatic steatosis during total parenteral nutrition and bowel rest in the rat. *J Parenter Enteral Nutr* 19:80–82.

Peden, V. H., C. L. Witzleben, and M. A. Skelton. 1971. Total parenteral nutrition. *J Pediatr* 78:180–181.

Quigley, E. M., M. N. Marsh, J. L. Shaffer, and R. S. Markin. 1993. Hepatobiliary complications of total parenteral nutrition. *Gastroenterology* 104:286–301.

Reddy, B. S., J. MacFie, M. Gatt, L. Farlane-Smith, K. Bitzopoulou, and A. M. Snelling. 2007. Commensal bacteria do translocate across the intestinal barrier in surgical patients. *Clin Nutr* 26:208–215.

Richardson, T. J., and D. Sgoutas. 1975. Essential fatty acid deficiency in four adult patients during total parenteral nutrition. *Am J Clin Nutr* 28:258–263.

Salvino, R., R. Ghanta, D. L. Seidner, E. Mascha, Y. Xu, and E. Steiger. 2006. Liver failure is uncommon in adults receiving long-term parenteral nutrition. *J Parenter Enteral Nutr* 30:202–208.

Schepens, M. A., H. M. Roelofs, W. H. Peters, and G. J. Wanten. 2006. No evidence for oxidative stress in patients on home parenteral nutrition. *Clin Nutr* 25:939–948.

Schneider, S. M., F. Joly, M. F. Gehrardt, A. M. Badran, A. Myara, F. Thuillier, C. Coudray-Lucas, L. Cynober, F. Trivin, and B. Messing. 2006. Taurine status and response to intravenous taurine supplementation in adults with short-bowel syndrome undergoing long-term parenteral nutrition: A pilot study. *Br J Nutr* 96:365–370.

Sondheimer, J. M., E. Asturias, and M. Cadnapaphornchai. 1998. Infection and cholestasis in neonates with intestinal resection and long-term parenteral nutrition. *J Pediatr Gastroenterol Nutr* 27:131–137.

Spencer, A. U., S. Yu, T. F. Tracy, M. M. Aouthmany, A. Llanos, M. B. Brown, M. Brown, R. J. Shulman, R. B. Hirschl, P. A. Derusso, J. Cox, J. Dahlgren, P. J. Strouse, J. I. Groner, and D. H. Teitelbaum. 2005. Parenteral nutrition-associated cholestasis in neonates: Multivariate analysis of the potential protective effect of taurine. *J Parenter Enteral Nutr* 29:337–343.

Spurr, S. G., L. J. Grylack, and N. R. Mehta. 1989. Hyperalimentation-associated neonatal cholestasis: Effect of oral gentamicin. *J Parenter Enteral Nutr* 13:633–636.

Suchy, F. J., J. C. Bucuvalas, A. L. Goodrich, M. S. Moyer, and B. L. Blitzer. 1986. Taurocholate transport and Na^+-K^+-ATPase activity in fetal and neonatal rat liver plasma membrane vesicles. *Am J Physiol* 251:G665–G673.

van Munster I. P., A. Tangerman, and F. M. Nagengast. 1994. Effect of resistant starch on colonic fermentation, bile acid metabolism, and mucosal proliferation. *Dig Dis Sci* 39:834–842.

Vileisis, R. A., R. J. Inwood, and C. E. Hunt. 1980. Prospective controlled study of paren-
    teral nutrition-associated cholestatic jaundice: Effect of protein intake. *J Pediatr*
    96:893–897.
Vina, J., M. Vento, F. Garcia-Sala, I. R. Puertes, E. Gasco, J. Sastre, M. Asensi, and F. V.
    Pallardo. 1995. L-Cysteine and glutathione metabolism are impaired in premature
    infants due to cystathionase deficiency. *Am J Clin Nutr* 61:1067–1069.
Wallis, K., D. A. Lloyd, and S. M. Gabe. 2007. Promoting intestinal adaptation. *Br J Hosp
    Med (Lond)* 68:11–14.
Wolfe, B. M., B. K. Walker, D. B. Shaul, L. Wong, and B. H. Ruebner. 1988. Effect of total
    parenteral nutrition on hepatic histology. *Arch Surg* 123:1084–1090.

Section II

**Steatosis and Metabolic
Liver Disease**

5 Lipid Metabolism and Control in Nonalcoholic Fatty Liver Disease

*Phunchai Charatcharoenwitthaya
and Keith D. Lindor*

CONTENTS

5.1   INTRODUCTION

Nonalcoholic fatty liver disease (NAFLD) is currently the most common chronic liver condition in the Western world. Clinical, epidemiological, and biochemical data strongly support the concept that NAFLD is the hepatic manifestation of the metabolic syndrome, the constellation of metabolic abnormalities including obesity, diabetes, dyslipidemia, and insulin resistance. NAFLD incorporates a spectrum of disease ranging from simple steatosis in its most benign form to an intermediate lesion, termed nonalcoholic steatohepatitis (NASH), and sometimes cirrhosis. The hallmark of NAFLD is hepatocyte accumulation of triglyceride. The mechanism responsible for an excessive amount of intrahepatic fat remains unclear but must involve an imbalance between the intrahepatic production of triglyceride (primarily derived from plasma fatty acids delivered to the liver that are not oxidized for fuel) and the removal of intrahepatic triglyceride [primarily exported from the liver within very low density lipoprotein (VLDL)]. To clarify the pathogenesis of NAFLD and identify potential therapeutic targets, an increased understanding of the dynamics of triglyceride metabolism in the liver in relation to whole-body metabolic status

67

TABLE 5.1

Key Facts of Lipid Metabolism

1. The metabolism of fat consists of catabolic processes that generate energy and anabolic processes that create biologically important molecules from fatty acids and other dietary carbon sources.
2. Defects in fat metabolism are responsible for development of fatty liver disease that may be due to imbalance in energy consumption and its combustion resulting in lipid storage or can be a consequence of peripheral resistance to insulin, whereby the transport of fatty acids from fat cells to the liver is increased.
3. Impairment or inhibition of several receptor molecules that control the enzymes responsible for the oxidation and synthesis of fatty acids appears to contribute toward fat accumulation.
4. A liver can remain fatty without disturbing liver function, but by varying mechanisms and possible insults to the liver may progress to outright inflammation of the liver.
5. When inflammation occurs in this setting, the condition is then called steatohepatitis, which may develop into cirrhosis up to 20% over time.
6. One debated mechanism proposes a "second hit," or further injury, enough to cause the disease to progress from one stage to the next by an increase in oxidative stress, hormonal imbalances, and mitochondrial abnormalities.

---

is warranted. Therefore, this chapter provides an overview of the fundamental principles of lipid metabolism, and its disturbance in insulin resistance relevant to understanding the mechanism of hepatic steatosis and lipotoxicity in NAFLD (Table 5.1).

5.2 HEPATIC LIPID HOMEOSTASIS

Long-chain fatty acids in simple nonesterified form are known as free fatty acids (FFAs). FFAs normally cycle between the liver and peripheral adipocytes without any appreciable accumulation of lipids within hepatocytes. Fatty acids serve several important and biologically diverse functions, which include serving as cell structural components in membrane phospholipids, providing an important source of caloric energy, playing a role in intracellular signaling, and the regulation of gene transcription. The various sources of FFAs include new synthesis within the liver via *de novo* lipogenesis from glucose and the circulation as shown in Figure 5.1. Fatty acids in the circulation derive from the hydrolysis of triglycerides in adipocytes in the postabsorptive state and, to a lesser extent, from the postprandial lipolysis of triglyceride-rich particles, chylomicrons. Carbohydrates provide two routes to formation of triglycerides: the glycerol backbone via triose phosphate and FFAs via acetyl coenzyme A. Fructose can directly contribute to both of these substrates, bypassing the regulated conversion of fructose 6-phosphate to fructose 1,6-diphosphate, and is thus a relatively unregulated source of substrate for triglyceride synthesis in the liver.

FFAs are transported to the liver packaged with albumin. Thereafter, FFAs dissociate from albumin in the space of Disse and cross the liver cell plasma membrane via two distinct pathways: the protein-mediated uptake and the passive, transmembraneous flip-flop of protonated FFAs (Bradbury and Berk, 2004; Pohl et al., 2004). Capillary-bound lipoprotein lipase, as produced by the liver, mediates the lipolysis of protein-bound triglycerides on the luminal surface of capillary endothelial cells

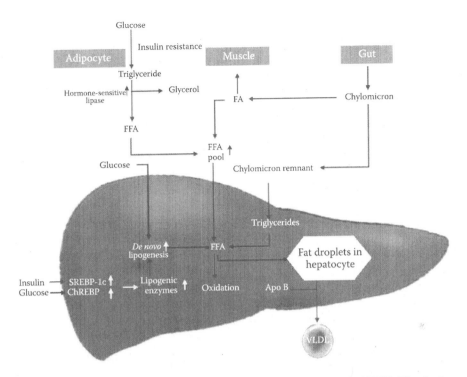

FIGURE 5.1 Lipid homeostasis in nonalcoholic fatty liver disease (NAFLD). The fundamental defect in insulin resistance is an increase in insulin-mediated suppression of lipolysis in adipose tissue, resulting in more free fatty acids (FFAs) delivery to the liver. Normally, hepatic lipid homeostasis is under the control of nuclear transcription factors, especially sterol regulatory element–binding protein (SREBP) and carbohydrate response element–binding protein (ChREBP). In NAFLD, an imbalance between the intrahepatic production of triglyceride (primarily derived from plasma fatty acids delivered to the liver that are not oxidized for fuel) and the removal of intrahepatic triglyceride [primarily exported from the liver within very low density lipoprotein (VLDL)] is the mechanism responsible for an excessive amount of intrahepatic fat.

(Heeren et al., 2002). This may be associated with a higher proportion of FFAs moving across the plasma membrane into or out of hepatocytes occurring by the passive nonsaturable pathway (Pohl et al., 2004; Hubbard et al., 2006). Several plasma membrane protein transporters are involved in the FFA uptake process; however, the main translocation process across the plasma membrane due to the saturable transport process involves members of the fatty acid transport protein (FATP) family (Hubbard et al., 2006). FATP5 is highly expressed in hepatocytes that reveal high-level FFA uptake for metabolism and storage.

Once taken up by the hepatocyte, FFAs then undergo oxidation within mitochondria, peroxisomes, or microsomes, or they become esterified into triglycerides, which are neutral lipids consisting of a glycerol backbone and three long-chain fatty acids. The β oxidation of mitochondrial FFAs is rate-limited by FFA uptake by mitochondria. Uptake requires the presence of the enzyme carnitine palmitoyl acyltransferase, which is inhibited by insulin and malonyl coenzyme A and stimulated by glucagon. FFA oxidation at other intracellular sites under physiologic conditions seems to make only a minor contribution to reducing the pool of hepatic FFAs. Triglyceride synthesis involves a series of steps; the final step is rate limiting and catalyzed by acetyl coenzyme A carboxylase (ACC): diacylglycerol acyltransferase (DGAT). Ultimately, triglycerides and other lipids are packaged in VLDL particles for transport to other organs. Indeed, the increased hepatic uptake and biosynthesis of FFAs are compensated through increased removal of lipids from the liver. The principal apolipoproteins for VLDL particle are apolipoprotein (Apo) B100, ApoE, ApoC-I, ApoC-II, and ApoC-III. ApoB100 is cotranslationally lipidated with triglycerides within the lumen of the endoplasmic reticulum by microsomal triglyceride transfer protein (Wetterau et al., 1997), which similarly lipidates ApoB48 in the intestinal epithelial cells. Within the circulation, the apoC-II of VLDL activates lipoprotein lipase within specific capillary beds, hydrolyzing the triglycerides, with release of glycerol and FFA. In adipose tissue, the released FFAs are taken up by the adipocytes and reesterified to triglycerides for storage. Most of the resulting VLDL remnants are cleared by receptor-mediated endocytosis in the liver.

5.3   REGULATION OF LIPID HOMEOSTASIS

The liver plays a major role in the regulation of glucose and lipid metabolism. Thus, the disruption of the normal mechanisms for synthesis, transport, and removal/metabolism of FFAs and triglycerides constitutes the basis for the development of fatty liver. Fat accumulation in hepatocytes is commonly associated with resistance to insulin's action to suppress hepatic gluconeogenesis and antilipolysis in adipocytes. However, the exact mechanisms that link hepatic lipid accumulation and insulin resistance remain unclear; increasing evidence suggests that nuclear transcription factors play important roles. Several nuclear transcription factors have emerged as dominant regulators of hepatocyte metabolic homeostasis, including the sterol regulatory element–binding proteins (SREBP), carbohydrate response element–binding protein (ChREBP), liver X–activated receptor (LXR), and the peroxisome proliferator–activated receptor (PPAR) as shown in Table 5.2. Moreover, increasing evidence suggests that cross-talk of these nuclear factors could play crucial roles in lipid metabolism.

SREBPs are a family of transcription factors that regulate lipid homeostasis by controlling the expression of a range of enzymes required for endogenous cholesterol, fatty acid, triglyceride, and phospholipid synthesis. SREBP-1a is highly expressed in tissues with a high capacity for cell proliferation, such as spleen and intestine, whereas SREBP-1c and SREBP-2 are the predominant isoforms expressed with especially high levels in liver, white adipose tissue, and skeletal muscle (Shimomura et al., 1997). Overexpression of SREBP-1a in mice liver markedly increases the expression of genes involved in cholesterol and triglyceride synthesis (Horton et al., 2003). SREBP-1c mediates insulin-directed lipogenic activity by increasing *de novo* lipogenesis via increased transcription and expression of several key lipogenic enzymes, including ATP citrate-lyase, ACC, fatty acid synthase (FAS), and steroyl coenzyme A desaturase. SREBP-1c also increases the expression of acetyl coenzyme

TABLE 5.2

Nuclear Transcription Factors Involved in Regulation of Lipid Homeostasis

Transcription Factor	Location	Function
Sterol regulatory element–binding protein 1c	Liver	Increase lipogenesis
Sterol regulatory element–binding protein 2	Liver	Increase cholesterol synthesis
Carbohydrate response element–binding protein	Liver	Increase lipogenesis
Liver X–activated receptor	Liver, intestines, adipose tissue	Regulate cholesterol metabolism, lipid biosynthesis, and glucose homeostasis
Peroxisome proliferators–activated receptor α	Liver	Promote β oxidation of fatty acids
Peroxisome proliferators activated receptor γ	Adipose tissue	Promote adipocyte differentiation with increasing in lipogenesis

A synthetase, which in turn increases production of acetyl coenzyme A, the starting point for lipogenesis (Magaña and Osborne, 1996). SREBP-1c further contributes to a positive triglyceride balance by inhibiting expression of microsomal triglycerides transfer protein, which decreases VLDL formation (Sato et al., 1999). SERBP-2 regulates 3-hydroxyl-3-methylglutaryl-CoA reductase and LDL receptor expression and has a major role in cholesterol homeostasis (Shimano, 2001).

The transcription factor ChREBP plays a pivotal role in the control of lipogenesis through the transcriptional regulation of lipogenic genes, including ACC and FAS. ChREBP is translocated to the nucleus and activated in response to high glucose concentrations in the liver, independently of insulin. ChREBP binds to its functional heterodimeric partner, Max-like protein X (Mlx), and induces the transcription of lipogenic and glycolytic genes containing a carbohydrate response element, such as those encoding ACC, FAS, and liver-type pyruvate kinase (Weickert and Pfeiffer, 2006). For most genes in the hepatocyte, both ChREBP-Mlx and SREBP are required for induction, and the two signaling pathways function in a highly synergistic manner to support the full transcriptional response for the hepatocyte to store excess carbohydrate nutrients as triglycerides. This overlapping regulatory control of lipogenesis may serve to ensure that lipogenesis, an energy-requiring process, does not occur under inappropriate physiological conditions (Ma et al., 2005).

LXRs are also recognized as important regulators of cholesterol metabolism, lipid biosynthesis, and glucose homeostasis. LXRs belong to a subclass of nuclear hormone receptors that form obligate heterodimers with retinoid X receptor and are activated by oxysterols. LXRs have been identified as a dominant activator of SERBP-1c promoter (Yoshikawa et al., 2001). Next, activated SREBP-1c stimulates the transcription of genes involved in *de novo* lipogenesis and interacts with regulatory elements in the promoters of various insulin-regulated genes. In addition to being a cholesterol sensor, LXR has a vital role in macrophage biology, inflammation, and innate immunity (Castrillo and Tontonoz, 2004). In response to stimulation with lipopoly-saccharide, LXR signaling inhibits macrophage expression of inducible nitric oxide synthase, cyclooxygenase 2, and interleukin 6 (Joseph et al., 2003).

PPARs, comprising a ligand-activated nuclear hormone receptor superfamily, are known to regulate the expression of numerous genes involved in fatty acid metabo-lism and adipocyte differentiation (Schoonjans et al., 1996). PPARs are differentially activated by a variety of saturated or unsaturated FFAs and lipid-like compounds. PPARs have three isoforms that have different patterns of tissue expression and func-tional activity. PPAR-α is primarily expressed in the liver, in which it has been shown to promote β oxidation of fatty acids. In the small intestine, PPAR-β/δ increase FFA binding proteins and have a role in intestinal adaptation to changes in dietary content (Poirier et al., 2001). PPAR-γ, preferentially expressed in adipose tissue, promotes adipocyte differentiation and lipoprotein lipase activity, thereby making triglyceride-derived FFA available for uptake. It also induces FFA transport protein and acetyl coenzyme A synthase, thereby increasing adipose tissue lipogenesis. PPARs also have important anti-inflammatory effects because they interfere with nuclear factor kappa B (NF-κB) and other proinflammatory pathway (Bocher et al., 2002).

Taken together, fatty acid metabolism in the liver is transcriptionally regulated by two reciprocal systems: PPAR-α controls fatty acid degradation, whereas SREBP-1c, activated by LXR, regulates fatty acid synthesis. The roles of these transcription factors in whole body physiology and metabolism can be best illustrated by com-paring two opposite nutritional states: fasted and refed states (Kersten et al., 1999; Leone et al., 1999). In the fasted liver, PPAR-α plays a major role in fatty acids being oxidized to acetyl-CoA and subsequently to ketone bodies. In contrast, expression of SREBP-1c is reduced during fasting. In the refed state, lipogenesis is induced through increased amount of SREBP-1, whereas PPAR-α is decreased. This coor-dinated reciprocal regulation of the two transcription factors is a key to nutritional regulation of fatty acids and triglycerides as an energy storage system and impli-cates the presence of a cross-talk between these factors. However, further studies are needed to evaluate the physiological relevance of the cross-talk between these and other nuclear transcription factors to harvest the net beneficial effects.

5.4 DEVELOPMENT OF HEPATIC STEATOSIS

Several lines of evidence indicate that NAFLD should be considered part of a multi-organ system derangement in insulin sensitivity. The amount of intrahepatic tri-glyceride is directly correlated with impaired insulin action in liver (suppression of glucose production), skeletal muscle (stimulation of glucose uptake), and adipose tissue (suppression of lipolysis), independent of percentage body fat and intra-abdominal adipose tissue volume (Korenblat et al., 2008). Systemic insulin resis-tance coupled with impaired insulin action in skeletal muscle, adipose tissue, and hepatocyte leads to high circulating FFA loads as a consequence of the inability of cells to handle both carbohydrate and fat loading. Normal handling of FFAs would result in increased glycogen storage, reduced lipogenesis, increased hepatic export of VLDL, and enhanced oxidation of FFAs (Parekh and Anania, 2007). The persistence of high circulating levels of FFAs and persistent hyperglycemia result in a series of changes in hepatic FFA metabolism that ultimately leads to hepatic steatosis. Fatty acid synthesized by the liver *de novo* is also increased in the insulin-resistant state, whereas decreased β oxidation of FFAs and impaired synthesis and secretion of ApoB reduces the secretion of triglycerides from the liver as VLDL (Korenblat et al., 2008). The consequence is net storage of hepatocyte storage of triglycerides or steatosis.

The key physiologic factors involved in the accumulation of excessive intrahepatic triglyceride in NAFLD have been carefully evaluated in nondiabetic obese subjects with NAFLD (Fabbrini et al., 2008). Excessive intrahepatic triglyceride content in obese subjects is associated with alterations in both adipose tissue and hepatic lipid metabolism; subjects with NAFLD have increased rates of adipose tissue triglyceride lipolysis and hepatic VLDL secretion. Increased intrahepatic triglyceride content is not simply a marker of altered hepatic metabolic function but is directly involved in the pathophysiology of NAFLD because the increase in VLDL secretion was caused by an increased incorporation of nonsystemic fatty acids into VLDL from lipolysis of intrahepatic and intra-abdominal fat and *de novo* lipogenesis (Fabbrini et al., 2008). Moreover, the increase in VLDL secretion is likely responsible for the increase in serum triglyceride concentrations commonly observed in patients with NAFLD. The dissociation in VLDL and VLDL-ApoB100 kinetics suggests that a failure to adequately increase the secretion rate of ApoB100, which provides the framework for triglyceride incorporation into VLDL, limits the liver's capacity to export triglyceride. These data underscore the complex metabolic interactions associated with NAFLD in obese persons.

5.5   PROGRESSION OF NAFLD

The precise mechanisms by which NAFLD develops into the steatohepatitis phenotype remain unknown. A "two-hit" hypothesis for the development and progression of NAFLD was proposed (Figure 5.2). Briefly, the first hit involves accumulation of triglyceride in hepatocytes. Once the presence of hepatic steatosis is established, progression to steatohepatitis involves a "second hit" and oxidative stress is thought to play a key role. The resulting accumulation of fat within the hepatocytes has several effects. FFAs impair insulin signaling and cause hepatic insulin resistance via mechanisms involving activation of protein kinase C, Jun N-terminal kinase, inhibitor kappa beta kinase β and NF-κB (Samuel et al., 2004; Cai et al., 2005). Finally, it appears that consequences of fat accumulation within the liver (fat-induced hepatic insulin resistance and up-regulation of PPAR-α–regulated genes) result in increased FFA oxidation. Mitochondrial and peroxisomal fatty acids oxidations are both capable of producing hepatotoxic free oxygen radicals that contribute to the development of oxidative stress (Chalasani et al., 2003; Reddy, 2001). These data suggest that insulin resistance could in fact deliver both "hits" in the pathogenesis of NAFLD.

As proposed above, accumulation of triglycerides within the liver previously was thought to represent the "first hit" in the progression of this disease. Consistent with this view, studies in animal models of steatosis have demonstrated improvements in hepatic steatosis and insulin sensitivity when triglyceride synthesis was inhibited (Yu et al., 2005). In an animal model of progressive NAFLD, however, suppression

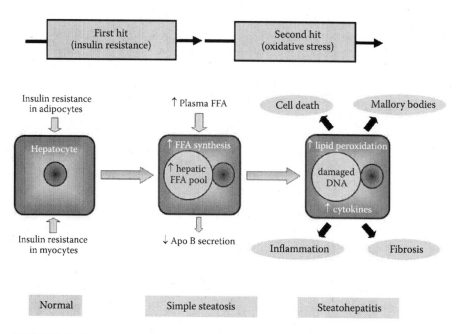

FIGURE 5.2 Pathophysiology of NAFLD. NAFLD is associated with peripheral and hepatic insulin resistance, which is the first hit that causes hepatic steatosis. Development of nonalcoholic steatohepatitis requires a second hit. Possible pathophysiologic processes involved in the second hit include lipid peroxidation, apoptosis, and inflammatory cytokines.

of DGAT2 expression at the final step of triglyceride synthesis improved hepatic steatosis but increased hepatic FFA content, up-regulated cytochrome P-450 2E1, exacerbated hepatic oxidative damage, and increased hepatocyte death, liver inflammation, and fibrosis (Yamaguchi et al., 2007). Liver disease progression occurred despite significant improvements in insulin sensitivity. These results suggest that triglyceride accumulation *per se* is not harmful in this model; but rather, triglyceride synthesis appears to provide a protective mechanism to buffer the harmful effects of FFA-induced lipotoxicity. Hence, liver damage accrued from the "invisible" lipids rather than from the "visible" fat (i.e., triglycerides) that was the basis for a diagnosis of NAFLD. Hepatic triglyceride accumulation may simply identify livers that are experiencing increased exposure to FFAs. Whether this results in liver damage seems to be determined, at least in part, by the ability of hepatocytes to detoxify FFAs by incorporating them into triglyceride. Thus, individual differences in the ability to inhibit the lipotoxic effects of FFA accumulation by up-regulating triglyceride synthesis may explain why only some people with steatosis develop progressive liver disease.

Currently, there is accumulating evidence that mitochondrial dysfunction, particularly respiratory chain deficiency, plays a key role in the physiopathology of NASH. Reactive oxygen species (ROS) generation in an environment enriched in lipids in turn induces lipid peroxidation, which releases highly reactive aldehydic derivatives (e.g., malondialdehyde) that have diverse detrimental effects on hepatocytes and other hepatic cells. In hepatocytes, ROS, reactive nitrogen species, and lipid peroxidation products further impair the respiratory chain, either directly or indirectly through oxidative damage to the mitochondrial genome. This consequently leads to the generation of more ROS and a vicious cycle occurs. ROS and lipid peroxidation products then increase the generation of several cytokines playing a key role in cell death, inflammation, and fibrosis. Moreover, oxidative stress also produces alterations in the production of adipokines and proinflammatory cytokines secreted by the adipose tissue as shown in Table 5.3. These hormones play a major role in modulating insulin resistance and have potential to influence the progression of NASH including the development of hepatic fibrosis (Parekh and Anania, 2007). In addition, a recent report (Adams et al., 2004) of a high frequency of NASH with rapid progression to cirrhosis in patients with panhypopituitarism who are deficient in dehydroepiandrosterone (DHEA) led to the hypothesis that relative deficiency of DHEA may play a role in the histological progression of NAFLD.

A cytokine imbalance, particularly in an increase in the ratio of tumor necrosis factor α (TNF-α) to adiponectin, may play an important role in the development of NASH. Gene expression of TNF-α and TNF receptors is increased in the liver of patients with NASH as compared with both normal liver and fatty liver, and

TABLE 5.3
Adipokines and Proinflammatory Cytokines Involved in Progression of Nonalcoholic Fatty Liver Disease

Factors	Source	Role in Development of Steatohepatitis
Tumor necrosis factor α	Kupffer cells, macrophages, hepatic stellate cells, hepatocytes, adipocytes	- Induction of lipid peroxidation and apoptosis - Release of other cytokines from activated Kupffer cells - Mitochondrial injury with release of reactive oxygen species and caspases
Adiponectin	Adipocytes	- Enhances hepatic lipid oxidation - Improves insulin sensitivity - Anti-inflammatory effects
Leptin	Adipocytes	- Regulates hepatic fibrosis by activation of stellate cell and modulation of Kupffer cell function - Up-regulates profibrogenic transforming growth factor β synthesis
Resistin	Adipocytes, monocytes, Kupffer cells	- Release of proinflammatory and fibrogenic cytokines
Interleukin 6	Kupffer cells, macrophages, hepatic stellate cells, endothelial cells, adipocytes	- Activates hepatic stellate cells to cause fibrosis - Mediates synthesis of acute phase proteins by hepatocytes
Interleukin 8	Inflammatory cells	- Mediates inflammatory response

the expression is higher in patients with more severe NASH (Crespo et al., 2001). Circulating TNF-α levels are significantly higher in patients with NASH as compared with control (Hui et al., 2004). However, the molecular mechanisms linking lipid accumulation in hepatocytes, increased TNF-α production, and liver damage remain poorly understood. Hepatocyte stimulation by FFAs leads to increased lysosomal permeability, and subsequently release of cathepsin B in the cytosol causes NF-κB translocation into the nucleus with increased production and release of TNF-α. Cathepsin B also causes mitochondrial dysfunction leading to hepatocyte apoptosis. In addition, TNF-α may further promote lysosomal destabilization, resulting in accentuating liver injury (Feldstein et al., 2004). Moreover, TNF-α may contribute to steatohepatitis by up-regulation of SREBP-1c and FAS mRNA levels (Endo et al., 2007).

Adiponectin, an insulin-sensitizing agent that decreases export of fatty acids from adipose depots, is closely implicated in the pathogenesis of NAFLD. It reduces lipid accumulation within hepatocytes by inhibiting fatty acid import and increasing fatty acid oxidation and export. These actions are exerted through activation of the cyclic adenosine 5'-monophosphate-dependent protein kinase. In human studies (Hui et al., 2004), serum adiponectin levels are inversely related to hepatic fat stores and are lower in patients with NASH than in persons with uncomplicated steatosis. In another study (Kaser et al., 2005), hepatic expression of adiponectin, and its type II receptor was less in NASH than in fatty liver. Moreover, adiponectin also exerts anti-inflammatory effects by opposing the synthesis and release of TNF-α from macrophages within adipose tissue in obesity (Masaki et al., 2004). It is therefore of great interest that administration of exogenous adiponectin reverses experimental forms of NAFLD and steatohepatitis (Yamauchi et al., 2003).

Leptin, discovered as a product of the obesity gene, has been shown to play an important role in partitioning energy stores, including fat and glucose by way of modulating insulin sensitivity. The high circulating leptin levels associated with obesity in humans suggest a role for leptin in NASH, especially since leptin exerts complex effects on insulin response in hepatocytes, stimulating glucose transport and turnover, consistent with an insulinotropic effect (Kamohara et al., 1997). Leptin increased transforming growth factor β mRNA in isolated sinusoidal endothelial cells and Kupffer cells, and augmented platelet-derived growth factor–dependent proliferation of hepatic stellate cells by enhancing downstream intracellular signaling pathways via mitogen-activated protein kinase and phosphatidylinositol 3-kinase (Ikejima et al., 2005). These findings indicate that leptin may be one of the key regulators for inflammation and progression of fibrosis in NASH. However, accumulated knowledge about leptin in the scheme of NASH has not completely proved the possibility that leptin influences fibrotic and ultimately functional severity in NASH.

DHEA is the most abundant steroid hormone and has been shown to influence sensitivity to oxidative stress, insulin sensitivity, expression of PPAR-α, and procollagen messenger RNA. Recently, our group has demonstrated that more advanced NAFLD, as indicated by the presence of NASH with advanced fibrosis stage, is strongly associated with low circulating sulfated DHEA (Charlton et al., 2008). A role of sulfated DHEA deficiency in histological progression of NAFLD is likely to involve effects on insulin sensitivity, hepatic susceptibility to oxidative stress injury, and/or stimulation of fibrosis. Although the literature concerning the role of DHEA in mediating insulin sensitivity in humans is conflicting, evidence generated from randomized controlled trials suggests that DHEA enhances insulin sensitivity (Kawano, 2000). In healthy humans (Mastrocola et al., 2003), DHEA and its metabolite reduce tissue susceptibility to oxidation of both lipids and proteins. Moreover, DHEA has been shown to directly inhibit procollagen type I synthesis at the transcriptional level *in vivo* and *in vitro* in animals and *in vitro* in human fibroblasts (Iwasaki et al., 2005). Finally, DHEA might exert a hepatoprotective effect in NAFLD through attenuation of ROS-mediated release of cytokines by Kupffer cells, adipose tissue, and hepatocytes. Thus, there are several potential mechanisms for DHEA deficiency to promote histological progression in NAFLD.

5.6 PRACTICAL APPLICATIONS

Over the past decade, there has been increasing knowledge on lipid metabolism and control in NAFLD by studies in different experimental models and humans with this condition. Although the exact mechanisms that link hepatic lipid accumulation and insulin resistance have not been elucidated, increasing evidence suggests that several nuclear transcription factors and cytokines secreted by the adipose tissue, in particular, TNF-α and adiponectin, appear to play a central role as regulators of insulin sensitivity and development of fatty liver, as well as in the inflammatory process and fibrogenesis. A better understanding of the role of these factors and their possible interactions to regulate hepatocyte metabolic homeostasis in NAFLD may help us to identify potential novel treatments to halt progression of the disease. Since NAFLD is the hepatic component of the metabolic syndrome, initial treatment should be directed at correcting coexisting comorbidities such as obesity, diabetes, hypertension, and dyslipidemia. Other than weight reduction, there is no proven effective therapy for NAFLD.

5.7 SUMMARY POINTS

- The fundamental principles of hepatic lipid metabolism in the normal state and the mechanisms of hepatic steatosis and its disturbance in the insulin-resistant state underlie the development of fatty liver.
- Regulation of nuclear transcription factors has an effect on hepatocyte metabolic homeostasis and possibly the evolution of fatty liver disease.
- Generation of reactive oxygen species in the liver likely influences progression of fatty liver disease.
- Adipokines and proinflammatory cytokines modulate insulin resistance and influence the progression of fatty liver disease.
- Hepatic lipotoxicity seen in animal and human research models of fatty liver disease may lead to NASH.

REFERENCES

Adams, L. A., A. Feldstein, K. D. Lindor, and P. Angulo. 2004. Nonalcoholic fatty liver disease among patients with hypothalamic and pituitary dysfunction. *Hepatology* 39: 909–914.

Bocher, V., I. Pineda-Torra, J. C. Fruchart, and B. Staels. 2002. PPARs: Transcription factors controlling lipid and lipoprotein metabolism. *Ann N Y Acad Sci* 967:7–18.

Bradbury, M. W., and P. D. Berk. 2004. Lipid metabolism in hepatic steatosis. *Clin Liver Dis* 8:639–671.

Cai, D., M. Yuan, D. F. Frantz, P. A. Melendez, L. Hansen, J. Lee, and S. E. Shoelson. 2005. Local and systemic insulin resistance resulting from hepatic activation of IKK-beta and NF-kappaB. *Nat Med* 11:183–190.

Castrillo, A., and Tontonoz. P. 2004. Nuclear receptors in macrophage biology: At the crossroads of lipid metabolism and inflammation. *Annu Rev Cell Dev Biol* 20:455–480.

Chalasani, N., J. C. Gorski, M. S. Asghar, A. Asghar, B. Foresman, S. D. Hall, and D. W. Crabb. 2003. Hepatic cytochrome P450 2E1 activity in nondiabetic patients with nonalcoholic steatohepatitis. *Hepatology* 37:544–550.

Charlton, M., P. Angulo, N. Chalasani, R. Merriman, K. Viker, P. Charatcharoenwitthaya, S. Sanderson, S. Gawrieh, A. Krishnan, and K. Lindor. 2008. Low circulating levels of dehydroepiandrosterone in histologically advanced nonalcoholic fatty liver disease. *Hepatology* 47:484–492.

Crespo, J., A. Cayón, P. Fernández-Gil, M. Hernández-Guerra, M. Mayorga, A. Domínguez-Díez, J. C. Fernández-Escalante, and F. Pons-Romero. 2001. Gene expression of tumor necrosis factor-alpha and TNF-receptors, p55 and p75, in nonalcoholic steatohepatitis patients. *Hepatology* 34:1158–1163.

Endo, M., T. Masaki, M. Seike, and H. Yoshimatsu. 2007. TNF-alpha induces hepatic steatosis in mice by enhancing gene expression of sterol regulatory element binding protein–1c (SREBP-1c). *Exp Biol Med (Maywood)* 232:614–621.

Fabbrini, E., B. S. Mohammed, F. Magkos, K. M. Korenblat, B. W. Patterson, and S. Klein. 2008. Alterations in adipose tissue and hepatic lipid kinetics in obese men and women with nonalcoholic fatty liver disease. *Gastroenterology* 134:424–431.

Feldstein, A. E., N. W. Werneburg, A. Canbay, M. E. Guicciardi, S. F. Bronk, R. Rydzewski, L. J. Burgart, and G. J. Gores. 2004. Free fatty acids promote hepatic lipotoxicity by stimulating TNFalpha expression via a lysosomal pathway. *Hepatology* 40:185–194.

Heeren, J., A. Niemeier, M. Merkel, and U. Beisiegel. 2002. Endothelial-derived lipoprotein lipase is bound to postprandial triglyceride-rich lipoproteins and mediates their hepatic clearance in vivo. *J Mol Med* 80:576–584.

Horton, J. D., N. A. Shah, J. A. Warrington, N. N. Anderson, S. W. Park, M. S. Brown, and J. L. Goldstein. 2003. Combined analysis of oligonucleotide microarray data from transgenic and knockout mice identifies direct SREBP target genes. *Proc Natl Acad Sci U S A* 100:12027–12032.

Hubbard, B., H. Doege, S. Punreddy, H. Wu, X. Huang, V. K. Kaushik, R. L. Mozell, J. J. Byrnes, A. Stricker-Krongrad, C. J. Chou, L. A. Tartaglia, H. F. Lodish, A. Stahl, and R. E. Gimeno. 2006. Mice deleted for fatty acid transport protein 5 have defective bile acid conjugation and are protected from obesity. *Gastroenterology* 130:1259–1269.

Hui, J. M., A. Hodge, G. C. Farrell, J. G. Kench, A. Kriketos, and J. George. 2004. Beyond insulin resistance in NASH: TNF-alpha or adiponectin? *Hepatology* 40:46–54.

Ikejima, K., K. Okumura, T. Lang, H. Honda, W. Abe, S. Yamashina, N. Enomoto, Y. Takei, and N. Sato. 2005. The role of leptin in progression of non-alcoholic fatty liver disease. *Hepatol Res* 33:151–154.

Iwasaki, T., K. Mukasa, M. Yoneda, S. Ito, Y. Yamada, Y. Mori, N. Fujisawa, T. Fujisawa, K. Wada, H. Sekihara, and A. Nakajima. 2005. Marked attenuation of production of collagen type I from cardiac fibroblasts by dehydroepiandrosterone. *Am J Physiol Endocrinol Metab* 288:1222–1228.

Joseph, S. B., A. Castrillo, B. A. Laffitte, D. J. Mangelsdorf, and P. Tontonoz. 2003. Reciprocal regulation of inflammation and lipid metabolism by liver X receptors. *Nat Med* 9:213–219.

Kamohara, S., R. Burcelin, J. L. Halaas, J. M. Friedman, and M. J. Charron. 1997. Acute stimulation of glucose metabolism in mice by leptin treatment. *Nature* 389:374–377.

Kaser, S., A. Moschen, A. Cayon, A. Kaser, J. Crespo, F. Pons-Romero, C. F. Ebenbichler, J. R. Patsch, and H. Tilg. 2005. Adiponectin and its receptors in non-alcoholic steato-hepatitis. *Gut* 54:117–121.

Kawano, M. 2000. Complement regulatory proteins and autoimmunity. *Arch Immunol Ther Exp (Warsz)* 48:367–372.

Kersten, S., J. Seydoux, J. M. Peters, F. J. Gonzalez, B. Desvergne, and W. Wahli. 1999. Peroxisome proliferator–activated receptor alpha mediates the adaptive response to fasting. *J Clin Invest* 103:1489–1498.

Korenblat, K. M., E. Fabbrini, B. S. Mohammed, and S. Klein. 2008. Liver, muscle, and adipose tissue insulin action is directly related to intrahepatic triglyceride content in obese subjects. *Gastroenterology* 134:1369–1375.

Leone, T. C., C. J. Weinheimer, and D. P. Kelly. 1999. A critical role for the peroxisome proliferator–activated receptor alpha (PPARalpha) in the cellular fasting response: The PPARalpha-null mouse as a model of fatty acid oxidation disorders. *Proc Natl Acad Sci U S A* 96:7473–7478.

Ma, L., N. G. Tsatsos, and H. C. Towle. 2005. Direct role of ChREBP·Mlx in regulating hepatic glucose-responsive genes. *J Biol Chem* 280:12019–12027.

Magaña, M. M., and T. F. Osborne. 1996. Two tandem binding sites for sterol regulatory element binding proteins are required for sterol regulation of fatty-acid synthase promoter. *J Biol Chem* 271:32689–32694.

Masaki, T., S. Chiba, H. Tatsukawa, T. Yasuda, H. Noguchi, M. Seike, and H. Yoshimatsu. 2004. Adiponectin protects LPS-induced liver injury through modulation of TNF-alpha in KK-Ay obese mice. *Hepatology* 40:177–184.

Mastrocola, R., M. Aragno, S. Betteto, E. Brignardello, M. G. Catalano, O. Danni, and G. Boccuzzi. 2003. Pro-oxidant effect of dehydroepiandrosterone in rats is mediated by PPAR activation. *Life Sci* 73:289–299.

Parekh, S., and F. A. Anania. 2007. Abnormal lipid and glucose metabolism in obesity: Implications for nonalcoholic fatty liver disease. *Gastroenterology* 132:2191–2207.

Pohl, J., A. Ring, R. Ehehalt, T. Herrmann, and W. Stremmel. 2004. New concepts of cellular fatty acid uptake: Role of fatty acid transport proteins and of caveolae. *Proc Nutr Soc* 63:259–262.

Poirier, H., I. Niot, M. C. Monnot, O. Braissant, C. Meunier-Durmort, P. Costet, T. Pineau, W. Wahli, T. M. Willson, and P. Besnard. 2001. Differential involvement of peroxisome-proliferator–activated receptors alpha and delta in fibrate and fatty-acid–mediated inductions of the gene encoding liver fatty-acid–binding protein in the liver and the small intestine. *Biochem J* 355:481–488.

Reddy, J. K. 2001. Nonalcoholic steatosis and steatohepatitis: III. Peroxisomal beta-oxidation, PPAR alpha, and steatohepatitis. *Am J Physiol Gastrointest Liver Physiol* 281:1333–1339.

Samuel, V. T., Z. X. Liu, X. Qu, B. D. Elder, S. Bilz, D. Befroy, A. J. Romanelli, and G. I. Shulman. 2004. Mechanism of hepatic insulin resistance in non-alcoholic fatty liver disease. *J Biol Chem* 279:32345–32353.

Sato, R., W. Miyamoto, J. Inoue, T. Terada, T. Imanaka, and M. Maeda. 1999. Sterol regulatory element–binding protein negatively regulates microsomal triglyceride transfer protein gene transcription. *J Biol Chem* 274:24714–24720.

Schoonjans, K., B. Staels, and J. Auwerx. 1996. The peroxisome proliferator activated receptors (PPARS) and their effects on lipid metabolism and adipocyte differentiation. *Biochim Biophys Acta* 1302:93–109.

Shimano, H. 2001. Sterol regulatory element–binding proteins (SREBPs): Transcriptional regulators of lipid synthetic genes. *Prog Lipid Res* 40:439–452.

Shimomura, I., H. Shimano, J. D. Horton, J. L. Goldstein, and M. S. Brown. 1997. Differential expression of exons 1a and 1c in mRNAs for sterol regulatory element binding protein–1 in human and mouse organs and cultured cells. *J Clin Invest* 99:838–845.

Weickert, M. O., and A. F. Pfeiffer. 2006. Signalling mechanisms linking hepatic glucose and lipid metabolism. *Diabetologia* 49:1732–1741.

Wetterau, J. R., M. C. Lin, and H. Jamil. 1997. Microsomal triglyceride transfer protein. *Biochim Biophys Acta* 1345:136–150.

Yamaguchi, K., L. Yang, S. McCall, J. Huang, X. X. Yu, S. K. Pandey, S. Bhanot, B. P. Monia, Y. X. Li, and A. M. Diehl. 2007. Inhibiting triglyceride synthesis improves hepatic steatosis but exacerbates liver damage and fibrosis in obese mice with nonalcoholic steatohepatitis. *Hepatology* 45:1366–1374.

Yamauchi, T., J. Kamon, Y. Ito, A. Tsuchida, T. Yokomizo, S. Kita, T. Sugiyama, M. Miyagishi, K. Hara, M. Tsunoda, K. Murakami, T. Ohteki, S. Uchida, S. Takekawa, H. Waki, N. H. Tsuno, Y. Shibata, Y. Terauchi, P. Froguel, K. Tobe, S. Koyasu, K. Taira, T. Kitamura, T. Shimizu, R. Nagai, and T. Kadowaki. 2003. Cloning of adiponectin receptors that mediate antidiabetic metabolic effects. *Nature* 423:762–769.

Yoshikawa, T., H. Shimano, M. Amemiya-Kudo, N. Yahagi, A. H. Hasty, T. Matsuzaka, H. Okazaki, Y. Tamura, Y. Iizuka, K. Ohashi, J. Osuga, K. Harada, T. Gotoda, S. Kimura, S. Ishibashi, and N. Yamada. 2001. Identification of liver X receptor–retinoid X receptor as an activator of the sterol regulatory element–binding protein 1c gene promoter. *Mol Cell Biol* 21:2991–3000.

Yu, X. X., S. F. Murray, S. K. Pandey, S. L. Booten, D. Bao, X. Z. Song, S. Kelly, S. Chen, R. McKay, B. P. Monia, and S. Bhanot. 2005. Antisense oligonucleotide reduction of DGAT2 expression improves hepatic steatosis and hyperlipidemia in obese mice. *Hepatology* 42:362–371.

6 Using Parenteral Fish Oil in NASH

Jonathan A. Meisel, Hau D. Le,
Vincent E. De Meijer,
Kathleen M. Gura, and Mark Puder

CONTENTS

6.1 INTRODUCTION

It is estimated that more than 1.1 billion adults worldwide are overweight, and 312 million of these adults are obese. Moreover, according to the International Obesity Task Force, at least 155 million children worldwide are overweight or obese as well (Haslam et al., 2005). Overweight is defined as body mass index (BMI) > 25 kg m^{-2}, and about one-third of overweight people are obese (BMI > 30 kg m^{-2}; Centers for Disease Control and Prevention). As the prevalence over the past decade has more than doubled, so have the health care–related costs. In the United States alone, direct and indirect costs of obesity have been estimated to exceed $100 billion annually (Weight-control Information Network, 2008). Evidence from multiple studies indicates that obesity is strongly associated with hypertension, hypercholesterolemia (Mokdad et al., 2003), diabetes, heart disease (Targher et al., 2007), and premature death (Allison et al., 1999).

One less publicized but equally significant medical condition directly related to the rate of obesity is nonalcoholic fatty liver disease (NAFLD). Mostly unrecognized before 1980 when it was first described by Ludwig et al. (1980), it is now estimated that up to 30% of the adult Western population, including the United States, has NAFLD (Browning et al., 2004). Today, NAFLD is the most common form of chronic liver disease in Western countries, and its prevalence is increasing with the current epidemic of obesity and the metabolic syndrome (Bellentani et al., 2000). Prevalence in non-Western countries is expected to increase as well, mainly due to globalization of the Western diet.

Patients with NAFLD not only have higher rates of morbidity and mortality from liver-related complications such as cirrhosis and hepatocellular carcinoma (Angulo, 2002), but this condition is closely related to the hallmark features of the metabolic syndrome such as obesity, diabetes, and cardiovascular disease (Hamaguchi et al., 2007). The main focus of this chapter is on a subset of NAFLD termed nonalcoholic steatohepatitis (NASH). It begins with a brief review of the pathophysiology of NASH, followed by a discussion of the current therapeutic options, and the role that diet plays on liver function. It will also investigate the use of fish oil and omega-3 fatty acids.

6.2 NASH: PATHOGENESIS AND CURRENT THERAPEUTIC OPTIONS

6.2.1 DEFINITION

NAFLD encompasses a histological spectrum ranging from simple steatosis, progressing to NASH, cirrhosis, and ultimately liver failure. In 2005, the Pathology Committee of the United States National Institutes of Health NASH Clinical Research Network designed and validated a scoring system comprising 14 histological features for NAFLD that encompasses the entire pathologic spectra of the disease. Microscopically, a diagnosis of NASH consists of accumulation of fatty acids and triglycerides in the liver, ballooning of hepatocytes ± Mallory bodies, inflammation, and fibrosis (Kleiner et al., 2005). Two clinical forms of NASH exist. The primary form, which occurs more frequently, is intimately associated with obesity and the metabolic syndrome. Secondary NASH is a result of a variety of hepatotoxic insults including drugs, industrial toxins, and as a complication from long-term parenteral nutrition (PN) (Chitturi et al., 2001). The latter is often termed parenteral nutrition–associated liver disease (PNALD) (Paquot et al., 2005). This will be discussed in further detail.

6.2.2   Epidemiology

NASH affects 3–6% of the U.S. and Western populations (Torres et al., 2008), approximately 3% of the lean population, and almost 50% of the morbidly obese (Angulo, 2002). The prevalence has been steadily increasing over the past several years, together with the rising incidence of obesity, and due to the invasive nature of the gold standard diagnosis (i.e., liver biopsy), it is thought that the prevalence may be underestimated. One in seven patients with NASH will develop cirrhosis in their lifetime (Paquot et al., 2005). Moreover, patients with NASH have a high incidence of progressing to end-stage liver disease and hepatocellular carcinoma (Torres et al., 2008), making early diagnosis of these patients critically important. NASH is ranked as one of the most common causes of cryptogenic cirrhosis in the United States, behind hepatitis C and alcoholic liver disease (Clark et al., 2003). Although not exclusively, NASH is often seen as a manifestation of the metabolic syndrome (Paquot et al., 2005). In most cases, primary NASH is seen in overweight or obese middle-aged adults. These individuals often suffer from diabetes mellitus, hypertension, and hyperlipidemia, although not every patient with these diseases will go on to develop NASH. Furthermore, some patients with NASH are not obese, nor do they have hypertension, diabetes, or hypercholesterolemia. Secondary NASH, as a complication from PN, is seen in both children and adults who receive PN for a prolonged period.

6.2.3   Pathophysiology

NASH is often a silent disease with few to no symptoms. Patients generally feel well in the early stages until the disease has reached a more advanced stage or cirrhosis develops. The progression of NASH can take years, typified by worsening inflammation, hepatocellular degeneration, scarring, and fibrosis of the liver (Paquot et al., 2005). As fibrosis worsens, cirrhosis develops, and the liver becomes irreversibly damaged. Although not every patient with NASH develops cirrhosis, there are no proven treatments to halt its progression.

Although NASH is becoming more common, the specific underlying mechanism for liver injury is still not fully elucidated. A "two-hit hypothesis" has been proposed to describe the pathogenesis of NASH (Day et al., 1998). First is the accumulation of excess fat in the liver (simple steatosis), followed by necroinflammation and fibrosis. Over the past several years, there have been many studies investigating the biochemical pathways responsible for the pathogenesis of NASH from simple steatosis. A study of gene expression in patients with cirrhosis showed that genes involved in reducing reactive oxygen species (ROS) and those involved in fatty acid and glucose metabolism were suppressed in patients with NASH (Sreekumar et al., 2003). Results from a recent analysis of more than 50,000 genes and various biological pathways in patients with NASH indicated that there are at least 15 different pathways involved in its pathogenesis (Yoneda et al., 2007). There is a growing consensus that the progression from steatosis to NASH is multifactorial, with oxidative stress, cytokines, genetics, and mitochondrial dysfunction all playing a significant role.

6.3 CURRENT TREATMENT REGIMENS FOR NASH

Currently, not one specific therapy for NASH exists. The standard of care involves a multimodality approach that mainly targets lifestyle modification, as studies using specific pharmacologic therapies have been inconclusive. See Table 6.1 for a summary of therapeutic options.

6.3.1 WEIGHT LOSS

Weight loss is the primary goal in patients with NAFLD and NASH. Even a modest 6% reduction in weight will improve insulin resistance and decrease hepatic steatosis (Sato et al., 2007). Liver histology and serum biomarkers may also improve as patients lose weight by reducing their caloric intake (Palmer et al., 1990; de Luis et al., 2008). Patients who have undergone bariatric surgery have actually had conflicting results in regards to histological improvement postoperatively. Some studies have shown a mild worsening of lobular fibrosis and inflammation after weight loss of more than 30 kg (Kral et al., 2004), whereas others have shown significant histological improvement (Barker et al., 2006).

TABLE 6.1
Practical Guidelines for Treatment of Patients with NASH: Treatment Options

Treatment Modality	Examples
Weight reduction	Lifestyle modification (diet and exercise)
	Bariatric surgery
Pharmacological Intervention	
Drug-induced weight loss	Orlistat, Sibutramine
Antioxidants	Vitamin E, Ascorbic acid
Lipid-lowering agents	
Statins	Atorvastatin, Simvastatin
Fibrates	Fenofibrate, Gemfibrozil
Bile acid sequestrants	Cholestyramine
Other	Ezetimibe
Insulin sensitizing medications	
Thiazoledinediones	Pioglitazone, Rosiglitazone
Biguanides	Metformin
Enteral fish oil	Dietary supplementation
Parenteral fish oil[a]	Omegaven® (for those dependent on parenteral nutrition)

[a] This therapeutic option is not currently approved by the Food and Drug Administration (FDA). Omegaven is currently undergoing clinical trials.

6.3.2 Pharmacologic Therapy

Clinical and biochemical studies have provided insight into possible specific pharmacological therapies for patients with NASH. To date, however, none of these studies have been conclusive. The most promising results have come from studies investigating insulin-sensitizing medications, particularly a class of drugs called thiazolidinediones. Thiazolidinediones, including rosiglitazone and pioglitazone, are peroxisome proliferator–activated receptor γ (PPAR-γ) agonists that have been shown to improve insulin resistance and glucose and lipid metabolism. Activation of PPAR-γ receptors reduces blood glucose levels and decreases hyperinsulinemia by regulation of insulin-responsive gene transcription that is involved in glucose production, transport, and utilization (Ioannides-Demos et al., 2005). PPAR-γ agonists activate these receptors, which impact the secretion of several substances from adipocytes that are involved in glucose metabolism and the regulation of insulin sensitivity, which include tumor necrosis factor α (TNF-α) and free fatty acids that may result in improved insulin signaling in insulin-sensitive tissues (Arner, 2003). In one short-term study, pioglitazone improved alanine transaminase (ALT) values, reduced hepatic steatosis, and decreased insulin resistance (Yoneda et al., 2007). Drugs targeting insulin sensitivity (i.e., metformin) by decreasing hepatic gluconeogenesis have also shown encouraging preliminary results (Bugianesi et al., 2005).

Orlistat belongs to the drug class known as lipase inhibitors and has shown promise in the treatment of NASH due to its ability to inhibit both gastric and pancreatic lipase. In 2006, patients with NAFLD diagnosed by ultrasound were randomly assigned to either orlistat or placebo. Patients receiving orlistat showed a significant reduction in ALT levels and reversal of steatosis. However, the observed beneficial effects were thought to be due to the weight loss effect of the drug (Zelber-Sagi et al., 2006).

6.3.3 Antioxidants

Patients with NASH have a depletion of antioxidants within hepatocytes, resulting in increased ROS (Mehta et al., 2002). Antioxidants can potentially be beneficial in NASH by reducing the ROS. Alpha tocopherol (vitamin E) and ascorbic acid (vitamin C) have both been extensively studied. One study evaluated the combination of the two in NASH patients who were given 1000 IU of vitamin E and 1000 mg of vitamin C daily for 6 months. These patients showed an improvement in hepatic fibrosis, but they showed no change in serum transaminases when compared to those receiving a placebo (Harrison et al., 2003).

6.3.4 Lipid-Lowering Agents

Lipid-lowering medications for the treatment of NASH have had mixed results. Statins, which inhibit 3-hydroxy-3-methylglutaryl-coenzyme-A reductase in the cholesterol biosynthesis pathway, have been studied the most. A pilot trial with atorvastatin in 2006 showed that it was safe and efficacious in treating hyperlipidemia in NAFLD patients (Gomez-Dominguez et al., 2006). However, a more recent study using simvastatin showed no improvement in insulin sensitivity in a group of patients with metabolic syndrome (Devaraj et al., 2007). Aside from statins, ezetimibe, an antihyperlipidemic drug that lowers cholesterol by inhibiting its absorption within the intestine, decreases hepatic steatosis and fibrosis in obese rats (Deushi et al., 2007).

6.3.5 Diet

Logically, diet is a main focus for the treatment of obesity, NAFLD, and NASH. Several studies have investigated the dietary intake of patients with NASH. When comparing the daily food intake of patients with NASH to that of healthy controls, patients with NASH consumed significantly more saturated and less polyunsaturated fatty acids (PUFAs) (Musso et al., 2003). Patients with NASH also showed significantly greater energy intake compared to controls (Capristo et al., 2005). Although there is evidence that consuming fish rich in omega-3 PUFAs can reduce the risk of NFALD, the benefit might not be seen in the morbidly obese patients. In a study of 70 morbidly obese patients, no relationship was found between dietary intake of various fatty acids with the degree of hepatic steatosis, inflammation, or fibrosis (Solga et al., 2004).

It may therefore be best to approach NASH in a multidisciplinary manner by combining education, nutritional counseling, and physical activity. In a trial of 16 patients undergoing this multidisciplinary treatment, there was significant improvement in both liver histological scores as well as weight reduction (Huang et al., 2005).

Recent investigation has turned toward fish oil, because of its high omega-3 content, and evaluation of its hepatoprotective effects. The next section discusses clinical and experimental studies in which omega-3 PUFAs are used as a treatment option for NASH.

6.4 OMEGA-6 VERSUS OMEGA-3 FATTY ACIDS

Interest in the field of omega-3 fatty acids is increasing because of their antiinflammatory properties as well as their potential beneficial effect on hepatic steatosis through an increase in beta oxidation (Ide et al., 1996) and a decrease in *de novo* lipogenesis (Alwayn et al., 2005).

Inflammation is essential in the diagnosis of NASH, and it is known that omega-6 (n-6) PUFAs, more specifically linoleic acid (LA) and arachidonic acid (AA) (see Figure 6.1), play a key role in inflammation through the up-regulation of multiple inflammatory mediators. LA activates nuclear factor–κB and increases the production of other inflammatory mediators such as interleukin 6 (IL-6) and TNF-α (Dichtl et al., 2002; Park et al., 2001). Similarly, AA activates the same proinflammatory factors (Camandola et al., 1996). In addition, AA is a key substrate for two-series prostaglandins, thromboxanes, and four-series leukotrienes, which are all recognized as potent proinflammatory mediators (Tilley et al., 2001). It has therefore been postulated that increased amounts of n-6 PUFAs can initiate or worsen inflammatory states.

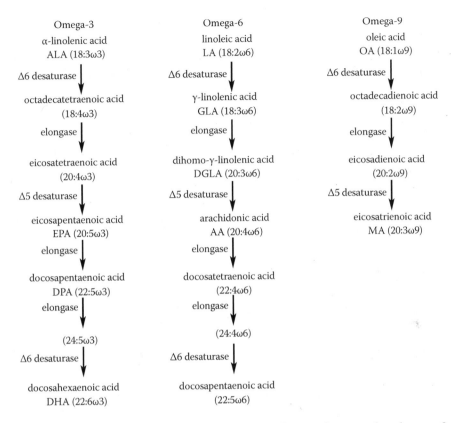

FIGURE 6.1 Pathway of metabolism and synthesis of omega-3, omega-6, and omega-9 PUFAs. Metabolism of omega-3, omega-6, and omega-9 fatty acids into their downstream products. PUFAs, polyunsaturated fatty acids.

TABLE 6.2
Key Facts of Fish and Fish Oil Including Its Perceived Benefits, How It Is Produced, and Potential Hazards

1. Fish oil is recommended as part of a healthy diet because it contains omega-3 fatty acids that have been shown to reduce inflammation.
2. Fish accumulate omega-3 fatty acids by eating microalgae that produce these fatty acids or by eating smaller prey fish that have consumed the algae.
3. The FDA recommends limiting the consumption of certain fish due to their high levels of toxins such as mercury (tuna, shark, swordfish).
4. Fish oil supplements have become popular among those wishing to increase their intake without eating more fish.
5. Fish oil should not be confused with cod liver oil. Although cod liver is an excellent source of EPA and DHA, it is a concentrated source of vitamins A and D, both of which become toxic at high doses.

The n-3 PUFAs are α-linolenic acid (ALA), docosahexaenoic acid (DHA), and eicosapentaenoic acid (EPA), and are contained in fish oils. Fish oil may have potential for anti-inflammatory effects by interfering with the AA pathway and producing anti-inflammatory eicosonoids (Chen et al., 1992). In 1997, Yeh et al. showed that n-3 PUFAs reduced superoxide dismutase and glutathione in rats receiving PN. This suggests that omega-3 FAs in fish oil play a role in reducing radicals that contribute to inflammation. This is consistent with several studies showing that fish oil could modulate inflammation through the inhibition of TNF-α and decreasing cytokines that trigger proinflammatory reactions (Rallidis et al., 2003; Novak et al., 2003).

Clinical studies investigating enteral fish oil in patients with NAFLD have also been performed. In 2001, Calder showed how consuming fish oil resulted in higher

TABLE 6.3
Levels of Omega-3 Fatty Acids in Various Common Fish

Fish	Omega-3 Fatty Acids (g/3 oz serving)
Catfish	
Farmed	0.15
Wild	0.2
Clam	0.24
Cod	0.19
Crab, Alaskan king	0.35
Flounder/sole	0.42
Haddock	0.2
Halibut	0.4–1
Herring	1.76
Lobster	0.07–0.41
Mackerel	0.34–1.57
Oyster	0.37–1.17
Salmon	
Atlantic, farmed	1.09–1.83
Atlantic, wild	0.9–1.56
Sardines	0.98–1.7
Scallop	0.17
Shrimp	0.27
Swordfish	0.97
Trout, rainbow	
Farmed	0.98
Wild	0.84
Tuna	
White, canned in water	0.73
Light, canned in water	0.26

Source: American Heart Association. 2008.

Note: Levels of fatty acids are rough estimates because oil content varies with species, season, packaging, and cooking method.

levels of DHA and EPA at the expense of AA and, in turn, lowered the production of prostaglandins, leukotrienes, and thromboxane-B2 by neutrophils (Lee et al., 1985). In a nonrandomized study in 2006, patients with NAFLD were given 1 g of fish oil per day for 1 year and were compared to controls who refused to take the fish oil capsules. After 1 year, liver steatosis was absent in 24% of the patients in the fish oil group. Liver transaminases and serum triacylglycerol levels improved as well (Capanni et al., 2006). Another study investigating enteral fish oil supplementation showed similar results (Spadaro et al., 2008). Complete regression of hepatic steatosis was seen in 33% of the patients taking fish oil, and an overall reduction was seen in half. In the group that did not receive fish oil, complete regression was not seen. Additional information regarding fish oil and the omega-3 fatty acid content present in common fish may be found in Tables 6.2 and 6.3.

6.5 SECONDARY NASH AS A COMPLICATION OF PN: PNALD

PN is a life-saving therapy for patients unable to absorb enteral nutrients secondary to insufficient intestinal length or function. Before the development of PN, patients with insufficient gastrointestinal absorptive capability commonly died of starvation and complications of malnutrition. Today, more than 30,000 patients in the United States are permanently dependent on PN for survival (Howard et al., 1995). Although lifesaving, long-term use of PN is associated with many complications, including septicemia and metabolic abnormalities (Buchman, 2001). The most serious and devastating complication associated with long-term PN use is PNALD. PNALD is a subtype of NAFLD, ranging from steatosis to cholestasis, cholelithiasis, fibrosis, and ultimately cirrhosis and liver failure (Kelly, 1998).

Despite years of extensive study, the etiology of PNALD remains unclear. Recent evidence suggests that the composition of the intravenous lipid emulsion administered with PN may contribute to this liver injury. Since the 1960s, these products have been used in PN as a source of essential fatty acids and as an alternative source of nonprotein calories (Edgren et al., 1963). Currently, in the United States, the only Food and Drug Administration–approved lipid emulsions are composed of either soybean oil alone (Intralipid®, Fresenius Kabi, and Liposyn III®, Hospira) or a combination of soybean and safflower oils (Liposyn II®, Hospira), which are rich in n-6 PUFAs. In 1998, a meta-analysis of PN with and without lipids showed the inclusion of lipids to be detrimental (Heyland et al., 1998). More specifically, lipid emulsions derived from soybean oil have been shown to cause liver injury both *in vitro* and *in vivo* in rodent models (Aksnes et al., 1996; Chen et al., 1996). Soybean oil–based emulsions have immunosuppressive effects in several *in vitro* (Calder et al., 1994) as well as clinical studies (Monson et al., 1988). In 2000, Furst and Kuhn hypothesized that the ratio of n-6 PUFAs to n-3 PUFAs in lipid emulsions needed to be decreased. The long-chain n-3 PUFAs found in fish oil (DHA and EPA) would replace the n-6 fatty acids in soybean oil, thus decreasing both the amount of LA as well as the n-6/n-3 ratio in the lipid emulsion. Benefits would result from having less proinflammatory mediators as well as more anti-inflammatory ones. Results from these and numerous other studies have prompted the investigation into alternative lipid emulsions such as those composed of fish oil (Alwayn et al., 2005).

6.6 PARENTERAL FISH OIL AND ITS PROTECTIVE EFFECT ON THE LIVER

Fish oil has been investigated as a source of fat in intravenous lipid emulsions for PN, but its use was hindered by skepticism that fish oil monotherapy might not provide enough essential fatty acids to prevent essential fatty acid deficiency and to enhance growth (Carlson et al., 1992). Despite this, many research groups began to look for an alternative to the conventional soybean oil in lipid emulsion. The main focus of the final section of this chapter will be on parenteral fish oil and its clinical use in patients with PN-induced NASH.

In the mid-1990s, Clarke et al. (1994) reported that dietary PUFAs were negative regulators of hepatic lipogenesis. Since that time, subsequent studies have demonstrated that the down-regulation of lipogenic enzymes is mediated by their reduction of sterol regulatory element–binding protein 1 (SREBP-1) in the liver (Kim et al., 1999). Additional research on the mechanism of hepatic protection of n-3 PUFAs on PNALD indicated that an increased clearance of triglycerides and reduced lipogenesis through suppression of the SREBP-1 enzyme likely plays a role (Park et al., 2003). A study in leptin-deficient *ob/ob* mice showed that hepatic steatosis improved with increased enteral PUFAs by down-regulation of SREBP-1 and hepatic lipogenesis (Sekiya et al., 2003).

In 2005, Alwayn et al. showed that a fish oil–based lipid emulsion both prevented and reversed PN-induced hepatic steatosis in an established murine model. Mice were exclusively fed a fat-free, high-carbohydrate diet for 19 days, and they consistently developed severe macrovesicular steatosis. Mice that received an intravenous fish oil–based lipid emulsion were shown to have significant reduction in their hepatic steatosis (Alwayn et al., 2005). Furthermore, they showed that the route of lipid administration played a significant role in affecting hepatic steatosis (Javid et al., 2005). Mice receiving a conventional intravenous soy-based emulsion developed hepatic steatosis, whereas mice receiving the emulsion enterally had normal livers. This suggests that the composition of the intravenous lipid emulsion administered with PN might be the cause of the liver injury, and the use of a fish oil–based lipid emulsion may help alleviate, reverse, and possibly even prevent PNALD.

Clinically, parenteral fish oil has also been extensively investigated for its hepatoprotective effects. Initially, combination lipid emulsions such as SMOFlipid® (Fresenius Kabi) or 50:50 mixtures of a soybean oil lipid (Intralipid, Baxter Healthcare, Fresenius Kabi) supplemented with a fish oil lipid (Omegaven, Fresenius Kabi) were investigated. Details regarding the composition of the different lipid emulsions are shown in Table 6.4. Results of these studies were promising. Patients receiving at least 50% fish oil were found to have lower rates of wound infections, shorter hospital stays, decreased need for mechanical ventilation, and a significantly lower mortality (Tsekos et al., 2004).

Studies have shown that administering a lipid emulsion comprising solely of fish oil lowered patients' production of leukotriene B4, C2, and thromboxane A2, all of which are derived from AA (Wachtler et al. 1997). Plasma concentrations of TNF-α and IL-6 were lower in patients receiving intravenous fish oil in another study (Weiss et al., 2002). Heller et al. (2004) showed that PN supplemented with fish oil

TABLE 6.4

Comparison and Characteristics of Four Commercial Parenteral Lipid Emulsions (100 g fat/L)

Product	Intralipid	Liposyn II	SMOFlipid	Omegaven
Manufacturer	Fresenius Kabi	Hospira	Fresenius Kabi	Fresenius Kabi
Oil source (g)				
Soybean	100	50	30	0
Safflower	0	50	0	0
MCT	0	0	30	0
Olive oil	0	0	25	0
Fish	0	0	15	100
Fat composition (%)[a]				
Linoleic	50	65	18.6	0.4
α-Linolenic	9	4	2.4	< 0.2
EPA	0	0	2.4	2.1
DHA	0	0	2.2	2.3
Oleic	26	17.7	27.7	1.0
Palmitic	10	8.8	9.1	0.6
Stearic	3.5	3.4	2.8	0.1
Arachidonic	0	0	0.5	0.3

Note: Data were provided by the manufacturer. MCT, medium chain triglyceride; EPA, eicosapentaenoic acid; DHA, docosahexaenoic acid.

[a] Values in Omegaven group represent means.

improved liver and pancreas function in patients recovering from abdominal surgery. Together, these studies support the concept that fish oil modulates the inflammation and improves liver function in patients postoperatively.

Parenteral fish oil in children has been studied as well, but to a lesser extent. In 2006, Gura et al. reported the reversal of PNALD in two infants with intestinal failure by substituting a fish oil–based lipid emulsion for the conventional soy-based emulsion. A subsequent report on 18 patients in the treatment of PNALD compared to historical controls showed similar promising results in the reversal of cholestasis (Gura et al., 2008). Over the next several years, with further prospective studies, it should be possible to draw more definitive conclusions regarding the efficacy of fish oil in treating NASH.

6.7 SUMMARY POINTS

- Obesity has become an epidemic, and its prevalence is steadily increasing. This has resulted in an increase in the number of patients with NAFLD and NASH.

- Although much research has been done, there is no ideal therapy for NASH. Current recommendations revolve around weight loss, improved nutrition, and increased physical activity to improve the features of the metabolic syndrome.
- Pharmacological therapy for NASH has been promising but inconclusive. Insulin-sensitizing medications, lipid-lowering agents, and antioxidants have all shown some improvement in liver function, but rarely any regression of the disease process.
- There are numerous studies showing the beneficial effects of n-3 PUFAs on inflammation and the immune system. These studies have generated much interest in the use of n-3 fatty acids in lipid emulsions for PN.
- Most recently, novel therapy for hepatic steatosis using fish oil has shown the most promising results. Both enteral and parenteral fish oil has been shown to improve hepatic steatosis in animal models of NAFLD.
- In children reliant on PN for survival, parenteral fish oil has been shown to reverse the NAFLD seen in these patients.
- Finally, parenteral fish oil is currently being investigated in a prospective randomized controlled trial to determine if it can prevent the liver injury caused by the current intravenous nutrition.

REFERENCES

Aksnes, J., et al. 1996. Lipid entrapment and cellular changes in the rat myocard, lung and liver after long-term parenteral nutrition with lipid emulsion. A light microscopic and ultrastructural study. *Apmis* 104:515–522.

Allison, D. B., et al. 1999. Annual deaths attributable to obesity in the United States. *JAMA* 282:1530–1538.

Alwayn, I. P., et al. 2005. Omega-3 fatty acid supplementation prevents hepatic steatosis in a murine model of nonalcoholic fatty liver disease. *Pediatr Res* 57:445–452.

American Heart Association. 2008. Fish, levels of mercury and omega-3 fatty acids. Accessed August 13, 2008 from http://www.americanheart.org/presenter.jhtml?identifier=3013797.

Angulo, P. 2002. Nonalcoholic fatty liver disease. *N Engl J Med* 346:1221–1231.

Arner, P. 2003. The adipocyte in insulin resistance: Key molecules and the impact of the thiazolidinediones. *Trends Endocrinol Metab* 14:137–145.

Barker, K. B., et al. 2006. Non-alcoholic steatohepatitis: Effect of Roux-en-Y gastric bypass surgery. *Am J Gastroenterol* 101:368–373.

Bellentani, S., et al. 2000. Prevalence of and risk factors for hepatic steatosis in Northern Italy. *Ann Intern Med* 132:112–117.

Browning, J. D., et al. 2004. Prevalence of hepatic steatosis in an urban population in the United States: Impact of ethnicity. *Hepatology* 40:1387–1395.

Buchman, A. L. 2001. Complications of long-term home total parenteral nutrition: Their identification, prevention and treatment. *Dig Dis Sci* 46:1–18.

Bugianesi, E., et al. 2005. A randomized controlled trial of metformin versus vitamin E or prescriptive diet in nonalcoholic fatty liver disease. *Am J Gastroenterol* 100:1082–1090.

Calder, P. C. 2001. Polyunsaturated fatty acids, inflammation, and immunity. *Lipids* 36:1007–1024.

Calder, P. C., et al. 1994. Inhibition of lymphocyte proliferation in vitro by two lipid emulsions with different fatty acid compositions. *Clin Nutr* 13:69–74.

Camandola, S., et al. 1996. Nuclear factor κB is activated by arachidonic acid but not by eicosapentaenoic acid. *Biochem Biophys Res Commun* 229:643–647.

Capanni, M., et al. 2006. Prolonged n-3 polyunsaturated fatty acid supplementation ameliorates hepatic steatosis in patients with non-alcoholic fatty liver disease: A pilot study. *Aliment Pharmacol Ther* 23:1143–1151.

Capristo, E., et al. 2005. Nutritional aspects in patients with non-alcoholic steatohepatitis (NASH). *Eur Rev Med Pharmacol Sci* 9:265–268.

Carlson, S. E., et al. 1992. First year growth of preterm infants fed standard compared to marine oil n-3 supplemented formula. *Lipids* 27:901–907.

Centers for Disease Control and Prevention [cited June 26, 2008]. Available from http://www.cdc.gov/nccdphp/dnpa/obesity/defining.htm.

Chen, M. F., et al. 1992. Effects of dietary supplementation with fish oil on prostanoid metabolism during acute coronary occlusion with or without reperfusion in diet-induced hypercholesterolemic rabbits. *Int J Cardiol* 36:297–304.

Chen, W. J., et al. 1996. Effects of fat emulsions with different fatty acid composition on plasma and hepatic lipids in rats receiving total parenteral nutrition. *Clin Nutr* 15:24–28.

Chitturi, S., et al. 2001. Etiopathogenesis of nonalcoholic steatohepatitis. *Semin Liver Dis* 21:27–41.

Clark, J. M., et al. 2003. Nonalcoholic fatty liver disease: An underrecognized cause of cryptogenic cirrhosis. *JAMA* 289:3000–3004.

Clarke, S. D., et al. 1994. Dietary polyunsaturated fatty acid regulation of gene transcription. *Annu Rev Nutr* 14:83–98.

Day, C. P., et al. 1998. Steatohepatitis: A tale of two "hits"? Gastroenterology 114:842–845.

de Luis, D. A., et al. 2008. Effect of a hypocaloric diet in transaminases in nonalcoholic fatty liver disease and obese patients, relation with insulin resistance. *Diabetes Res Clin Pract* 79:74–78.

Deushi, M., et al. 2007. Ezetimibe improves liver steatosis and insulin resistance in obese rat model of metabolic syndrome. *FEBS Lett* 581:5664–5670.

Devaraj, S., et al. 2007. Simvastatin (40 mg/day), adiponectin levels, and insulin sensitivity in subjects with the metabolic syndrome. *Am J Cardiol* 100:1397–1399.

Dichtl, W., et al. 2002. Linoleic acid–stimulated vascular adhesion molecule–1 expression in endothelial cells depends on nuclear factor–kappaB activation. *Metabolism* 51:327–333.

Edgren, B., et al. 1963. The theoretical background of the intravenous nutrition with fat emulsions. *Nutr Dieta Eur Rev Nutr Diet* 13:364–386.

Furst, P., and K. S. Kuhn. 2000. Fish oil emulsions: What benefits can they bring? *Clin Nutr* 19:7–14.

Gomez-Dominguez, E., et al. 2006. A pilot study of atorvastatin treatment in dyslipemid, non-alcoholic fatty liver patients. *Aliment Pharmacol Ther* 23:1643–1647.

Gura, K. M., et al. 2006. Reversal of parenteral nutrition–associated liver disease in two infants with short bowel syndrome using parenteral fish oil: Implications for future management. *Pediatrics* 118:e197–e201.

Gura, K. M., et al. 2008. Safety and efficacy of a fish-oil–based fat emulsion in the treatment of parenteral nutrition–associated liver disease. *Pediatrics* 121:e678–e686.

Hamaguchi, M., et al. 2007. Nonalcoholic fatty liver disease is a novel predictor of cardiovascular disease. *World J Gastroenterol* 13:1579–1584.

Harrison, S. A., et al. 2003. Vitamin E and vitamin C treatment improves fibrosis in patients with nonalcoholic steatohepatitis. *Am J Gastroenterol* 98:2485–2490.

Haslam, D. W., et al. 2005. Obesity. *Lancet* 366:1197–1209.

Heller, A. R., et al. 2004. Omega-3 fatty acids improve liver and pancreas function in post-operative cancer patients. *Int J Cancer* 111:611–616.

Heyland, D. K., et al. 1998. Total parenteral nutrition in the critically ill patient: A meta-analysis. *JAMA* 280:2013–2019.

Howard, L., et al. 1995. Current use and clinical outcome of home parenteral and enteral nutrition therapies in the United States. *Gastroenterology* 109:355–365.

Huang, M. A., et al. 2005. One-year intense nutritional counseling results in histological improvement in patients with non-alcoholic steatohepatitis: A pilot study. *Am J Gastroenterol* 100:1072–1081.

Ide, T., et al. 1996. Stimulation of the activities of hepatic fatty acid oxidation enzymes by dietary fat rich in alpha-linolenic acid in rats. *J Lipid Res* 37:448–463.

Ioannides-Demos, L. L., et al. 2005. Pharmacotherapy for obesity. *Drugs* 65:1391–1418.

Javid, P. J., et al. 2005. The route of lipid administration affects parenteral nutrition–induced hepatic steatosis in a mouse model. *J Pediatr Surg* 40:1446–1453.

Kelly, D. A. 1998. Liver complications of pediatric parenteral nutrition—epidemiology. *Nutrition* 14:153–157.

Kim, H. J., et al. 1999. Fish oil feeding decreases mature sterol regulatory element–binding protein 1 (SREBP-1) by down-regulation of SREBP-1c mRNA in mouse liver. A possible mechanism for down-regulation of lipogenic enzyme mRNAs. *J Biol Chem* 274:25892–25898.

Kleiner, D. E., et al. 2005. Design and validation of a histological scoring system for nonalcoholic fatty liver disease. *Hepatology* 41:1313–1321.

Kral, J. G., et al. 2004. Effects of surgical treatment of the metabolic syndrome on liver fibrosis and cirrhosis. *Surgery* 135:48–58.

Lee, T. H., et al. 1985. Effect of dietary enrichment with eicosapentaenoic and docosahexaenoic acids on in vitro neutrophil and monocyte leukotriene generation and neutrophil function. *N Engl J Med* 312:1217–1224.

Ludwig, J., et al. 1980. Nonalcoholic steatohepatitis: Mayo Clinic experiences with a hitherto unnamed disease. *Mayo Clin Proc* 55:434–438.

Mehta, K., et al. 2002. Nonalcoholic fatty liver disease: Pathogenesis and the role of anti-oxidants. *Nutr Rev* 60:289–293.

Mokdad, A. H., et al. 2003. Prevalence of obesity, diabetes, and obesity-related health risk factors, 2001. *JAMA* 289:76–79.

Monson, J. R., et al. 1988. Total parenteral nutrition adversely influences tumour-directed cellular cytotoxic responses in patients with gastrointestinal cancer. *Eur J Surg Oncol* 14:935–943.

Musso, G., et al. 2003. Dietary habits and their relations to insulin resistance and postprandial lipemia in nonalcoholic steatohepatitis. *Hepatology* 37:909–916.

Novak, T. E., et al. 2003. NF-kappa B inhibition by omega-3 fatty acids modulates LPS-stimulated macrophage TNF-alpha transcription. *Am J Physiol Lung Cell Mol Physiol* 284:L84–L89.

Palmer, M., et al. 1990. Effect of weight reduction on hepatic abnormalities in overweight patients. *Gastroenterology* 99:1408–1413.

Paquot, N., et al. 2005. Fatty liver in the intensive care unit. *Curr Opin Clin Nutr Metab Care* 8:183–187.

Park, H. J., et al. 2001. Linoleic acid–induced VCAM-1 expression in human microvascular endothelial cells is mediated by the NF-kappa B-dependent pathway. *Nutr Cancer* 41:126–134.

Park, Y., et al. 2003. Omega-3 fatty acid supplementation accelerates chylomicron triglyceride clearance. *J Lipid Res* 44:455–463.

Rallidis, L. S., et al. 2003. Dietary alpha-linolenic acid decreases C-reactive protein, serum amyloid A and interleukin-6 in dyslipidaemic patients. *Atherosclerosis* 167:237–242.

Sato, F., et al. 2007. Effects of diet-induced moderate weight reduction on intrahepatic and intramyocellular triglycerides and glucose metabolism in obese subjects. *J Clin Endocrinol Metab* 92:3326–3329.

Sekiya, M., et al. 2003. Polyunsaturated fatty acids ameliorate hepatic steatosis in obese mice by SREBP-1 suppression. *Hepatology* 38:1529–1539.

Solga, S., et al. 2004. Dietary composition and nonalcoholic fatty liver disease. *Dig Dis Sci* 49:1578–1583.

Spadaro, L., et al. 2008. Effects of n-3 polyunsaturated fatty acids in subjects with nonalcoholic fatty liver disease. *Dig Liver Dis* 40:194–199.

Sreekumar, R., et al. 2003. Hepatic gene expression in histologically progressive nonalcoholic steatohepatitis. *Hepatology* 38:244–251.

Targher, G., et al. 2007. Prevalence of nonalcoholic fatty liver disease and its association with cardiovascular disease among type 2 diabetic patients. *Diabetes Care* 30:1212–1218.

Tilley, S. L., et al. 2001. Mixed messages: Modulation of inflammation and immune responses by prostaglandins and thromboxanes. *J Clin Invest* 108:15–23.

Torres, D. M., et al. 2008. Diagnosis and therapy of nonalcoholic steatohepatitis. *Gastroenterology* 134:1682–1698.

Tsekos, E., et al. 2004. Perioperative administration of parenteral fish oil supplements in a routine clinical setting improves patient outcome after major abdominal surgery. *Clin Nutr* 23:325–330.

Wachtler, P., et al. 1997. Influence of a total parenteral nutrition enriched with omega-3 fatty acids on leukotriene synthesis of peripheral leukocytes and systemic cytokine levels in patients with major surgery. *J Trauma* 42:191–198.

Weight-control Information Network 2008 [cited June 26, 2008]. Available from http://win.niddk.nih.gov/statistics/index.htm.

Weiss, G., et al. 2002. Immunomodulation by perioperative administration of n-3 fatty acids. *Br J Nutr* 87 Suppl 1:S89–S94.

Yeh, S. L., et al. 1997. Effects of n-3 and n-6 fatty acids on plasma eicosanoids and liver antioxidant enzymes in rats receiving total parenteral nutrition. *Nutrition* 13:32–36.

Yoneda, M., et al. 2007. Life style-related diseases of the digestive system: Gene expression in nonalcoholic steatohepatitis patients and treatment strategies. *J Pharmacol Sci* 105:151–156.

Zelber-Sagi, S., et al. 2006. A double-blind randomized placebo-controlled trial of orlistat for the treatment of nonalcoholic fatty liver disease. *Clin Gastroenterol Hepatol* 4:639–644.

7 Iron Overload in Nonalcoholic Fatty Liver Disease: Implications for Nutrition

Richard Kirsch and Ralph E. Kirsch

CONTENTS

7.1   INTRODUCTION

Nonalcoholic fatty liver disease (NAFLD) is emerging as the most common liver condition in developed countries, and its prevalence is increasing worldwide. NAFLD, which affects 20–30% of the adult population in Western countries, is strongly associated with the metabolic syndrome. The spectrum of NAFLD includes simple steatosis (fatty liver), nonalcoholic steatohepatitis (NASH), and cirrhosis. Most people with NAFLD have simple steatosis, a generally benign condition. NASH, the more severe form of NAFLD, is less common, affecting 2–3% of the population. It is characterized by hepatocyte injury, inflammation, and fibrosis, and progresses to cirrhosis in 15–25% of patients (de Alwis and Day, 2008; Younossi, 2008). The pathogenesis of NASH is thought to involve "multiple" hits. Insulin resistance (IR) is usually the first hit leading to steatosis, which can, in turn, worsen hepatic IR. Further hits include oxidative stress, endotoxins, cytokines, and environmental toxins. Potential sources of oxidative stress in NAFLD include products of mitochondrial and peroxisomal fatty acid oxidations, cytochrome P450 activity, cytokine-mediated inflammation, apoptosis, and iron. Oxidative stress promotes lipid peroxidation of hepatocyte membranes, resulting in hepatocyte injury, secretion of proinflammatory cytokines, and stellate cell activation leading to fibrosis (Edmison and McCullough, 2007; London and George, 2007).

Patients with NAFLD frequently show features of hyperferritinemia and/or iron overload. The interplay between these conditions has generated much interest over the past decade. Attention has focused on the relationship between NAFLD and hemochromatosis gene (*HFE*) mutations, the potential role of iron in NAFLD progression and iron-overload-IR interplay. This chapter reviews the literature in this field and its implications for nutrition (Table 7.1).

TABLE 7.1
Key Facts and Concepts of Iron Overload in Patients with NAFLD

NAFLD	• Most common liver condition in developed countries; its prevalence is increasing worldwide
	• Associated with features of the metabolic syndrome including IR
	• Frequently associated with hyperferritinemia and/or iron overload
Iron overload and NAFL	Iron's ability to cause cellular damage and fibrosis has raised concern that iron overload may exacerbate NAFLD
	However, most human studies have shown no relationship between hepatic iron overload and fibrosis severity in NAFLD
Hemochromatosis and NAFLD	The prevalence and significance of hemochromatosis gene (*HFE*) mutations in NAFLD have been the subject of conflicting reports
IR-HIO	• Characterized by hyperferritinemia, normal transferrin saturation, and features of IR
	• Most common cause of iron overload in NAFLD
Iron-insulin relationship	• Excess iron increases IR
	• Iron depletion enhances insulin sensitivity
	• Insulin promotes increased iron stores
	• Phlebotomy may improve insulin sensitivity and NAFLD
	• Copper deficiency is prevalent in NAFLD and may be related to iron overload; further studies are required to clarify this relationship

NAFLD, nonalcoholic fatty liver disease; IR, insulin resistance; IR-HIO, IR-associated hepatic iron overload.

7.2 HEPATIC IRON METABOLISM AND OVERLOAD

Knowledge of human iron homeostasis has advanced considerably with the identification and characterization of new molecules related to iron absorption and transport. This has led to a more precise classification of hepatic iron overload.

7.2.1 IRON HOMEOSTASIS

Because daily iron loss is limited and not dictated by the level of iron stores, intestinal absorption is the only step in extracellular iron homeostasis that can be regulated. The pathway of iron absorption and export by the duodenal enterocyte is

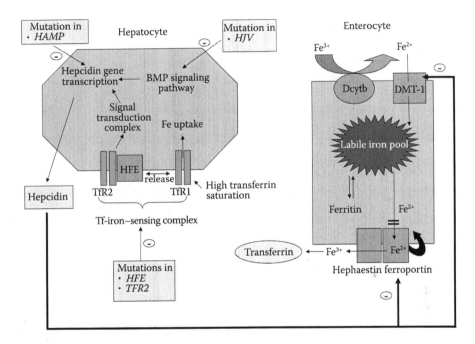

FIGURE 7.1 Schematic representation of current concepts in iron absorption and regulation. Ferric iron (Fe^{3+}) is reduced to the ferrous iron (Fe^{2+}) by ferric reductases [e.g., duodenal cytochrome b ferric reductase (Dcytb)] on the luminal aspect of enterocytes. Fe^{2+} is taken up by divalent metal transporter 1 (DMT-1), enters the labile iron pool, and is either stored intracellularly as ferritin or exported across the basolateral membrane by ferroportin. Hephaestin reoxidizes Fe^{3+} to Fe^{2+}, which is bound by circulating transferrin. Hepatic regulation of this process is proposed to occur as follows: HFE protein [normally sequestered by transferrin receptor 1 (TfR1)] is released at increased transferrin saturation and binds TfR2. Through a cytoplasmic signal transduction complex, this induces synthesis and secretion of hepcidin. Hepcidin promotes internalization and degradation of ferroportin and reduces DMT-1 expression, thereby blocking iron export. Additional upstream regulators include hemojuvelin (HJV) and bone morphogenetic protein (BMP) coreceptor. Mutations in the *HFE, TFR2, HJV, HAMP* (hepcidin) genes result in decreased hepcidin levels and hereditary iron overload syndromes (Based on Deugnier, Y., Brissot, P., and Loreal, O., *J Hepatol*, 48, S113–S123, 2008; Sebastiani, G. and Walker, A. P., *J Gastroenterol*, 13, 4673–4689, 2007).

1. $Fe^{3+} + O_2^- \rightarrow Fe^{2+} + O_2$ (Haber–Weiss reaction)

2. $Fe^{2+} + H_2O_2 \rightarrow Fe^{3+} + OH^- + OH^-$ (Fenton reaction)

FIGURE 7.2 The Fenton–Haber–Weiss reaction. First reaction: Superoxide anion (O_2^-) reduces ferric iron (Fe^{3+}) to the ferrous state (Fe^{2+}) (Haber–Weiss reaction). Second reaction: Fe^{2+} and hydrogen peroxide (H_2O_2) react to generate the highly reactive hydroxyl (OH^-) radical (Fenton reaction).

illustrated in Figure 7.1. Dietary ferric iron (Fe^{3+}) is reduced a ferrous iron (Fe^{2+}) state by ferric reductases expressed on the luminal surfaces of enterocytes. Ferrous iron is taken up by divalent metal transporter 1 and enters the labile iron pool. Iron is then stored intracellularly as ferritin or exported across the basolateral membrane by the transmembrane iron exporter, ferroportin. Hephaestin, a membrane bound, copper-containing ferroxidase, reoxidizes exported iron to the ferric state, which is avidly bound by circulating transferrin. The liver plays a central regulatory role in this process through the secretion of the iron-regulatory peptide, hepcidin. Hepcidin interacts with ferroportin, leading to its internalization and degradation, thereby blocking cellular iron export. Hepcidin production is up-regulated by iron overload and inflammation and down-regulated by hypoxia and anemia. This is mediated by upstream regulators including HFE, hemojuvelin (HJV), bone morphogenetic protein coreceptor, and transferrin receptor 2 (TfR-2) (Figure 7.2). Mutations in genes encoding these proteins are associated with decreased hepcidin levels and hereditary iron overload syndromes (Deugnier et al., 2008; Sebastiani and Walker, 2007).

Intracellular iron homeostasis is tightly controlled by iron regulatory proteins (IRP) 1 and 2, which regulate ferritin expression through the recognition of specific sequences on iron responsive elements. When the intracellular iron concentration is low, IRPs bind iron response elements with high affinity resulting in the down-regulation of ferritin expression. When the cell has sufficient iron, IRPs lose their affinity for iron responsive elements, permitting ferritin expression. These mechanisms prevent iron toxicity through the rapid modification of gene expression in response to fluctuations in intracellular iron (Baptista-Gonzalez et al., 2008).

7.2.2 CLASSIFICATION OF IRON OVERLOAD

Hepatic iron storage disorders are classified into hereditary (primary) and acquired (secondary) hepatic iron overload (Table 7.2). Hereditary iron overload disorders are divided into hemochromatotic and nonhemochromatotic forms based on pathophysiological, molecular, and phenotypic characteristics. Hereditary hemochromatosis (HH) is defined by normal erythropoiesis, increased transferrin saturation, parenchymal distribution of iron deposition, and genetic mutations resulting in impaired production and/or regulation and/or activity of hepcidin (Pietrangelo, 2007). As such, HH consists of five distinct genetic disorders related to abnormalities in *HFE*, *HJV*, *HAMP* (hepcidin), *TfR2*, and *SCL40A1* (ferroportin) genes (Deugnier et al., 2008). *HFE*-HH (type 1 HH), which accounts for > 90% of these disorders, is the paradigm of severe iron overload. This autosomal recessive disorder with low clinical

TABLE 7.2
Classification of Hepatic Iron Overload Disorders

Disorder	Gene
Primary (genetic) iron overload (HH)	
1. Hemochromatotic	
HFE HH	*HFE* gene
Juvenile hemochromatosis	*HJV* or *HAMP* (hepcidin)
TfR2-related hemochromatosis	*TFR2*
Ferroportin disease type B	*SLC40A1*
2. Nonhemochromatotic	
Ferroportin disease type A	*SLC40A1*
A(hypo)ceruloplasminemia	Ceruloplasmin
A(hypo)transferrinemia	Transferrin
Secondary (acquired) iron overload	
1. Iron loading anemias	
Thalassemia major	
Sideroblastic anemia	
Chronic hemolytic anemias	
2. Chronic liver disease	
Chronic viral hepatitis	
Alcoholic liver disease	
Insulin resistance associated hepatic iron overload	
Advanced cirrhosis	
3. Excessive iron supply	
Dietary iron overload in sub-Saharan Africa	
Iron overload due to excessive iron supplementation (parenteral)	
Transfusional overload	
4. Miscellaneous	
Porphyria cutanea tarda	
Neonatal iron overload	
Anemia of inflammation	

Source: Based on Deugnier, Y., Brissot, P., and Loreal, O., *J Hepatol*, 48, S113–S123, 2008; Sebastiani, G. and Walker, A. P., *J Gastroenterol*, 13, 4673–4689, 2007.

Note: HH, hereditary hemochromatosis.

penetrance is the most common monogenic disorder in Celtic populations (Sebastiani and Walker, 2007). The C282Y and H63D mutations in *HFE* account for the vast majority of cases. C282Y homozygosity accounts for a high proportion of HH cases with a prevalence of about 1 in 300 in people of Northern European decent. (C282Y heterozygosity occurs in roughly 1 in 10.) The H63D mutation is more common (approximately 1 in 5 Europeans are H63D heterozygotes), but H63D homozygotes mostly develop only mild iron overloads. Compound H63D/C282Y heterozygotes, however, may develop overt HH (Sebastiani and Walker, 2007). Patients with HH manifest increased deposition of iron in parenchymal cells of the liver, heart, joints, pancreas, and other endocrine organs. If untreated, this may lead to hepatocellular injury, stellate cell activation, and fibrosis (Adams et al., 2000). Non-*HFE* forms of HH are much rarer and were recently reviewed (Deugnier et al., 2008).

Acquired hepatic iron overload includes iron overload secondary to chronic liver diseases (e.g., cirrhosis, alcoholic liver disease, viral hepatitis C, NAFLD, porphyria cutanea tarda) (Deugnier et al., 2008; Sebastiani and Walker, 2007), hematological diseases (e.g., thalassemia, sickle cell disease), or excessive dietary intake (e.g., sub-Saharan African iron overload) (Bothwell et al., 1964). Here, the hepatic iron concentration is lower than that seen in HH (Sebastiani and Walker, 2007). Recently, a syndrome of hepatic iron overload occurring in patients with IR and NAFLD was described. Termed "IR-associated hepatic iron overload" (IR-HIO), this condition is now considered the leading cause of mild to moderate hepatic iron overload in patients with NAFLD (Mendler et al., 1999).

7.2.3 Iron and Oxidative Stress

Under physiological conditions, mitochondria, peroxisomes, and microsomes generate a variety of reactive oxygen species (ROS), the levels of which are tightly controlled by enzymic and nonenzymic antioxidants (Pietrangelo, 2003). However, in iron overload, excess free iron can catalyze the conversion of ROS into highly reactive and toxic hydroxyl radicals via the Fenton–Haber–Weiss reaction (Figure 7.2). Here, O_2^- reduces Fe^{3+} to Fe^{2+}, which then reacts with H_2O_2 to form highly reactive hydroxyl radicals (Baptista-Gonzalez et al., 2008). The latter result in lipid peroxidation, oxidation of amino acid side chains, cross-linking of proteins, protein fragmentation, DNA damage, and strand breaks (Sies, 1991). Once initiated, free iron promotes additional lipid peroxidation, thereby perpetuating the process (Emerit et al., 2001). Lipid peroxidation of cell membranes results in functional and structural modifications and the generation of by-products including highly reactive aldehydes from oxidative breakdowns of polyunsaturated fatty acids (Esterbauer, 1996). These by-products may further damage the cell through the formation of protein adducts (Pietrangelo, 2003).

7.2.4 Iron and Fibrogenesis

The mechanisms by which iron overload leads to hepatic fibrosis are unclear. Excess iron has been shown to induce hepatic stellate cell activation and collagen production *in vitro* and *in vivo* (Pietrangelo et al., 1994; Ramm et al., 1995). Hepatic injury in humans with untreated hemochromatosis is relatively mild and progression to cirrhosis is slow. Iron appears to unleash its full pathogenic potential when acting as a cofactor in the setting of underlying chronic liver disease or together with other hepatotoxins (Barton et al., 1995; Pietrangelo, 2003). The contribution of iron to fibrogenesis in NAFLD is considered below.

7.3   IRON OVERLOAD AND NAFLD

The relationship between NAFLD and iron overload has been the subject of intense debate. Early studies examining the relationship among NAFLD, HFE mutations, and fibrogenesis in NAFLD produced conflicting results. Later, attention turned to the relationship between IR and hepatic iron overload following the description of the IR-HIO syndrome. Recently, attention has been focused on the mechanisms underlying iron's influence on insulin sensitivity and the effects of insulin in iron homeostasis. Results of these studies are discussed below.

7.3.1   NAFLD AND HFE MUTATIONS

Many studies have investigated the prevalence of *HFE* mutations in NAFLD. Over-representation of *HFE* mutations in patients with NASH was first reported by an Australian center with a special interest in iron overload. Out of 51 patients with NASH, 31% were either heterozygous or homozygous for the C282Y mutation compared to only 13% of controls. Increased stainable iron on liver biopsy was present in 41% of patients with NASH and correlated significantly with C282Y mutations and fibrosis (George et al., 1998). A subsequent American study reported a significant increase in H63D heterozygosity in 36 patients with NASH compared to controls (44.4% vs. 26.6%). For C282Y, heterozygosity was not different between patients and controls (17.5% vs. 11%) but did correlate significantly with hepatic fibrosis in NASH patients (Bonkovsky et al., 1999). A prospective study conducted in Italy including 263 patients with NAFLD (167 with liver biopsies) found the prevalence of C282Y and H63D mutations to be similar to the general population, and *HFE* mutations were not associated with iron overload or fibrosis (Bugianesi et al., 2004). Studies from Brazil, India, the United States, and Turkey also failed to demonstrate a relationship between *HFE* mutations and NASH (Deguti et al., 2003; Duseja et al., 2005; Nelson et al., 2007; Neri et al., 2008; Simsek et al., 2006). Furthermore, a large number of studies found no relationship among hepatic iron accumulation, *HFE* mutations, and the severity of liver disease in patients with NAFLD (Angulo et al., 1999; Bacon et al., 1994; Bugianesi et al., 2004; Chitturi et al., 2002; Deguti et al., 2003; Duseja et al., 2005; Mendler et al., 1999; Neri et al., 2008; Yamauchi et al., 2004; Younossi et al., 1999). Potential explanations for these conflicting results include ascertainment bias, genetic differences in the populations studied, and statistically underpowered studies (Nelson et al., 2007; Sebastiani and Walker, 2007). In an attempt to overcome these limitations, six North American centers examined the relationship between *HFE* mutations and liver fibrosis in 126 patients with NASH. The overall prevalence of *HFE* mutations did not differ significantly from that in the general population. However, among Caucasian patients, those with the C282Y mutation were significantly more likely to have bridging fibrosis or cirrhosis (44% vs. 21%) compared to patients with other genotypes (Nelson et al., 2007). It is clear from the above data that the relationship among iron overload, *HFE* mutations, and NAFLD remains unsettled. Large, multicenter, prospective studies are needed to clarify this important issue.

7.3.2   IR-HIO SYNDROME

In 1997, a French group reported a new syndrome of hepatic iron overload characterized by hyperferritinemia, normal transferrin saturation, and features of IR.

They showed, by HLA typing and later by genotyping for *HFE* mutations that this syndrome was unrelated to hemochromatosis (Moirand et al., 1997; Mendler et al., 1999). In a series of 161 patients with unexplained hepatic iron overload, they found 94% of patients to have one or more features of the IR syndrome and 52% to have histological evidence of NAFLD (half had NASH). They coined the term "IR associ-ated hepatic iron overload" to describe this condition (Mendler et al., 1999). Several studies have confirmed the relationship between hyperferritinemia, iron overload, IR, type II diabetes mellitus (Bozzini et al., 2005; Fargion et al., 2001; Fernandez-Real et al., 1998), and NAFLD (Fargion et al., 2001; Mendler et al., 1999; Turlin et al., 2001). IR-HIO is characterized by hyperferritinemia with normal or high normal-transferrin saturation (Fargion et al., 2001; Mendler et al., 1999). Histologically, iron accumulates in both hepatocytes and sinusoidal cells in contrast to HH in which iron deposition is largely hepatocellular (Figure 7.3) (Turlin et al., 2001). Isolated hyper-ferritinemia is a nonspecific finding in inflammation, liver necrosis, and alcoholic liver disease and does not imply iron overload (Bell et al., 1994). However, increased ferritin levels may serve as a marker of more severe liver disease in patients with

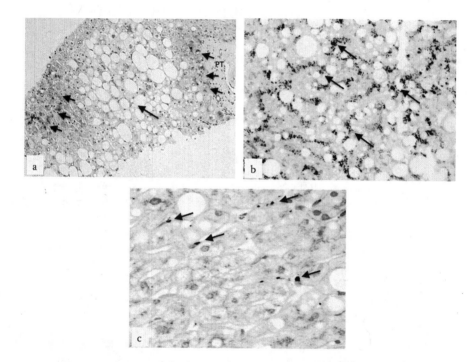

FIGURE 7.3 Liver biopsies from patients with nonalcoholic fatty liver disease (NAFLD) and iron overload. (a) Liver biopsy from a patient with NAFLD and iron overload. Iron gran-ules (small arrows) show a distinct zonal distribution around portal tracts (PT) and is located primarily in hepatocytes, characteristic of HFE-related iron overload. Note the steatosis (long arrow). (b) Higher magnification of (a). (c) Liver biopsy from a patient with NAFLD and mild iron overload associated with insulin resistance. Iron deposition is mild and involves Kupffer cells (short arrows) in addition to hepatocytes. (Perls' Prussian blue stain, a–c.)

NAFLD (Bugianesi et al., 2004; Fargion et al., 2001). Interestingly, hyperferritinemia in patients with NAFLD and IR-HIO may be reversed by a low caloric diet (Fargion et al., 2001; Piperno et al., 1998). The apparent relationship between iron overload, IR, and NAFLD has prompted studies evaluating the effect of iron depletion on these conditions. Preliminary evidence suggests a beneficial effect. Phlebotomy has been reported to improve insulin sensitivity, reduce hyperglycemia, and improve liver transaminases in patients with diabetes and NAFLD (Aigner et al., 2008a; Facchini, 1998; Facchini et al., 2002; Fargion et al., 2005; Piperno et al., 1998; Sumida et al., 2006; Valenti et al., 2007). Moreover, regular blood donors have increased insulin sensitivity compared to matched controls (Fernandez-Real et al., 2005).

7.3.3   IRON STORES AND INSULIN SENSITIVITY: INTERPLAY AND UNDERLYING MECHANISMS

Recently, attention has focused on mechanisms underlying the relationship between iron stores and insulin sensitivity. Iron chelation by desferrioxamine increases insulin sensitivity and glucose uptake in HepG2 cells, whereas iron supplementation has the opposite effect. Iron depletion appears to increase insulin receptor binding activity and signaling and increases expression of genes involved in glucose uptake (Dongiovanni et al., 2008; Fargion et al., 2005). Iron overload may also interfere with insulin signaling through the generation of ROS, which may impair glucose uptake through a direct effect on insulin receptor function, or by inhibiting the translocation of GLUT4 to the plasma membrane (Bertelsen et al., 2001). In addition, decreased hepatic extraction and metabolism of insulin due to iron accumulation in hepatocytes may contribute to hyperinsulinemia (Niederau et al., 1984).

The interaction between iron and insulin works both ways, with insulin exerting several effects on iron homeostasis. Insulin stimulates ferritin synthesis and induces a rapid and pronounced increase in iron uptake by cultured adipocytes through increased TfR externalization (Davis et al., 1986). The colocalization of TfRs with glucose transporters and insulin such as growth factor II receptor in microsomal membranes of adipocytes suggests that regulation of iron uptake by insulin may occur in parallel with glucose uptake (Tanner and Lienhard, 1989). Animal studies also suggest a regulatory effect for insulin on iron homeostasis. Genetically obese insulin-resistant *ob/ob* mice showed a twofold increase in iron absorption and significantly higher hemoglobin levels than lean control mice (Failla et al., 1988). Similarly, rats rendered obese/IR by a high fat/high energy diet showed elevated hemoglobin levels associated with higher transferrin levels, lower transferrin saturation, and lower hepcidin mRNA expression than lean controls. Hepatic and splenic iron stores in IR animals were decreased relative to controls, and duodenal levels were unchanged. Taken together, these findings point toward a higher iron requirement in IR animals, perhaps driven by increased erythropoiesis (Le Guenno et al., 2007). The results of this animal study differ from the human situation in which IR is often associated with increased iron stores. Recent evidence suggests that iron accumulation in NAFLD may, at least in part, be due to reduced iron export due to down-regulation of ferroportin 1 (FP-1) and impaired hepatic iron sensing due to low HJV expression. Increased hepcidin levels in NAFLD patients likely reflect the physiological response of the liver to iron accumulation, since increased hepcidin expression is reported only in NAFLD patients with iron overload but not those without (Aigner et al., 2008a).

7.3.4 PRACTICAL APPLICATIONS: THEORETICAL ASPECTS

This section evaluates iron stores as a potential target for improved insulin sensitivity and improvement of NAFLD. Both dietary iron intake and iron removal are considered. The first question is whether excessive dietary iron may be detrimental in NAFLD. Intake of iron beyond physiological requirements is endemic in many parts of the world. Many countries fortify foods with iron to reduce iron-deficiency anemia. In addition, approximately 40% of American adults use multivitamins and mineral supplements containing ferrous sulfate (Ervin et al., 2004). Iron fortification and iron supplementation may place some sectors of the population at increased risk of iron overload (Swanson, 2003). With increasing awareness of the role of dietary pro-oxidants in chronic disease, the potential health risks associated with excess iron intake have come under increasing scrutiny (Arosio and Levi, 2002). Dietary iron, once absorbed, is not actively excreted and absorption of iron remains the critical determinant of body iron stores. Normally, this process is tightly controlled and healthy individuals are unlikely to accumulate excess iron through fortified food or iron supplements (Beard, 2002). However, feedback mechanisms may not protect all populations from iron accumulation. A study including 614 participants aged 68–93 years from the Framingham Heart Study Cohort demonstrated a relationship between iron intake and iron stores. Iron stores correlated with iron supplement use, frequent consumption of red meat, and frequent intake of fruit or fruit juices (Fleming and Sly, 2002). Others have failed to demonstrate a relationship between iron intake and iron stores in the elderly (Garry et al., 2000) and the precision with which the homeostatic feedback loop regulates iron absorption in the elderly remains an open question. The effect of excess dietary iron has also been evaluated in heterozygotes for C282Y mutations. In a study conducted before the availability of C282Y genotyping, iron absorption was evaluated in children and siblings of HH patients who shared a single HLA haplotype. These presumed heterozygotes showed no difference in nonheme iron absorption from a hamburger meal compared to controls. However, after fortification of the meal with 20 mg of ferrous sulfate and 100 mg of vitamin C, they absorbed 2.5 times as much nonheme iron as controls (Lynch et al., 1989). This observation fueled concern over fortification in countries where *HFE* mutations are fairly common. However, studies performed after C282Y genotyping became available were unable to confirm these findings. The conflicting findings of the initial and subsequent studies might be explained in part by the possible misclassification of heterozygotes before the availability of genotyping (some may have been compound heterozygotes) as well as differences in the doses and dosing schedules used. Although this issue remains unresolved, it seems that dietary iron intake including fortified foods has a minor effect, if any at all, on iron absorption in C282Y heterozygotes (Singh et al., 2006).

A second question is whether reduction of iron stores, either by dietary restriction or iron removal (e.g., phlebotomy), has the potential to enhance insulin sensitivity and improve NAFLD. A study of iron stores and insulin sensitivity in 30 lacto-ovo vegetarians and 30 adult, lean, and glucose-tolerant meat eaters found lacto-ovo vegetarians to have lower serum ferritin levels and to be more insulin-sensitive than their meat-eating counterparts. Lowering of serum ferritin levels by phlebotomy in six meat eaters reproduced the improvement in insulin sensitivity observed in lacto-ovo vegetarians (Hua et al., 2001). Preliminary evidence suggests that phlebotomy may have beneficial effects on IR and possibly a subset of patients with NAFLD. Phlebotomy has been reported to improve insulin sensitivity, reduce hyperglycemia, and improve liver transaminases in patients with diabetes and NAFLD (Aigner et al., 2008a; Facchini, 1998; Facchini et al., 2002; Fargion et al., 2005; Piperno et al., 1998; Sumida et al., 2006; Valenti et al., 2007), whereas regular blood donors have been found to have increased insulin sensitivity compared to matched controls (Fernandez-Real et al., 2005). The limited data regarding phlebotomy in NAFLD patients come mostly from small studies without adequate controls (Facchini et al., 2002; Guillygomarc'h et al., 2001; Valenti et al., 2003). A recent case control study compared 64 NAFLD patients with hyperferritinemia undergoing phlebotomy compared to 64 matched NAFLD controls. Both groups received standard nutritional/lifestyle counseling. Iron depletion resulted in a significantly greater reduction in IR compared to just nutritional and lifestyle counseling alone, independent of changes in body mass index, baseline homeostatic metabolic assessment IR index, or the presence of metabolic syndrome (Valenti et al., 2007). Although these findings are promising, large randomized studies evaluating liver histology endpoints are needed before this therapy can be considered outside of the research setting.

Finally, a recent study suggested that a significant proportion of NAFLD patients are copper deficient. Patients with low serum and liver copper levels were found to have higher serum ferritin levels, an increased prevalence of siderosis in liver biopsies, and a ±3-fold increase in hepatic iron concentration compared to NAFLD patients who were not copper deficient. Low copper bioavailability caused increased hepatic iron stores via decreased FP-1 expression and ceruloplasmin ferroxidase activity, thereby blocking liver iron export in copper-deficient patients (Aigner et al., 2008b). Interestingly, patients with a genetic deficiency in ceruloplasmin (a copper containing ferroxidase catalyzing the oxidation of ferrous to ferric iron, an essential step for the release of iron to plasma transferrin) develop hepatic iron overload (Hellman et al., 2000). These findings should prompt prospective studies determining whether normalization of copper levels improves iron status and liver histology in these patients. If so, this may have implications for nutritional therapy in NAFLD patients with iron overload.

In summary, preliminary data suggest that iron depletion may have beneficial effects on IR and NAFLD, particularly in the setting of hyperferritinemia. Large randomized controlled studies are needed before the true benefits of such interventions are known and evidence-based guidelines can be formulated. Current guidelines for the management of NAFLD do not include any specific recommendations regarding iron intake or iron removal (de Alwis and Day, 2008; Younossi, 2008). The potential effect of copper deficiency on iron overload in NAFLD merits further study.

7.4 SUMMARY POINTS

- NAFLD is strongly associated with the metabolic syndrome.
- Patients with NAFLD frequently show hyperferritinemia and/or iron overload.
- Iron's ability to promote oxidative stress has raised concern that iron overload may exacerbate NAFLD.
- Most human studies have shown no relationship between hepatic iron overload and fibrosis severity in NAFLD.
- The prevalence and significance of *HFE* mutations in NAFLD have been the subject of conflicting reports.
- IR-HIO syndrome is the most common cause of iron overload in NAFLD.
- Excess iron increases IR whereas iron depletion enhances insulin sensitivity.
- Insulin promotes increased iron stores.
- Phlebotomy may improve insulin sensitivity and NAFLD.
- Copper deficiency is prevalent in NAFLD and may be related to iron overload. Further studies are required to clarify this relationship.
- Evidence-based recommendations for nutritional intervention in NAFLD-associated iron overload are currently lacking.

REFERENCES

Adams, P., P. Brissot, and L. W. Powell. 2000. EASL International Consensus Conference on Haemochromatosis. *J Hepatol* 33:485–504.

Aigner, E., I. Theurl, M. Theurl, et al. 2008a. Pathways underlying iron accumulation in human nonalcoholic fatty liver disease. *Am J Clin Nutr* 87:1374–1383.

Aigner, E., I. Theurl, H. Haufe, et al. 2008b. Copper availability contributes to iron perturbations in human nonalcoholic fatty liver disease. *Gastroenterology* 135:680–688.

Angulo, P., J. C. Keach, K. P. Batts, and K. D. Lindor. 1999. Independent predictors of liver fibrosis in patients with nonalcoholic steatohepatitis. *Hepatology* 30:1356–1362.

Arosio, P., and S. Levi. 2002. Ferritin, iron homeostasis, and oxidative damage. *Free Radic Biol Med* 33:457–463.

Bacon, B. R., M. J. Farahvash, C. G. Janney, and B. A. Neuschwander-Tetri. 1994. Nonalcoholic steatohepatitis: An expanded clinical entity. *Gastroenterology* 107:1103–1109.

Baptista-Gonzalez, H., N. C. Chavez-Tapia, D. Zamora-Valdes, et al. 2008. Importance of iron and iron metabolism in nonalcoholic fatty liver disease. *Mini Rev Med Chem* 8:171–174.

Barton, A. L., B. F. Banner, E. E. Cable, and H. L. Bonkovsky. 1995. Distribution of iron in the liver predicts the response of chronic hepatitis C infection to interferon therapy. *Am J Clin Pathol* 103:419–424.

Beard, J. 2002. Dietary iron intakes and elevated iron stores in the elderly: Is it time to abandon the set-point hypothesis of regulation of iron absorption? *Am J Clin Nutr* 76:1189–1190.

Bell, H., A. Skinningsrud, N. Raknerud, and K. Try. 1994. Serum ferritin and transferrin saturation in patients with chronic alcoholic and non-alcoholic liver diseases. *J Intern Med* 236:315–322.

Bertelsen, M., E. E. Anggard, and M. J. Carrier. 2001. Oxidative stress impairs insulin internalization in endothelial cells in vitro. *Diabetologia* 44:605–613.

Bonkovsky, H. L., Q. Jawaid, K. Tortorelli, et al. 1999. Non-alcoholic steatohepatitis and iron: Increased prevalence of mutations of the HFE gene in non-alcoholic steatohepatitis. *J Hepatol* 31:421–429.

Bothwell, T. H., H. Seftel, P. Jacobs, J. D. Torrance, and N. Baumslag. 1964. Iron overload in Bantu subjects; Studies on the availability of iron in Bantu beer. *Am J Clin Nutr* 14:47–51.

Bozzini, C., D. Girelli, O. Olivieri, et al. 2005. Prevalence of body iron excess in the metabolic syndrome. *Diabetes Care* 28:2061–2063.

Bugianesi, E., P. Manzini, S. D'Antico, et al. 2004. Relative contribution of iron burden, HFE mutations, and insulin resistance to fibrosis in nonalcoholic fatty liver. *Hepatology* 39:179–187.

Chitturi, S., M. Weltman, G. C. Farrell, et al. 2002. HFE mutations, hepatic iron, and fibrosis: Ethnic-specific association of NASH with C282Y but not with fibrotic severity. *Hepatology* 36:142–149.

Davis, R. J., S. Corvera, and M. P. Czech. 1986. Insulin stimulates cellular iron uptake and causes the redistribution of intracellular transferrin receptors to the plasma membrane. *J Biol Chem* 261:8708–8711.

de Alwis, N. M., and C. P. Day. 2008. Non-alcoholic fatty liver disease: The mist gradually clears. *J Hepatol* 48 Suppl 1:S104–S112.

Deguti, M. M., A. M. Sipahi, L. C. Gayotto, et al. 2003. Lack of evidence for the pathogenic role of iron and HFE gene mutations in Brazilian patients with nonalcoholic steatohepatitis. *Braz J Med Biol Res* 36:739–745.

Deugnier, Y., P. Brissot, and O. Loreal. 2008. Iron and the liver: Update 2008. *J Hepatol* 48 Suppl 1:S113–S123.

Dongiovanni, P., L. Valenti, A. Ludovica Fracanzani, et al. 2008. Iron depletion by deferoxamine up-regulates glucose uptake and insulin signaling in hepatoma cells and in rat liver. *Am J Pathol* 172:738–747.

Duseja, A., R. Das, M. Nanda, et al. 2005. Nonalcoholic steatohepatitis in Asian Indians is neither associated with iron overload nor with HFE gene mutations. *World J Gastroenterol* 11:393–395.

Edmison, J., and A. J. McCullough. 2007. Pathogenesis of non-alcoholic steatohepatitis: Human data. *Clin Liver Dis* 11:75–104, ix.

Emerit, J., C. Beaumont, and F. Trivin. 2001. Iron metabolism, free radicals, and oxidative injury. *Biomed Pharmacother* 55:333–339.

Ervin, R. B., J. D. Wright, and D. Reed-Gillette. 2004. Prevalence of leading types of dietary supplements used in the Third National Health and Nutrition Examination Survey, 1988–94. *Adv Data* 9:1–7.

Esterbauer, H. 1996. Estimation of peroxidative damage. A critical review. *Pathol Biol (Paris)* 44:25–28.

Facchini, F. S. 1998. Effect of phlebotomy on plasma glucose and insulin concentrations. *Diabetes Care* 21:2190.

Facchini, F. S., N. W. Hua, and R. A. Stoohs. 2002. Effect of iron depletion in carbohydrate-intolerant patients with clinical evidence of nonalcoholic fatty liver disease. *Gastroenterology* 122:931–939.

Failla, M. L., M. L. Kennedy, and M. L. Chen. 1988. Iron metabolism in genetically obese (*ob/ob*) mice. *J Nutr* 118:46–51.

Fargion, S., P. Dongiovanni, A. Guzzo, et al. 2005. Iron and insulin resistance. *Aliment Pharmacol Ther* 22 Suppl 2:61–63.

Fargion, S., M. Mattioli, A. L. Fracanzani, et al. 2001. Hyperferritinemia, iron overload, and multiple metabolic alterations identify patients at risk for nonalcoholic steatohepatitis. *Am J Gastroenterol* 96:2448–2455.

Fernandez-Real, J. M., A. Lopez-Bermejo, and W. Ricart. 2005. Iron stores, blood donation, and insulin sensitivity and secretion. *Clin Chem* 51:1201–1205.

Fernandez-Real, J. M., W. Ricart-Engel, E. Arroyo, et al. 1998. Serum ferritin as a component of the insulin resistance syndrome. *Diabetes Care* 21:62–68.

Fleming, R. E., and W. S. Sly. 2002. Mechanisms of iron accumulation in hereditary hemochromatosis. *Annu Rev Physiol* 64:663–680.

Garry, P. J., W. C. Hunt, and R. N. Baumgartner. 2000. Effects of iron intake on iron stores in elderly men and women: Longitudinal and cross-sectional results. *J Am Coll Nutr* 19:262–269.

George, D. K., S. Goldwurm, G. A. MacDonald, et al. 1998. Increased hepatic iron concentration in nonalcoholic steatohepatitis is associated with increased fibrosis. *Gastroenterology* 114:311–318.

Guillygomarc'h, A., M. H. Mendler, R. Moirand, et al. 2001. Venesection therapy of insulin resistance-associated hepatic iron overload. *J Hepatol* 35:344–349.

Hellman, N. E., M. Schaefer, S. Gehrke, et al. 2000. Hepatic iron overload in aceruloplasminaemia. *Gut* 47:858–860.

Hua, N. W., R. A. Stoohs, and F. S. Facchini. 2001. Low iron status and enhanced insulin sensitivity in lacto-ovo vegetarians. *Br J Nutr* 86:515–519.

Le Guenno, G., E. Chanseaume, M. Ruivard, B. Morio, and A. Mazur. 2007. Study of iron metabolism disturbances in an animal model of insulin resistance. *Diabetes Res Clin Pract* 77:363–370.

London, R. M., and J. George. 2007. Pathogenesis of NASH: Animal models. *Clin Liver Dis* 11:55–74, viii.

Lynch, S. R., B. S. Skikne, and J. D. Cook. 1989. Food iron absorption in idiopathic hemochromatosis. *Blood* 74:2187–2193.

Mendler, M. H., B. Turlin, R. Moirand, et al. 1999. Insulin resistance–associated hepatic iron overload. *Gastroenterology* 117:1155–1163.

Moirand, R., A. M. Mortaji, O. Loreal, et al. 1997. A new syndrome of liver iron overload with normal transferrin saturation. *Lancet* 349:95–97.

Nelson, J. E., R. Bhattacharya, K. D. Lindor, et al. 2007. HFE C282Y mutations are associated with advanced hepatic fibrosis in Caucasians with nonalcoholic steatohepatitis. *Hepatology* 46:723–729.

Neri, S., D. Pulvirenti, S. Signorelli, et al. 2008. The HFE gene heterozygosis H63D: A cofactor for liver damage in patients with steatohepatitis? Epidemiological and clinical considerations. *Intern Med J* 38:254–258.

Niederau, C., M. Berger, W. Stremmel, et al. 1984. Hyperinsulinaemia in non-cirrhotic haemochromatosis: Impaired hepatic insulin degradation? *Diabetologia* 26:441–444.

Pietrangelo, A. 2003. Iron-induced oxidant stress in alcoholic liver fibrogenesis. *Alcohol* 30:121–129.

Pietrangelo, A. 2007. Hemochromatosis: An endocrine liver disease. *Hepatology* 46:1291–1301.

Pietrangelo, A., R. Gualdi, G. Casalgrandi, et al. 1994. Enhanced hepatic collagen type I mRNA expression into fat-storing cells in a rodent model of hemochromatosis. *Hepatology* 19:714–721.

Piperno, A., M. Sampietro, A. Pietrangelo, et al. 1998. Heterogeneity of hemochromatosis in Italy. *Gastroenterology* 114:996–1002.

Ramm, G. A., S. C. Li, L. Li, et al. 1995. Chronic iron overload causes activation of rat lipocytes in vivo. *Am J Physiol* 268:G451–G458.

Sebastiani, G., and A. P. Walker. 2007. HFE gene in primary and secondary hepatic iron overload. *World J Gastroenterol* 13:4673–4689.

Sies, H. 1991. Oxidative stress: From basic research to clinical application. *Am J Med* 91:31S–38S.

Simsek, H., Y. H. Balaban, H. Sumer, E. Yilmaz, and G. Tatar. 2006. HFE mutations analysis of Turkish patients with nonalcoholic steatohepatitis. *Dig Dis Sci* 51:1723–1724.

Singh, M. et al. 2006. Risk of iron overload in carriers of genetic mutations associated with hereditary haemochromatosis: UK Food Standards Agency workshop. *Br J Nutr* 96:770–773.

Sumida, Y., K. Kanemasa, K. Fukumoto, et al. 2006. Effect of iron reduction by phlebotomy in Japanese patients with nonalcoholic steatohepatitis: A pilot study. *Hepatol Res* 36:315–321.

Swanson, C. A. 2003. Iron intake and regulation: Implications for iron deficiency and iron overload. *Alcohol* 30:99–102.

Tanner, L. I., and G. E. Lienhard. 1989. Localization of transferrin receptors and insulin-like growth factor II receptors in vesicles from 3T3-L1 adipocytes that contain intracellular glucose transporters. *J Cell Biol* 108:1537–1545.

Turlin, B., M. H. Mendler, R. Moirand, et al. 2001. Histologic features of the liver in insulin resistance–associated iron overload. A study of 139 patients. *Am J Clin Pathol* 116:263–270.

Valenti, L., A. L. Fracanzani, P. Dongiovanni, et al. 2007. Iron depletion by phlebotomy improves insulin resistance in patients with nonalcoholic fatty liver disease and hyperferritinemia: Evidence from a case-control study. *Am J Gastroenterol* 102:1251–1258.

Valenti, L., A. L. Fracanzani, and S. Fargion. 2003. Effect of iron depletion in patients with nonalcoholic fatty liver disease without carbohydrate intolerance. *Gastroenterology* 124:866; author reply 866–867.

Yamauchi, N., Y. Itoh, Y. Tanaka, et al. 2004. Clinical characteristics and prevalence of GB virus C, SEN virus, and HFE gene mutation in Japanese patients with nonalcoholic steatohepatitis. *J Gastroenterol* 39:654–660.

Younossi, Z. M. 2008. Review article: Current management of non-alcoholic fatty liver disease and non-alcoholic steatohepatitis. *Aliment Pharmacol Ther* 28:2–12.

Younossi, Z. M., T. Gramlich, B. R. Bacon, et al. 1999. Hepatic iron and nonalcoholic fatty liver disease. *Hepatology* 30:847–850.

8 Nutritional and Clinical Strategies on Prevention and Treatment of NAFLD and Metabolic Syndrome

*Ana R. Dâmaso, Aline de Piano,
Lian Tock, and Rajaventhan Srirajaskanthan*

CONTENTS

8.1 INTRODUCTION

The term nonalcoholic fatty liver disease (NAFLD) has been used to describe a larger spectrum of steatosis liver diseases commonly associated with metabolic syndrome (MS) and represents a constellation of related health diseases. However, obesity-associated NAFLD was first described nearly 50 years ago, and was only partially confirmed recently due to the complexity of the biochemical machine that plays an important role between the inflammatory process and cellular mechanisms of NAFLD-related diseases (Zivkovic et al., 2007).

Nowadays, NAFLD is regarded as the hepatic manifestation of MS including the multifactorial disease involving a complex interaction of genetics, diet, and lifestyle, and is defined as the accumulation of lipids, primarily in the form of triacylglycerol in individuals who do not consume significant amounts of alcohol (20 g ethanol/day) (de Piano et al., 2007).

In this manner, imbalances in major lipid signaling pathways that are highly interconnected contribute to disease progression in chronic inflammation, autoimmunity, allergy, cancer, atherosclerosis, hypertension, heart hypertrophy, as well as metabolic and degenerative diseases. The resulting commonality of various different signaling components means that different diseases share common points of intervention (Wymann and Schneiter, 2008).

Given the close relationship among obesity, MS, and the development of NAFLD, it is not surprising that many NAFLD patients have multiple components of MS. Thus, management strategies for such patients need to be predominantly supported by diet therapy to promote weight loss as well as improve related comorbidities; however, experiences with multidisciplinary approaches, including clinical, exercise, and psychological counseling, are recommended for the long-term success of dietary and lifestyle interventions.

This chapter reviews the clinical strategies used in the treatment of MS and NAFLD with emphasis on a multidisciplinary approach and focus on nutrition.

8.2   PROCEDURES AND TREATMENT REGIMENS

8.2.1   CONCEPTS OF MULTIDISCIPLINARY INTERVENTION IN NAFLD AND MS

Despite the increasing prevalence of NAFLD, its pathogenesis and clinical significance remain poorly defined and there is no ideal treatment. However, as mentioned above and considering the multifactor altered mechanisms associated with NAFLD etiology, it would be expected to play a role in integrated health intervention.

In this sense, 5 years ago we started, as suggested by the World Health Organization (WHO) (2000) and inspired by the Adipositas Rehabilitation Zentrum, INSULA—Therapy Model from Germany (Siegfried et al., 2006), a multidisciplinary approach with the objective of primarily treating obesity. In subsequent years, it was observed that about 50% of obese adolescents had a positive ultrasonography (US) diagnostic for NAFLD and 28% presented MS by WHO criteria. Although the prevalence of NAFLD was reduced (from 50% to 29%) after short-term therapy, as well as MS (from 28% to 8%) after long-term therapy, some obese adolescents continued to show altered metabolic and hormonal analyzed parameters (Tock et al., 2006; Caranti et al., 2007).

The next step is keeping in mind the importance of promoting the best way to control these comorbidities, as part of the clinical approach of metformin use associated with lifestyle changes, with the specific purpose of normalizing insulin resistance, creating good health expectations for patients as long as possible, and improving their quality of life (data not published).

Another noteworthy question about therapeutic strategies is the relevance of the integrated approach between nutritional therapy and psychological counseling, considering in particular several eating disorders (e.g., bulimia, anorexia) as well as altered behaviors (e.g., anxiety, depression). When dealing with undesirable conditions such as metabolic and hormonal disorders, which result in imbalances between food intake and energy expenditure, one of the most important targets is to treat obesity, MS, and NAFLD. This clearly induces an amplification of the empowerment-based approach to control comorbidities, which sometimes delay the expected beneficial effects on patients' lives.

Finally, the relationship between nutritional therapy and exercise therapy is essential to enable appropriate calorific control and induces professionals (dieticians, physiotherapists) to work closely together. Through this consensus, one of the most promising means of treating these pathologies is integrated.

In fact, in a recent review published in *Hepatology*, Bellentani et al. (2008) concluded that although very few studies have tested the effectiveness of intensive behavior therapy in NAFLD, aimed at lifestyle modifications to produce stable weight loss by reduced calorie intake and increased physical activity, it is important that behavior therapy should simultaneously address all clinical and biochemical defects. Indeed, Bellentani et al. suggest that there is a need for multidisciplinary teams (nutritionists, psychologists, and physical activity supervisors) to treat patients with NAFLD.

8.2.2 Clinical Therapy

8.2.2.1 Medical Program

To accomplish their health and clinical goals, patients with NAFLD and MS need to undergo a long-term weight loss multidisciplinary program. The main foci of clinical treatment are as follows: identified genetic, metabolic, or endocrine disease; chronic alcohol consumption; previous drug utilization; enteral and parenteral diets; fast weight loss; viral hepatic diseases; and other causes of liver steatosis. Examination of NAFLD obese patient presents some distinct challenges for the clinician, including increased size and limited mobility, which create a barrier in the performance of physical examination: increased chest wall abdominal fat may impair effective auscultation and palpitation of these anatomical areas; increased risk for a host of diseases, many of which will not be recognized before the clinical evaluation because they are clinically difficult to detect and require appropriate screening for early detection (e.g., diabetes, hyperlipidemia). Finally, physicians must keep in mind those primary eating disorders (e.g., bulimia) as well as psychosocial related conditions (e.g., depression, loss of self-esteem) that are increasingly present in obese NAFLD patients and may have an important impact on subsequent medical therapy. These conditions can affect successful weight management and produce adverse health consequences in their own right. In this manner, the clinical examination includes the usual elements of patient history and physical conditions as well as the recognition of comorbid conditions and diseases that are more prevalent in NAFLD patients, which are necessary to accomplish this goal.

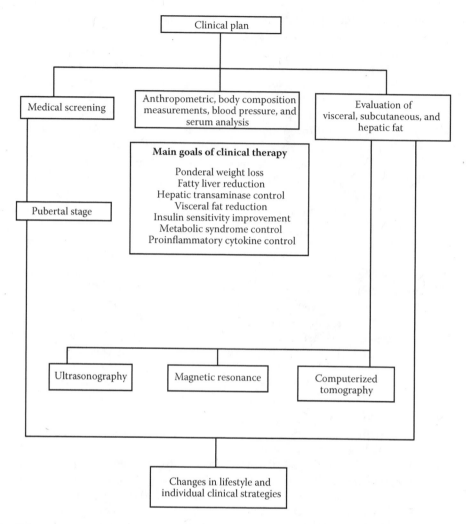

FIGURE 8.1 Organogram of clinical plan to be established at baseline and after short- and long-term multidisciplinary therapy.

At the beginning, after undergoing short- and long-term multidisciplinary therapy, the patients must be evaluated in all parameters included in the medical screening organogram presented in Figure 8.1. During the routine, the patients visit the clinician once a month.

8.2.2.1.1 Anthropometric and Body Composition Measurements

At the beginning and throughout the course of treatment, the weight, height, and body mass index, calculated as body weight (wt) divided by height (ht) squared (wt/ht²), plus anthropometric measurements of the subjects must be recorded. Body composition may be estimated by plethismography in the BOD POD body composition system. The advantage of this method over dual-energy x-ray absorptiometry is that it allows the operator to estimate the body compositions of patients with larger body habitus (up to 140 kg); however, it does not incorporate the measurement of body fat distribution (Fields et al., 2004). Considering the limitations as well as variations between body compositions, it is suggested to use two or three methods in the same subjects as part of the multidisciplinary therapy. The choice of method, naturally, depends on the objectives that the health team wants to attain during disease control.

8.2.2.1.2   Laboratory Studies

Based on the clinical history and a physical examination, laboratory testing is often driven by clinical suspicion. A fasting blood sample should be part of the routine screening panel for insulin resistance, hypothyroidism, dyslipidemia, hepatic transaminases altered profile [alanine aminotransferase (ALT), aspartate aminotransferase (AST), and γ-glutamyl transferase (GGT)], as well as other risks for inflammatory processes related to NAFLD, including proinflammatory [tumor necrosis factor α (TNF-α), leptin, protein C reactive, interleukin-6] and anti-inflammatory cytokine profiles (adiponectin), which contribute to the knowledge about NAFLD development and control (Schwimmer et al., 2003). Blood samples for all these analyzed parameters must be repeated after short- and long-term therapy.

8.2.2.2   NAFLD Image Diagnostic

8.2.2.2.1   Hepatic Steatosis, Visceral, and Subcutaneous Adiposity Measurements

NAFLD diagnosis and treatment can be accomplished by laboratory methods, including US, computerized tomography (CT), and magnetic resonance (MR). Although CT and MR offer somewhat smaller errors in hepatic and visceral fat estimations compared to US, this method is more useful in clinical routines because of its low cost and easy application. Future studies using these methods in the same NAFLD patients are essential for the proper assessment of compositional change with weight loss in a clinical trial (Saadeh et al., 2002; Dâmaso et al., 2008).

8.2.3   Psychological Therapy

A diagnosis must be established via validated questionnaires considering some psychological problems caused by obesity and MS described in the literature, such as depression, disturbances of body image, anxiety, and decrease in self-esteem. Considering the high prevalence of obese patients with NAFLD (about 60%), these questions were included as part of the therapy for all subjects in treatment (de Piano et al., 2007). During the multidisciplinary intervention, the psychologist must discuss with patients about body image and eating disorders (e.g., bulimia, anorexia nervosa); binge eating, their signals, symptoms, and consequences for health; the relation between feelings and food; familiar problems such as alcoholism; and other important topics to improve each behavior disturbance related to obesity, MS, as well as NAFLD.

An individual psychological therapy was recommended when behavior and nutritional problems were identified. After both short- and long-term multidisciplinary therapy and 12 months of intervention, patients must be reevaluated. Figure 8.2 shows the psychological algorithm suggested for this type of intervention.

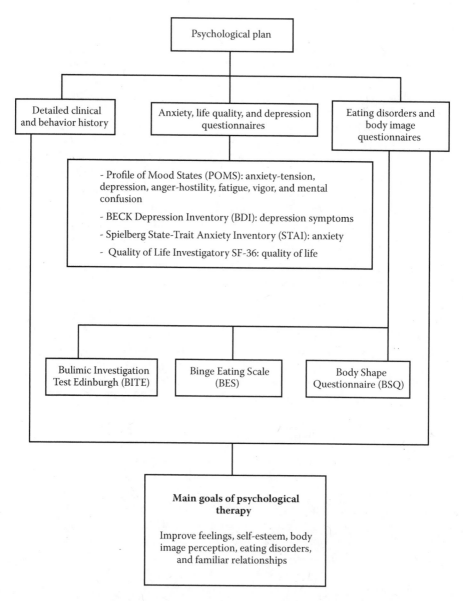

FIGURE 8.2 Organogram of psychological plan to be established at baseline and after short- and long-term multidisciplinary therapy.

8.2.4 Exercise Therapy

The main aim of exercise therapy is to promote lifestyle changes to motivate NAFLD patients to incorporate physical activity into their regimen as well as maintain a negative energy balance and, consequently, stable weight loss.

An exercise program should be realistic and should focus on long-term weight loss after inquiring about the medical background, exercise history, and preferences of the subject. NAFLD patients may need a personalized aerobic training and/or one composition session with aerobic exercise plus resistance training, including a 60-minute session, three times a week (180 min/week), under the supervision of a sports therapist. Each program needs to be based on the results of an initial oxygen uptake test for aerobic exercises (cycle ergometer and treadmill). The intensity may be set at a workload corresponding to a ventilatory threshold of 1 (50–70% of oxygen uptake test) according to recommendations on the type and amount of physical activity that will produce health benefits, focusing on the idea of accumulating moderate-intensity activity throughout the day (Matsudo and Matsudo, 2006).

At the end of short- and long-term multidisciplinary therapy, aerobic tests must be performed to assess physical capacities and adjust the physical training intensity for each individual. During aerobic and resistance sessions, the patient's heart rate needs to be monitored. The suggested exercise program was based on the American College of Sports Medicine (2001) recommendations. Information about lifestyle changes related to activity must also ensure that routine physical activity (walking, stair climbing, etc.) is encouraged.

In NAFLD and MS management, it was suggested that patients have theories of relationship between exercise effects and these diseases. Table 8.1 identifies the main topics to be encouraged in exercise classes.

Figure 8.3 shows exercise therapy as a suggested organogram.

TABLE 8.1
Main Exercise Topics Suggested for MS and NAFLD Long-Term Multidisciplinary Intervention

Exercise Class	Themes
1	General concepts for lifestyle changes
2	Hormonal regulation of energy balance
3	Different exercises and energy expenditures
4	Aerobic vs. strength training effects on obesity and comorbidities
5	Effects of exercise and nutrition on MS control
6	Effects of exercise and nutrition on NAFLD control
7	Effects of exercise and nutrition on immune system
8	Effects of exercise and nutrition on type II diabetes control
9	Effects of exercise and nutrition on weight loss management
10	Effects of exercise and nutrition on eating disorders
11	Yo-yo effects of rapid weight loss
12	Short- and long-term effects of exercise and nutrition on obesity and comorbidities

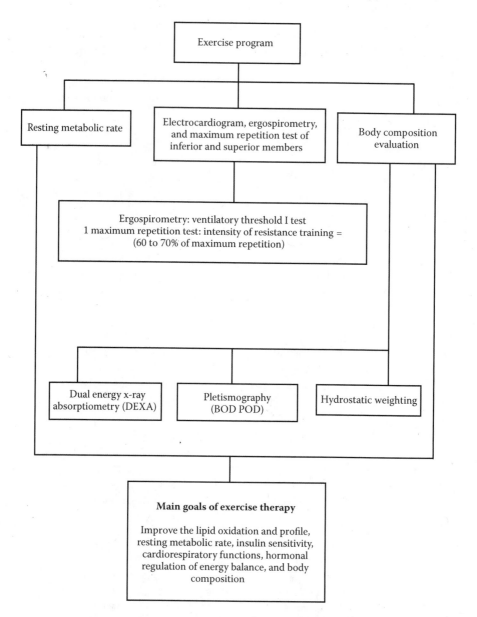

FIGURE 8.3 Organogram of exercise program to be established at baseline and after short- and long-term multidisciplinary therapy.

8.2.5 NUTRITIONAL THERAPY

As described at the beginning of this chapter, considering the strong association among obesity, MS, and the development of NAFLD, management strategies in the prevention and treatment of these diseases need to be based on a long-term multidisciplinary therapy including all associated comorbidities. The nutritional plan must consider strategies to promote gradual weight loss, glycemic control, reduction in low-density lipoprotein cholesterol (LDL-c), triglycerides, and very low-density lipoprotein cholesterol (VLDL-c) serum concentrations, mainly reduction in visceral adiposity. A recent study verified the correlation between visceral fat accumulation with increased degree and risk of developing NAFLD (Dâmaso et al., 2008).

Dietary standards recommend specific nutrients, but not the foods that contain them. To apply these standards to food choices, a better plan with options in terms of food groups or exchange lists is needed to support the patients in relation to which nutrients they require. The most commonly used tool in planning the daily menu is the food guide pyramid. Nutritional intervention is essential in evaluating food intake, deficiencies, or excess nutrients. Most methods of evaluating dietary intake involve different tools, such as 24-hour recall, 3-day food diary, food frequency, and diet history (Table 8.2).

A nutritional plan must be based on the levels recommended by the Dietary Reference Intake (DRI) according to age and gender (National Research Council, 2002). Patients with NAFLD and MS need to be encouraged to reduce their food intake and follow a balanced diet.

At the beginning of a multidisciplinary approach, diet history, 24-hour recall, 3-day dietary record, and food frequency questionnaires should be completed by each patient. It is important to observe that obese people can underreport their food consumption. The degree of underreporting may be substantial. However, this is a validated method to evaluate nutrition consumption (Hill and Davis, 2001). Portions need to be measured in terms of familiar volumes and sizes and with reference to an atlas of local food portions. These dietary data must be fed into a computer by the same dietician; thus, nutrient composition is analyzed by a computerized nutritional program to establish an adequate meal plan.

For NAFLD and MS control, it was suggested that patients undergo weekly dietetics lessons (food pyramid, recordatory inquiry, weight loss diets, diet vs. light,

---

TABLE 8.2
Nutritional Tools to Identify Eating Patterns in NAFLD and MS Patients

Method	Definition
24-Hour recall	Conducted by a trained interviewer who asks the individuals to recall exactly what they ate in the preceding 24-hour period.
Food diary	Individuals are instructed to record all food and drink they consume during a defined period ranging from 1 to 7 days. At least one weekend should be included since most people eat differently.
Food frequency	Presents a list of foods or food categories. Individuals respond to questions from a trained observer regarding how often each food is consumed per day, week, or month.
Diet history	A typical diet history could include some essential questions, such as familiar diseases history, age beginning to gain weight, habits foods, and all information to provide a more accurate picture of the individual's typical intake.

TABLE 8.3

Main Nutritional Topics for MS and NAFLD Long-Term Multidisciplinary Intervention

Nutritional Classes	Themes
1	Food guide pyramid, portion sizes, behavior food habits, and food as a social phenomenon
2	24-Hour recall (identifying potential problems)
3	Obesity and the "miracle diets"
4	Fat intake (types, sources, and substitute foods)
5	Food labels, dietetic, free fat, and low-calorie foods (food marketing and advertising)
6	Fast-food calories and nutritional compositions
7	Good nutritional choices on special occasion (parties, barbecues, holidays, and vacation)
8	Healthy sandwiches (practical class in an experimental kitchen)
9	How to fill out the 3-day food diary
10	Shakes and products promoting weight loss
11	Functional food
12	Decisions about food choices (what are your nutritional goals and what information is needed to achieve your nutritional goals?)

fat and cholesterol, nutrition facts) (de Piano et al., 2007). Table 8.3 shows the main topics suggested for nutritional classes in the treatment of MS and NAFLD.

Finally, complementary nutritional intervention must be improved by holding practical classes in an experimental kitchen to stimulate NAFLD patients to prepare their foods, introduce variety in their diet, and adopt habits that promote best life quality for a long time. However, treatment of NAFLD depends on the characteristics of each patient and may reflect the end results obtained after therapy. Thus, individual nutritional plan are an important tool in the management of NAFLD and MS. The organogram of a diet plans is illustrated in Figure 8.4.

Studies have shown that restrictive diets can aggravate NAFLD; they are associated with higher inflammation and degree of fibrosis in the liver because these diets promote a quick and intense weight loss through a high influx of free fatty acids to the liver (Bellentani et al., 2008). Another point that must be evaluated in diet composition is that both excessive carbohydrate and excessive fat intake could play a role in increasing blood glucose, free fatty acids, or insulin concentrations, independently or simultaneously (Zivkovic et al., 2007).

8.2.5.1   Establishing a Meal Plan

8.2.5.1.1   Calories

A proper nutritional plan must be individualized according to nutritional necessity and energy expenditure. A target of 5–10% of baseline weight is often used as an initial weight loss goal. According to the literature, every 0.250 kg of fat mass is equivalent

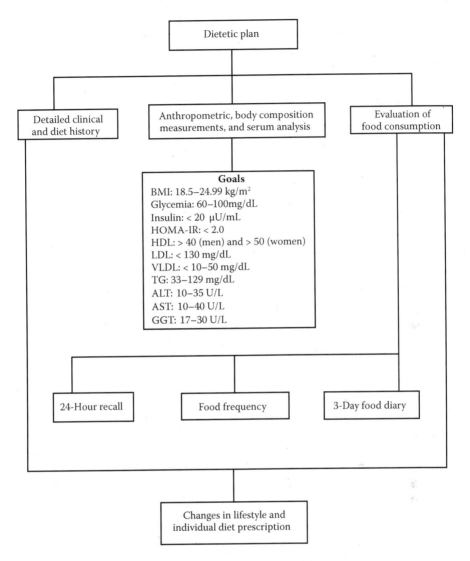

FIGURE 8.4 Organogram of a dietetic plan to be established at baseline and after short- and long-term multidisciplinary therapy.

to 3500 kcal. Thus, to achieve a weight loss of 0.500–1 kg/week, it is necessary to promote an energetic deficit of 1000 kcal/day (0.500 kg = 1000 kcal × 7 days/week) (Melby and Hickey, 2006). First of all, it is necessary to calculate the energy expenditure and the average energy consumption by 3 days' recordatory. Next, the nutritionist needs to calculate the energy intake by subtracting 500–1000 kcal from the estimated total daily calories previously calculated (using specific formulas according to age and gender), always incorporating new adequate food habits and stimulating an increase in the energy expenditure by a change in physical activity.

For example, according to the DRI (2002) specific formula, using the individual anthropometric measurements (including height and ideal average weight) and age:

Macronutrient Distribution

First step: Considering that basal energy expenditure (BEE) = 1800 kcal

Second step: Multiply by the appropriate activity factor: BEE × 1.3 (light activity) = 1800 kcal × 1.3 = 2340 kcal

Third step: Subtract 500–1000 kcal to create a deficit predicting 0.5–1 kg of weight loss per week = 2340 – 1000 = 1340 kcal/day

---

8.2.5.1.2   Carbohydrates

Solga et al. (2004) showed that high carbohydrate intake was associated with greater levels of inflammation in obese patients with NAFLD. High carbohydrate intake, mainly sucrose, glucose, fructose, and foods with a high glycemic index, cause an increase in *de novo* lipogenesis, which leads to an increased conversion of glucose to fatty acids. Indeed, high glycemic index carbohydrates lead to a quick increase with a subsequent decrease in insulin levels and an increase in glucagon and ghrelin, which are orexigenic hormones (Zivkovic et al., 2007).

The glycemic index describes the difference in the impact of ranking carbohydrates on the body according to their effects on blood glucose levels. A low glycemic index carbohydrate, which produces small fluctuations of blood glucose and insulin levels, is an important and coadjuvant tool in promoting long-term health, reducing the risk of NAFLD and improving some parameters of MS (Anderson et al., 2004).

The glycemic effect of foods depends on a number of factors: type of starch (amylose vs. amylopectin), fat, protein, and organic acid content of the food, as well as salts in the meal. Although food rich in lipids can present a low glycemic index, ingestion of this type of food must be limited. To control NAFLD and MS, it is important to evaluate the glycemic index and the glycemic load, which represents the effect on blood glucose considering the quantity and quality of carbohydrate amount per serving (Table 8.4).

Patients' diets must include foods rich in fiber, particularly soluble fiber dissolved in water. This type of fiber is very viscous when dissolved in the stomach and slows

---

TABLE 8.4

Reference Values to Glycemic Index and Glycemic Load Classifications

	Glycemic Index	Glycemic Load
High	≥ 70	≥ 20
Medium	56–69	11–19
Low	≤ 55	≤ 10

Source: University of Sydney, Glycemic Index, www.glycemicindex.com.

---

down the speed of digestion in the digestive tract, stabilizing blood glucose and insulin levels. The ideal amount of fiber required for NAFLD treatment has yet to be defined, but according to the American Diabetes Association (2004), the recommended total daily fiber intake is 25–30 g, of which 20–30% should come from soluble fiber.

Recently, the effects of high-fiber and low-glycemic index carbohydrates on glycemia and lipid profile were described in a meta-analysis (Anderson et al., 2004). In this manner, the choice of healthy sources of carbohydrates might be responsible for the beneficial effects on NAFLD and MS patients (Esposito et al., 2004).

8.2.5.1.3 Proteins

There is little information on the effect of protein quantity, quality, and composition on the pathophysiology of NAFLD and NASH. However, it is known that protein deficiency or malnutrition can cause steatosis. A normoproteic diet, representing 15–20% of the total energy intake, is therefore recommended (Zivkovic et al., 2007).

8.2.5.1.4 Saturated Fats

High saturated fat intake is associated with liver dysfunction caused by an increased production of reactive oxygen species, which leads to damage in the mitochondria of hepatocytes. In fact, lipotoxicity caused by long-chain fatty acids has been implicated in the development of numerous obesity-related diseases, including NAFLD. Indeed, high saturated fat intake (more than 10% of total energy) promotes insulin resistance, which plays a key role in the NAFLD genesis. Therefore, these data suggest that saturated fat intake must be limited in NAFLD patients (Cave et al., 2007).

However, the literature is rather unclear about the exact minimum amount of saturated fat intake that should be recommended to promote beneficial effects. Clinical evidence suggesting that this nutrient intake should be < 7% of total energy and > 10% of energy may be suboptimal for NAFLD patients (German and Dillard, 2004).

8.2.5.1.5 Monounsaturated Fatty Acids

Oleaginous, olive oil, nuts, and avocados are good sources of monounsaturated fatty acids (MUFAs). Studies have demonstrated their beneficial effects on cardiovascular disease risk factors and blood lipid profiles. In patients with type II diabetes, this type of fatty acid reduces VLDL-c and triacylglycerol without reducing high-density lipoprotein cholesterol (HDL-c), suggesting that an MUFA-rich diet could bring benefits to NAFLD patients (Rodriguez-Villar et al., 2004).

8.2.5.1.6 Polyunsaturated Fatty Acids

Low hepatic n-6 and n-3 polyunsaturated fatty acids (PUFAs) may contribute to steatosis and steatohepatitis and can be affected by diet and oxidative stress (Allard et al., 2008).

The two series of PUFAS, n-3 and n-6, and their derived products, are provided in *cis*-linoleic and linolenic acids, respectively. The main compounds of PUFA are arachidonic acids derived from n-6, and docosahexaenoic acids and eicosapentanoic derived from n-3. These nutrients present an anti-inflammatory action by decreasing the inflammatory mediators (Martin et al., 2006).

The ratio of n-6 to n-3 fatty acids seems to be important in determining the effect of PUFAs on various lipid and nonlipid indexes. The main sources of n-3 are fish and fish oil, and good sources of n-6 are vegetable oils. It was verified that 1–2 g of fish oil/day supplementation promotes decreased blood triacylglycerol, hepatic enzymes, fasting glucose, TNF-α, and steatosis regression in NAFLD patients (Capanni et al., 2006; Spadaro et al., 2006). These data suggest that consumption of n-3 fatty acids found in fish oils and walnuts is likely to improve blood lipid profiles and

TABLE 8.5
Different Dietetic Plans for NAFLD Control and Their Effectiveness in Some Clinical Parameters

Authors	Diet	Results
Yamamoto et al. (2007)	126 kJ/kg/day of energy, a fat energy fraction of 20%, ≤ 6 mg/day iron, and 1.1–1.2 g/kg/day of protein	↓ ALT, AST, ferritin, body weight, BMI
Capanni et al. (2006)	1 g fish oil/day supplementation for 12 months	↓ blood triacylglycerol concentrations, hepatic enzymes, fasting glucose, and steatosis in NAFLD
Spadaro et al. (2006)	2 g fish oil/day supplementation for 6 months	↓ blood triacylglycerol concentrations, hepatic enzymes, TNF-α, and steatosis regression
McAuley et al. (2005)	< 20% carbohydrate, 25–30% protein, 55–65% fat, 20% saturated, 10% MUFA, 300–600 cholesterol	↓ body weight, waist circumference, insulin sensitivity, triacylglycerol, and ↑ steatosis, total cholesterol, and LDL
Huang et al. (2005)	40–45% from carbohydrates, with emphasis on complex carbohydrates with fiber; 35–40% from fat with emphasis on monounsaturated and polyunsaturated fats; 15–20% from protein for 12 months	Histological improvement in 60% of NASH patients
Daubioul et al. (2005)	Oligofructans given for 8 weeks	↓ ALT and serum insulin
Esposito et al. (2004)	50–60% carbohydrates, 15–20% protein, and total fat = 30%	↓ Body weight, BMI, waist circumference, inflammatory markers, glucose, total cholesterol, triacylglycerol, and insulin resistance, as well as improving endothelial function and ↑ HDL-c concentrations
Solga et al. (2004)	Diet with higher carbohydrate intake	Higher odds of inflammation

Note: Clinical results from different dietetic plans.
ALT, alanine aminotransferase; AST, aspartate aminotransferase; BMI, body mass index; HDL-c, high-density lipoprotein; LDL, low-density lipoprotein; NAFLD, nonalcoholic fatty liver disease; TNF-α, tumor necrosis factor α; NASH, nonalcoholic steatohepatitis.

reduce inflammation, steatosis, and liver damage in NAFLD patients (Zivkovic et al., 2007).

8.2.5.1.7 Trans Fatty Acids

Trans fatty acids can be naturally found in dairy products as a result of bacterial metabolism in ruminant animals and industrialized foods—margarines, biscuits, ice creams, some breads, fried potatoes (fast food), cake shops, cakes—as a result of hydrogenation (Chiara et al., 2003).

It is essential to note that the *trans* fatty acids used in food processing act as risk factor to cardiovascular diseases, increased inflammatory markers, induced endothelial dysfunction and a worse blood lipid profile, increases in the LDL-c, and decreases in the HDL-c. Based on these findings, in 2006 the Food and Drug Administration ruled that manufactured foods are required to include the content of *trans* fatty acids on nutrition labels according to serving portion. The recommendation urges consumers to avoid the intake of *trans* fatty acids of less than 2 g/day.

Several studies featuring different diets for the treatment of MS and NAFLD offer better choices in nutritional therapy, considering the initial screening each patient presents at the beginning of the therapy. Table 8.5 shows the diet composition and its results.

In a previous study, visceral fat was defined as a good predictor of NAFLD development (Dâmaso et al., 2008). In fact, a positive correlation was observed among energy intake, lipid consumption (%), and saturated fatty acid ingestion with visceral fat accumulation in obese adolescents with NAFLD (data not shown). These findings suggest that diet composition has a strong influence on the genesis and treatment of NAFLD because excessive saturated fatty acid intake is a determining factor in the increase of the prevalence of NAFLD. In consideration of these facts, the nutritional plan must be based on a balanced and individualized diet, giving priority to complex carbohydrates, including fiber, and decreasing lipid consumption, mainly the sources of saturated fatty acids (Tables 8.6 and 8.7).

TABLE 8.6
Suggested Nutritional Plan for Prevention and Treatment of NAFLD and MS

Nutrients	Description
Calories	Basal energy expenditure × activity factor – 1000 kcal
Carbohydrates	45–60% of total energetic value, mainly from grains, fruits, and vegetables
Fibers	25–30 g (about 20–30% = soluble fiber)
Proteins	10–20% of total energetic value
Lipids	20–30% of total energetic value
Saturated fats	< 7% of total energetic value
Monounsaturated fats	10% of total energetic value
Polyunsaturated fats	10 % of total energetic value
Trans fatty acids	< 2 g/day
Dietetic cholesterol	< 200 mg

TABLE 8.7

Five Essential Recommendations for Prevention and Treatment of NAFLD and MS

1. Individual nutritional plan to promote gradual weight loss and maintenance of ideal weight
2. Changes in inadequate food habits
3. Reduction of simple carbohydrates intake and with high glycemic index, substituting them with complex carbohydrates, mainly with low glycemic index and load (Table 8.4)
4. Incorporation of fibers in the daily menu, such as fruits, vegetables, and oats, mainly soluble fibers that slow down the gastric emptying, promoting a maintenance of glycemic rate
5 Reduction of saturated and *trans* fatty acids, substituting with monounsaturated and polyunsaturated fatty acids, which decrease the risk of heart disease and improve insulin sensitivity

8.2.6 PRACTICAL APPLICATIONS

It is important to note that, based on our understanding of the disease pathogenesis, it seems logical that a multidisciplinary approach to addressing the underlying MS and obesity is required to effectively treat patients with NAFLD and serves as a potential weapon in our line of defense against correlated diseases.

8.3 SUMMARY POINTS, POLICY MAKERS, AND FUTURE RESEARCH

- NAFLD should be recognized as part of MS and should be managed by a multidisciplinary approach addressing liver disease in the context of risk factors for diabetes and premature cardiovascular disease.
- Lifestyle changes are the first line and mainstay of management. The basal universal approach consists of clinical, nutritional, exercise, and psychological counseling.
- It is important to identify the cutoff points of visceral fat on NAFLD and MS development as well as the relation to proinflammatory cytokines, with the aim of creating new clinical and nutritional strategies in the prevention and treatment of these diseases and their comorbidities.
- Future research is needed to discover possible specific liver drugs and deal with NAFLD and comorbidities related to obesity, MS, and associated chronic diseases, especially during the early stages of life.

REFERENCES

ACSM position stand on the appropriate intervention strategies for weight loss and prevention of weight regain for adults. 2001. *Med Sci Sports Exerc* 33:2145–2156.
American Diabetes Association. 2004. Nutrition principles and recommendations in diabetes. *Diabetes Care* 27:S36.

Allard, J. P., E. Aghdassi, S. Mohammed, et al. 2008. Nutritional assessment and hepatic fatty acid composition in non-alcoholic fatty liver disease (NAFLD): A cross-sectional study. *J Hepatol* 48:300–307.

Anderson, J. W., K. M. Randles, C. W. Kendall, et al. 2004. Carbohydrate and fiber recommendations for individuals with diabetes: A quantitative assessment and meta-analysis of the evidence. *J Am Coll Nutr* 23:5–17.

Bellentani, S., R. Dalle Grave, A. Suppini, et al. 2008. Fatty Liver Italian Network. Behavior therapy for non-alcoholic fatty liver disease: The need for a multidisciplinary approach. *Hepatology* 47:746–754.

Capanni, M., F. Calella, M. R. Biagini, et al. 2006. Prolonged n-3 polyunsaturated fatty acid supplementation ameliorates hepatic steatosis in patients with non-alcoholic fatty liver disease: A pilot study. *Aliment Pharmacol Ther* 23:1143–1151.

Caranti, D. A., M. T. de Mello, W. L. Prado, et al. 2007. Short- and long-term beneficial effects of a multidisciplinary therapy for the control of metabolic syndrome in obese adolescents. *Metabolism* 56:1293–1300.

Cave, M., I. Deaciu, C. Mendez, et al. 2007. Nonalcoholic fatty liver disease: Predisposing factors and the role of nutrition. *J Nutr Biochem* 18:184–195.

Chiara, V. L., R. Sichieri, and T. S. F. Carvalho. 2003. Teores de ácidos graxos trans de alguns alimentos consumidos no Rio de Janeiro. *Rev Nutr* 16:227–233.

Dâmaso, A. R., W. L. do Prado, A. de Piano, et al. 2008. Relationship between nonalcoholic fatty liver disease prevalence. *Dig Liver Dis* 40:132–139.

Daubioul, C. A., Y. Horsmans, P. Lambert, et al. 2005. Effects of oligofructans on glucose and lipid metabolism in patients with non-alcoholic steatohepatitis: Results of a pilot study. *Eur J Clin Nutr* 59:723–726.

de Piano, A., W. L. Prado, D. A. Caranti, et al. 2007. Metabolic and nutritional profile of obese adolescents with non-alcoholic fatty liver disease. *J Pediatr Gastroenterol Nutr* 44:446–452.

Esposito, K., R. Marfella, M. Ciotola, et al. 2004. Effect of a Mediterranean style diet on endothelial dysfunction and markers of vascular inflammation in the metabolic syndrome: A randomized trial. *JAMA* 292:1440–1446.

Fields, D. A., P. B. Higgins, and G. R. Hunter. 2004. Assessment of body composition by air-displacement plethismography: Influence of body temperature and moisture. *Dyn Med* 13:3.

German, J. B., and C. J. Dillard. 2004. Saturated fats: What dietary intake? *Am J Clin Nutr* 80:550–559.

Hill, R. J., and P. S. Davies. 2001. The validity of self-reported energy intake as determined using the doubly labeled water technique. *Br J Nutr* 85:415–430.

Huang, M. A., J. K. Greenson, C. Chao, et al. 2005. One-year intense nutritional counseling results in histological improvement in patients with non-alcoholic steatohepatitis: A pilot study. *Am J Gastroenterol* 100:1072–1081.

Martin, C. A., V. V. Almeida, M. R. Ruiz, et al. 2006. Ácidos graxos poliinsaturados ômega-3 e ômega-6: Importância e ocorrência em alimentos. *Rev Nutr* 19:761–770.

Matsudo, S. M., and V. R. Matsudo. 2006. Coalitions and networks: Facilitating global physical activity promotion. *Promot Educ* 13:133–138, 158–163.

McAuley, K. A., C. M. Hopkins, K. J. Smith, et al. 2005. Comparison of high-fat and high-protein diets with a high-carbohydrate diet in insulin-resistant obese women. *Diabetologia* 48:8–16.

Melby, C., and M. Hickey. 2006. Balanço energético e regulação do peso corporal. *Gatorade Sports Sci Inst* 48:1–6.

National Research Council. 2002. *Dietary Reference Intakes (DRI): Applications in Dietary Assessment.* Washington DC: National Academy Press.

Rodriguez-Villar, C., A. Perez-Heras, I. Mercade, et al. 2004. Comparison of a high-carbohydrate and a high-monounsaturated fat, olive oil–rich diet on the susceptibility of LDL to oxidative modification in subjects with type 2 diabetes mellitus. *Diabet Med* 21:142–149.

Saadeh, S., Z. M. Younossi, E. M. Remer, et al. 2002. The utility of radiological imaging in nonalcoholic fatty liver disease. *Gastroenterol* 123:745–750.

Schwimmer, J. B., R. Deutsch, J. B. Rauch, et al. 2003. Obesity, insulin resistance, and other clinicopathological correlates of pediatric nonalcoholic fatty liver disease. *J Pediatr* 143:500–505.

Siegfried, W., K. Kromeyer-Hauschild, G. Zabel, et al. 2006. Long-term inpatient treatment of extreme juvenile obesity: An 18-month catamnestic study. *MMW Fortschr Med* 148:39–41.

Solga, S., A. R. Alkhuraishe, J. M. Clark, et al. 2004. Dietary composition and nonalcoholic fatty liver disease. *Dig Dis Sci* 49:1578–1583.

Spadaro, L., O. Magliocco, D. Spampinato, et al. 2006. 738 Omega-3 polyunsaturated fatty acids: A pilot trial in non-alcoholic fatty liver disease. *J Hepatol* 44:S264.

Tock, L., W. L. Prado, D. A. Caranti, et al. 2006. Nonalcoholic fatty liver disease decrease in obese adolescents after multidisciplinary therapy. *Eur J Gastroenterol Hepatol* 18:1241–1245.

World Health Organization (WHO). 2000. *Obesity: Preventing and Managing the Global Epidemic*, WHO Obesity Technical Report Series 894. Geneva, Switzerland: World Health Organization.

Wymann, M. P., and R. Schneiter. 2008. Lipid signalling in disease. *Nat Rev Mol Cell Biol* 9:162–176.

Yamamoto, M., M. Iwasa, K. Iwata, et al. 2007. Restriction of dietary calories, fat and iron improves non-alcoholic fatty liver disease. *Hepatology* 22:498–503.

Zivkovic, A. M., J. B. German, and A. J. Sanyal. 2007. Comparative review of diets for the metabolic syndrome: Implications for nonalcoholic fatty liver disease. *Am J Clin Nutr* 86:285–300.

9 Emerging Nutritional Treatments for Nonalcoholic Fatty Liver Disease

Mariangela Allocca and Carlo Selmi

CONTENTS

9.1   INTRODUCTION

Nonalcoholic fatty liver disease (NAFLD) is the hepatic manifestation of the metabolic syndrome and is currently among the most prominent causes of chronic liver
disease in the United States, being found in up to 30% of the general population
(Browning et al., 2004). Although most patients with simple liver steatosis will not
progress, an NAFLD subtype with inflammatory features, coined nonalcoholic
steatohepatitis (NASH; estimated to affect 5% of the general population), does progress to cirrhosis and its complications.

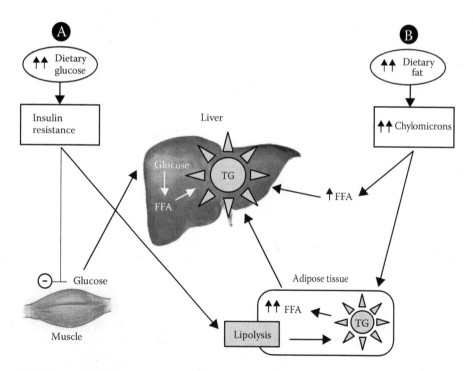

FIGURE 9.1   Mechanisms of insulin resistance and NAFLD establishment. (A) The increase
in dietary carbohydrates leads to insulin resistance and the increase of muscle-derived glucose efflux to the liver where it is transformed into free fatty acids (FFA) and triglycerides
(TG). In a complementary fashion, (B) the increase in fat intake increases FFA both directly
and through the adipose tissue, thus ultimately increasing liver TG.

Insulin resistance is considered a key factor in the development of NAFLD and NASH, as illustrated in Figure 9.1. Overnutrition or an excessive intake of carbohydrate and/or fat (e.g., an inappropriate diet) are thought to lead to chronically elevated glucose, insulin, and free fatty acid (FFA) plasma levels. These diet-induced conditions contribute to the development of resistance to insulin-stimulated glucose uptake by the adipose tissue and skeletal muscle as well as resistance to insulin-inhibited lipolysis in the adipose tissue. The resistance to insulin inhibition of lipolysis in the adipose tissue and the continuous stimulation of lipoprotein lipase–mediated hydrolysis of fats ultimately lead to an increased FFA flux to the liver. Glucose uptake in the liver is insulin independent, and increased glucose concentrations in the blood lead to the shunting of glucose to the liver, where it is converted to either glycogen or FFA through insulin-stimulated *de novo* lipogenesis, and to the stimulation of the production of free cholesterol. As a result, the triacylglycerols and cholesterol esters accumulate in the liver. In healthy individuals, elevated lipid concentrations in the liver lead to increased very low density lipoprotein (VLDL) production and secretion, whereas the impairments in lipid export via VLDL secretion, β oxidation of FFA, or other metabolic pathways observed in patients with NAFLD result in an inability to maintain fat balance and prevent fatty liver. The current "two-hit hypothesis" of

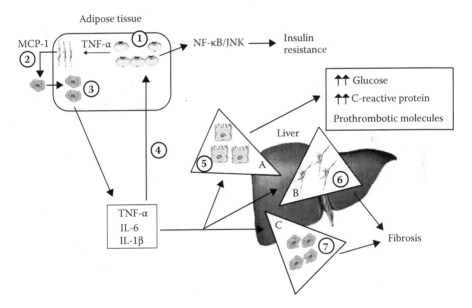

FIGURE 9.2 Inflammatory features of the metabolic syndrome. In obese subjects, mature adipocytes (1) secrete inflammatory mediators (e.g.., TNF-α), which (2) stimulate the production of monocyte chemotactic protein 1 (MCP-1) by preadipocytes. MCP-1, in turn, (3) acts to recruit macrophages, which secrete proinflammatory cytokines such as TNF-α, interleukin 6, and interleukin 1β. These mediators help perpetuate the mechanism by (4) stimulating adipocytes while also (5) act on hepatocytes to increase glucose production, inflammatory mediators, and prothrombotic molecules. Lastly, macrophage-derived cytokines activate liver-resident stellate cells (6) and Kupffer cells (7) to induce fibrosis.

TABLE 9.1

Effect of Macronutrients and Correlated Foods on Major Metabolic Syndrome Features

	Food	Action
SFA	Lard, butter, coconut oil, palm oil	↑ LDL
MUFA	Olive oil, nuts, avocados, peanut butter, peanut oil	↓ LDL
		↓ Triacylglycerol
		↑ HDL
PUFA (n-3)	Fish oil, walnuts, salmon, shellfish	↓ FFA, glucose, insulin
		↓ Triacylglycerol, LDL
		↑ HDL
		↓ TNF-α
Trans-fatty acid	Fast foods, baked goods, deep fried foods, margarine	↑ LDL
		↑ Inflammatory markers
Fiber	Whole grains, fruits, and vegetables	↑ Insulin resistance
		↓ LDL, triacylglycerol
Fructose	Sweetened drinks, sodas, candy	↓ Insulin resistance

NASH onset states that the lipid accumulation in the liver constitutes the first hit (Day and James 1998), whereas oxidative stress from mitochondrial reactive oxygen species with lipid peroxidation would produce the second hit, thus ultimately leading to the secretion of proinflammatory cytokines and stellate cell activation. Moreover, other mechanisms may also be implicated and include inflammation (Figure 9.2). The increased secretion of tumor necrosis factor α (TNF-α) and other proinflammatory cytokines may be also originated from adipocytes and infiltrating macrophages as suggested by the resulting systemic inflammation as well as obesity-associated insulin resistance (Diehl, 2004). From a nutritional standpoint, however, it is important to note the different impact of single dietary components (summarized in Table 9.1) on the onset of NAFLD and NASH.

9.2   ROLE OF INDIVIDUAL DIETARY COMPONENTS ON THE DEVELOPMENT OF NAFLD AND NASH

9.2.1   SATURATED FATTY ACIDS

Saturated fatty acids (SFAs) are known to promote endoplasmic reticulum stress as well as hepatocyte injury in rat models and their daily intake correlates with the risk of cardiovascular disease (Lichtenstein, 2006), thus suggesting that such an intake should be limited in NAFLD patients. It is not clear, however, what saturated fat intake should be recommended. We cannot exclude the existence of a threshold intake below which adverse effects may occur or that a minimum SFA intake may be essential to health, yet current data encourage us to limit SFA to constitute 7–10% of daily energy intake in patients with NAFLD.

9.2.2 Monounsaturated Fatty Acids

Monounsaturated fatty acids (MUFAs) significantly decrease oxidized low-density lipoprotein (LDL), LDL cholesterol, total cholesterol, and triacylglycerol concentrations but do not lead to a decrease in high-density lipoprotein (HDL) as seen with general low-fat diet (Kris-Etherton et al., 1999). In clinical practice, a diet rich in MUFA, particularly if poor in SFA and carbohydrates, should be encouraged in patients with NAFLD.

9.2.3 Polyunsaturated Fatty Acids

Polyunsaturated fatty acids (PUFAs) include essential n-6 and n-3 fatty acids such as α-linolenic acid, which is a precursor for the long-chain docosahexaenoic acid and eicosapentaenoic acid. Deficiencies in essential fatty acids may be involved in the development and progression of NAFLD (Werner et al., 2005) by decreasing lipid export from the liver. PUFAs from fish oil ultimately decrease the risk of heart disease and the severity of NAFLD as well illustrated by Dr. Puder elsewhere in this book. Similarly, a diet rich in walnuts is rich in α-linolenic acid and leads to increased plasma HDL and decreased plasma LDL in patients with diabetes (Tapsell et al., 2004) and hypercholesterolemia (Ros et al., 2004).

9.2.4 Trans-Fatty Acids

Trans-fatty acids (TFAs) are characterized by at least one double bond in the trans configuration formed during the hydrogenation of either vegetable or fish oils for plasticity and chemical stability in the food industry. Hydrogenated oils have been found to increase inflammatory markers, induce endothelial dysfunction, and increase the LDL/HDL and triacylglycerol/HDL ratios (Mozaffarian, 2006). In the absence of solid data, we may hypothesize that TFAs from hydrogenated oils should be minimized in NAFLD patients.

9.2.5 Carbohydrates and the Glycemic Index

Glycemic index (GI) is a ranking of carbohydrates on a scale from 0 to 100 according to the extent to which they raise blood sugar levels after ingestion. High-GI foods are rapidly digested and absorbed and result in marked fluctuations in blood sugar levels, whereas low-GI ones are characterized by a slow digestion and absorption leading to gradual rises in blood sugar and insulin levels. In 1999, the World Health Organization and the Food and Agriculture Organization recommended that people in industrialized countries base their diets on low-GI foods to prevent coronary heart disease (CHD), diabetes, and obesity. To improve the reliability of predicting the glycemic response of a given diet, glycemic load has been proposed to take into account the effect of a typical amount of carbohydrates in a portion on blood levels. The glycemic load of a food is the product of the GI of the food and the amount of carbohydrate in a serving. Given the close relation among obesity, diabetes mellitus, the metabolic syndrome, and the development of NAFLD, it seems reasonable to conclude that a low-GI and low-glycemic load diet should be encouraged in patients with insulin resistance and NAFLD.

9.2.6 FIBER

Dietary fibers are the indigestible portion of plant foods and can be water-soluble or water-insoluble. The latter (cellulose, lignans) has passive water-attracting properties that increase the bulk, soften stools, and shorten the intestinal transit time. Soluble fiber (pectins, natural gums, inulins) undergoes metabolic processing via fermentation in the large intestine, producing gas and short-chain fatty acids. Fermentable fiber reduces blood levels of LDL cholesterol, triacylglycerol, and glucose, and a recent meta-analysis demonstrated the effects of a high-fiber diet on reducing the glycemic response and cholesterol levels in patients with diabetes (Anderson et al., 2004). Taken together, the available data support the advice of a high-fiber diet in patients with NAFLD and insulin resistance.

9.2.7 FRUCTOSE

Most soft drinks are sweetened with sugars such as sucrose or high-fructose corn syrup, both containing 50–55% fructose. The worldwide consumption of sugar-sweetened soft drinks has been increasing throughout the past decades, rising from 3.9% of total energy intake in 1977 to 9.2% of total energy intake in 2001, and this has been associated with weight gain (Schulze et al., 2004). These drinks are typically consumed as additional calories and lead to an excess 150–300 kcal daily intake, thus contributing to the onset of the metabolic syndrome. The administration of an 18-day diet with 25% of total energy as sucrose results in a rise in aminotransferase levels (Porikos and Van Itallie, 1983), and an increased fructose intake may result in an increased lipid accumulation in the liver along with insulin resistance and elevated plasma triacylglycerol levels. A recent study on animals demonstrated that chronic fructose consumption led to fatty liver development and increased endotoxin levels in portal plasma and that concomitant treatment of fructose-fed mice with nonresorbable antibiotics blocked hepatic lipid accumulation (Bergheim et al., 2008). Patients with NAFLD manifest increased liver fructokinase levels compared to controls, and taken altogether, the available experimental and human data strongly support the notion that fructose avoidance should be encouraged in the prevention and treatment of NAFLD.

9.3 PRACTICAL APPLICATIONS AND TREATMENT REGIMENS

To date, no unique treatment regimen has been approved for NAFLD. However, a somehow intuitive cornerstone of any strategy in such patients is a significant decrease in body weight, and a bewildering array of diets have been recommended for the prevention and treatment of the metabolic syndrome while their impact on NAFLD remains, in most cases, poorly defined (Table 9.2). We note that all approaches may be strengthened by cognitive-behavioral therapies that significantly enhance the probability of long-term success of lifestyle and diet changes.

TABLE 9.2
Relative Amounts of Nutrients in Major Proposed Dietary Regimens

Diet	Carbohydrate (%)	Fat (%)	Protein (%)	SFA (%)	MUFA (%)	PUFA (%)	Cholesterol (mg/day)	Fiber (g/day)
ADA	55–65	20–30	15	< 10	–	–	< 300	–
AHA	50–60	25–35	15	7–10	–	–	< 300	25
NCEP I	50–60	30	15	< 10	20	10	< 300	20–30
TLC	50–60	25–35	15	< 7	20	10	< 200	20–30
DASH	50–60	25–35	15	< 7	–	–	–	20–30
American Diabetic Association	55–65	20–30	15	< 7	–	–	< 200	20–30
Mediterranean	55	30	15	< 10	15	5	200	20
Ornish	70–75	10	15–20	< 1	–	–	5	–
Atkins	< 20	55–65	25–30	20	10	5	300–600	5
Zone	40	30	30	12	10	5	200–300	15
South Beach	10–28	39–62	28–33	12	10	5	200–300	15
Weight Watchers	55–65	20–30	15	< 10	–	–	< 300	20–30

9.3.1 DIETARY GUIDELINES

9.3.1.1 American Dietetic Association

The American Dietetic Association (ADA) guidelines are intended for the metabolic syndrome and include a first tier with weight loss and exercise. The former is achieved through a suggested 100 kcal reduction of daily energy intake and a reduction in the intake of total fat, SFA, and trans fat. On the contrary, the ADA advises to increase the intakes of PUFA, in particular n-3 fatty acids, and MUFA along with the inclusion of plant sterols or stanol esters to reduce intestinal cholesterol absorption and, subsequently, LDL cholesterol. A nonsecondary question of the ADA recommendations raises some concern. In fact, we are not convinced of the safety profile of increasing the amount of plant stanols or sterols in the diet based on observations that only 5% of dietary plant sterols are absorbed, whereas in rare cases, the ability of the liver to excrete plant sterols into the bile is impaired. The accumulation of plant sterols in the body results in a condition called sitosterolemia associated with CHD (Salen et al., 2002) and, without further evidence of the safety profile, high intakes of plant sterols should not be recommended for the general population. On the other hand, this should be advocated in high-risk patients in whom benefit will outweigh potential risks.

9.3.1.2 American Heart Association

According to the American Heart Association (AHA), patients with NAFLD and features of the metabolic syndrome should be treated to reduce their risk of cardiovascular disease. The AHA guidelines recommend to eat fish twice a week, avoid trans fats, limit SFA intake to < 10% of total calories, and limit cholesterol to < 300 mg/day. In addition, it advises to avoid simple sugars and, on the contrary, to prefer foods with lower GI. The AHA/National Heart, Lung and Blood Institute joint scientific statement on the Diagnosis and Management of the Metabolic Syndrome further recommended to decrease the SFA intake to < 7% of total calories, although this raises some concerns for reasons previously illustrated.

9.3.1.3   National Cholesterol Education Program

The Step I and Step II National Cholesterol Education Program (NCEP) diets were created by the Expert Panel on Detection, Evaluation, and Treatment of High Blood Cholesterol in Adults through two subsequent guideline reports, the Adult Treatment Panel I and II. The Step I diet was a strategy for the prevention of heart diseases in patients with LDL concentration ≥ 160 mg/dL or in those with LDL concentration between 130 and 159 mg/dL in the presence of two or more additional risk factors (cigarette smoking, hypertension, low HDL, family history of premature CHD, age ≥ 45 years for men or ≥ 55 for women). This diet restricts total daily fat intake to ≤ 30%, SFA intake to < 10% of total calories, and cholesterol to < 300 mg/day. The Step II diet was then recommended to patients with CHD or who were already following the Step I diet, without achieving the major goals. This diet further restricts SFA intake to < 7% of total calories and cholesterol to < 200 mg/day. Currently, the Step I diet is still recommended for the general public, whereas the Step II diet has been renamed the Therapeutic Lifestyle Changes (TLC) diet.

9.3.1.4   Therapeutic Lifestyle Change

As mentioned above, the ATP II recommendations for lifestyle approach to reduce the risk of CHD has been designated TLC. This includes a decrease in SFA to 7% of daily calories, a reduction in total fat intake to 25–35% of daily calories and daily cholesterol to < 200 mg, intake of PUFA up to 10% of daily calories and MUFA up to 20% of total calories, intake of carbohydrate 50–60% of calories, protein at 15% of calories, Na+ < 2400 mg/day, and ultimately balance energy intake and expenditure to maintain the target body weight and prevent further weight gain. If the LDL cholesterol goal is not achieved in this manner, other therapeutic options for lowering LDL will include the addition of plant sterols and stanols (2 g/day) and viscous and soluble fiber (20–30 g/day). Based on its fat content, the TLC diet should not be recommended for patients with NAFLD only.

9.3.1.5   Dietary Approaches to Stop Hypertension

Dietary Approaches to Stop Hypertension (DASH) recommend a reduction in daily sodium intake to 2.4 g and preliminary evidence suggests that this advice may also apply to subjects with NAFLD and arterial hypertension (Marchesini et al., 2003).

9.3.1.6   American Diabetes Association

The Medical Nutrition Therapy is important in all three levels of diabetes clinical features by preventing its onset, achieving and maintaining its metabolic control, and delaying and managing its long-term complications (Bantle et al., 2008). We will review below some of the major nutrition recommendations and interventions presented by the American Diabetes Association position statement with the corresponding levels of evidence also reported. Given the close relationship between diabetes and NAFLD, these suggestions, with some issues that we have previously addressed, should be regarded as extremely valuable for patients with NAFLD or NASH.

9.3.1.6.1 Energy Balance, Overweight, and Obesity

1. In overweight and obese insulin-resistant individuals, weight loss is recommended by either low-carbohydrate or low-fat calorie-restricted diets, which may be effective in the short term (up to 1 year) (A-level evidence).
2. Physical activity and behavior modification are important components of all weight loss programs and are most helpful in maintenance of weight loss (B-level evidence).

9.3.1.6.2 Primary Prevention

1. Among individuals at high risk for developing type 2 diabetes, a 7% weight loss and 150 min/week of physical activity should be recommended. Dietary strategies include a reduced income of calories and fats (A-level evidence). Both the Finnish Diabetes Prevention study and the Diabetes Prevention Program focused on a reduced intake of calories by reduced dietary fat as a dietary intervention. The reduced intake of fats, particularly saturated fats, may reduce risk for diabetes both by producing an improvement in insulin resistance and promoting weight loss.
2. Individuals at high risk for type 2 diabetes should be encouraged to increase the intake of whole grains (one-half of grain intake) and dietary fiber (14 g/1000 kcal) (B-level evidence). Several studies have provided evidence for reduced risk of diabetes and insulin resistance with an increased intake of fiber and whole grain.
3. At the present status of knowledge, there are not sufficient data to conclude that low-GI and low-glycemic load diets reduce the risk for diabetes. Nevertheless, low-GI foods should be encouraged (E-level evidence).

9.3.1.6.3 Secondary Prevention

1. The use of GI and load may provide a limited additional benefit over that observed when total carbohydrate alone is considered (B-level evidence). Since dietary carbohydrate is the major determinant of postprandial glucose levels, low-carbohydrate diets may be the most effective approach to lowering postprandial glucose. However, glucose is the primary fuel used by the central nervous system, and the minimum daily requirement for providing glucose without reliance on glucose production from ingested protein or fat should be set at 130 g. Furthermore, foods containing carbohydrate are an important source of many nutrients, including water-soluble vitamins and minerals as well as fiber.
2. Limit saturated fat to < 7% of total calories (A-level evidence).
3. Intake of trans fat should be minimized (E-level evidence).

4. Limit dietary cholesterol to < 200 mg/day (E-level evidence).
5. Two or more servings of fish per week are recommended (B-level evidence).

9.3.2 POPULAR DIETS AND THEIR POTENTIAL USE IN NAFLD AND NASH

9.3.2.1 Mediterranean Dietary Pattern

The Mediterranean dietary pattern emphasizes the inclusion of particular foods rather than the limitation of specific macronutrients. This diet is characterized by a high intake of vegetables, legumes, fruits and nuts, and cereals and a high intake of olive oil with a low intake of saturated lipids, a moderately high intake of fish, a low to moderate intake of dairy products, a low intake of meat and poultry, and a regular but moderate intake of wine. Several recent reviews concluded that adherence to the Mediterranean diet leads to improvements in lipoprotein indexes, insulin sensitivity, endothelial function, and cardiovascular mortality. A randomized study comparing the effects of a Mediterranean diet with a generic low-fat diet demonstrated that in the Mediterranean group a higher proportion of patients no longer had features of the metabolic syndrome after 2 years of follow-up (Esposito et al., 2004). Similarly, a population-based cohort study in Greece reported that a higher degree of adherence to the Mediterranean diet was associated with a reduction in total mortality, CHD, and cancer without significant associations with food groups contributing to the Mediterranean diet score (Trichopoulou et al., 2003). It is likely that individual components may have a limited impact that emerges only when the components are integrated together. There seems to be convincing cumulative evidence that the combination of high MUFA and high fiber intakes, a low GI, and the emphasis on lean protein sources may also be a good option in patients with NAFLD. In addition, the Mediterranean diet is easy to understand and follow and is highly palatable, which may lead to a higher adherence among dieters in the long term.

9.3.2.2 Ornish Diet

The Ornish diet is a vegetarian diet containing 10% of calories from fats. The diet allows the unlimited consumption of fruits, vegetables, grains, beans, and legumes and restricts the intake of all meats (including fish), oils and fats, nuts, avocados, dairy products, sugar, simple carbohydrates, and alcohol. Multiple studies reported the effectiveness of the Ornish diet in preventing and even reversing coronary disease (Ornish et al., 1998). On the other hand, one of the main criticisms in using the Ornish diet in NAFLD treatment is the severe restriction of all fats, including n-3 fats and MUFAs, which have been associated with improvements in metabolic measures related to NAFLD. Furthermore, this diet may be too drastic and limiting for most patients in the long term, thus making its long-term impact less significant.

9.3.2.3 Atkins Diet

The Atkins diet is a low-carbohydrate diet with high protein and high fat intake. More specifically, carbohydrate intake is limited to 20 g/day during the first 2 weeks, whereas it is later gradually increased by 5 g/week until the weight loss goal is achieved. This "carbohydrate daily equilibrium" may range between 25 and 90 g of carbohydrates. In obese patients, weight loss appears to be more significant with the Atkins diet than with other diets in the short term, but not in the long term (McAuley et al., 2005). The long-term effects of this type of diet remain debated, especially in terms of CHD risk and possible effects on renal function. The possible increase in LDL, the high SFA intake, which may induce insulin resistance, and the low intake of fiber associated with the Atkins diet make this option not optimal for NAFLD.

9.3.2.4 Zone Diet

In the Zone diet, the proportion at each meal of carbohydrates, fats, and proteins are to be kept constant at 40%, 30%, and 30%, respectively, within three small meals and two intermediate snacks. The diet also emphasizes the daily supplementation with 4 g/day of fish oil. The Zone diet may be an option for reducing weight, insulin resistance, and the risk for CHD in some patients with NAFLD, but more evidence is awaited.

9.3.2.5 South Beach Diet

The South Beach diet is based on low-GI and MUFA-rich foods in three meals and two snacks in between per day. In the first phase, there is a very low intake of carbohydrates, which are replaced at each meal by meat, fish, eggs, shellfish, vegetables, cheese, nuts, and salad vegetables. In the second phase, carbohydrates are gradually reintroduced by adding one low-GI, high-fiber serving to one meal per week. The third phase is a maintenance phase. Although some characteristics of this diet may be attractive to patients with NAFLD, the high intake of fat (from 40% to 60%) should not be overlooked and no conclusive data are available.

9.3.2.6 Weight Watchers Diet

The Weight Watchers diet promotes a reduced intake of calories within an intensive support community, which constitutes its main advantage and the basis of the high success rates. The critical role of this support strategy is supported by the poor adherence to the diet in the long term.

9.3.3 DIETARY SUPPLEMENTS IN THE MANAGEMENT AND TREATMENT OF NAFLD AND NASH

The beneficial effects of nutritional supplements have been suggested by several studies using the reduction of blood lipids and/or the antioxidant effects as main endpoints. The majority of available data were obtained from observational studies or animal models, whereas few attempts have been made to prospectively study adequate patient populations with appropriate controls. In the case of NAFLD and NASH, moreover, the need for histology to define cases makes a therapeutic approach less feasible. We have some degree of evidence for multiple dietary supplements based on different mechanisms of action (as illustrated in Figure 9.3). Data are debated for probiotics (Lirussi et al., 2007), which possibly exert an anti-inflammatory effect on TNF-mediated mechanisms, although only in animal models (Li et al., 2003). Similarly, sesame oil leads to a significant reduction in the lipid

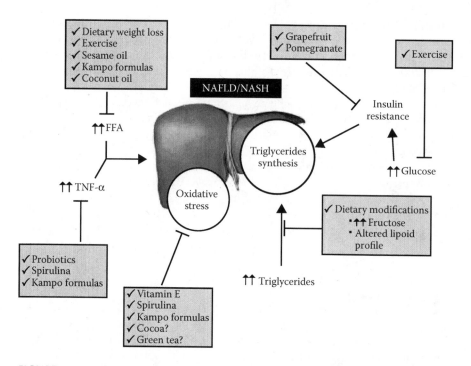

FIGURE 9.3 Sites of action for proposed supplements and alternative treatments in NAFLD and NASH. As illustrated in the text, we note that the vast majority of data are obtained from animal models or in vitro experiments, while solid data from human studies are awaited.

and glucose alterations of experimental diabetes, whereas coconut water signifi-cantly reduces steatosis in the liver in a model of metabolic syndrome (Sandhya and Rajamohan, 2006). The impact of coconut components was also observed in a small human study in which 25% coconut flakes led to an 11% reduction of plasma total cholesterol levels in 14 weeks of supplementation (Trinidad et al., 2004). Additional studies on human subjects have suggested that spirulina (Samuels et al., 2002) and grapefruit (Fujioka et al., 2006) or pomegranate (Esmaillzadeh et al., 2004) juices may be helpful in the management of metabolic syndrome. The use of spirulina is of particular interest based on the multiple pathways influenced by of this supple-ment and the growing amount of data supporting its beneficial effects in chronic inflammation or oxidative stress, both encountered in NASH. Vitamin E is the only supplement that has been widely investigated in multiple human and experimen-tal studies, yet no agreement on its efficacy has been reached. One randomized, placebo-controlled trial of vitamin E supplementation demonstrated a significant amelioration in terms of histological liver inflammation and fibrosis in patients with NASH (Harrison et al., 2003), whereas previous smaller studies with biochemical endpoints failed to demonstrate any benefits (Kugelmas et al., 2003). Most recently, traditional herbal compounds or Kampo formulas (Fujimoto et al., 2008) are gath-ering promising experimental data in animal models and should not be overlooked in future studies. Finally, there are no data on the impact of cocoa extracts or green tea on NAFLD. This is particularly surprising considering that cocoa (Selmi et al., 2006) and green tea (Wolfram et al., 2006) flavanols have been demonstrated to exert beneficial effects in several components of the metabolic syndrome and have important scavenging properties.

9.4   THE NAFLD PLANET IN THE METABOLIC SYNDROME GALAXY

"What is the best nutritional approach for the treatment of NAFLD and NASH" remains an elusive question. We may be convinced that the first logical approach would be to promote weight loss through diet and exercise. We should note that the total caloric intake must be appropriate to weight management goals. Individualization of the macronutrient composition will then depend on the metabolic status of the patient, taking into account all possible adverse events and available dietary regimens manifest variable degrees of effectiveness but are also burdened by potential adverse events in subjects with NAFLD. The media continuously propose original dietary approaches, and in some cases, these indeed reduce body weight. However, a study comparing the Atkins, Ornish, Weight Watchers, and Zone diets in overweight or obese patients with one or more risk factors for CHD demonstrated that each diet modestly reduced body weight and several risk factors at 1 year with low overall dietary adherence rates, particularly for the Atkins and Ornish diets, which the patients found to be too extreme (Dansinger et al., 2005). These data support that a sustained adherence to diet rather than the actual diet type is the major predictor of weight loss, and different dietary options may be combined considering both the preference of the patient and the cardiovascular risk profile. As an example, a growing body of research suggests that a low-carbohydrate diet and a low-fat diet may have significantly different effects on the cardiovascular risk, with low-carbohydrate diets increasing HDL cholesterol and low-fat diets decreasing LDL cholesterol concentrations. The ideal regimen for NAFLD has not been determined. Excess SFAs promote endoplasmic reticulum stress, hepatic steatosis, and inflammation in animal models. However, it remains uncertain if a minimum intake of SFA is required for optimal metabolism (Wang et al., 2006). A higher proportion of PUFAs in the diet in lieu of SFA has been advocated to promote significant cardiovascular benefits (Laaksonen et al., 2005), with the ratio of n-6 to n-3 fatty acids being important in predicting insulin resistance. An excessive amount of n-6 PUFA with a high n-6/n-3 ratio was observed in 45 patients with NASH compared to 856 controls (Cortez-Pinto et al., 2006). Furthermore, dietary fish oil may also be beneficial in NAFLD with improvement in serum triacylglycerol concentrations, fasting glucose, liver enzyme levels, and hepatic steatosis (Capanni et al., 2006). Dietary TFA should be avoided, since the intake of hydrogenated fats increases inflammatory markers and the LDL/HDL ratio (Mozaffarian, 2006). The increased intake of sucrose and fructose also plays a negative role in the development of NAFLD based on human studies and population-based epidemiological data. On the other hand, the scenario of dietary supplements in NAFLD remains quite elusive and should be the focus of rigorous research efforts in the future, based on the capillary diffusion of some popular supplements and their likelihood to be ineffective or to overcome the need for weight loss.

9.5   SUMMARY POINTS

1. NAFLD is rapidly becoming the main cause of chronic liver disease throughout the world, and in an undetermined proportion of cases, NAFLD has steatohepatitis features (NASH) and progresses to liver cirrhosis.
2. NASH is expected to become the leading etiology of liver cirrhosis requiring transplantation in the next decade.
3. NAFLD belongs to the corollarium of conditions characterizing the metabolic syndrome and recognizes insulin resistance as the *primum movens*.
4. The majority of nutritional studies and guidelines have been dedicated to obesity and insulin resistance without accounting for changes in fatty liver disease.
5. Available data seem to support the beneficial impact of such guidelines and weight loss also on NAFLD, but the ideal regimen for NAFLD has not been determined.
6. Individualization of the macronutrient composition should depend on the metabolic status of the patient, taking into account all possible adverse events and available dietary regimens manifest variable degrees of effectiveness but are also burdened by potential adverse events in subjects with NAFLD.
7. The efficacy of dietary supplements in NAFLD remains under debate and should be the focus of rigorous research efforts in the future. As an example, dietary fish oil seems beneficial in NAFLD.

REFERENCES

Anderson, J. W., K. M. Randles, C. W. Kendall, and D. J. Jenkins. 2004. Carbohydrate and fiber recommendations for individuals with diabetes: A quantitative assessment and meta-analysis of the evidence. *J Am Coll Nutr* 23:5–17.
Bantle, J. P., J. Wylie-Rosett, A. L. Albright, et al. 2008. Nutrition recommendations and interventions for diabetes: A position statement of the American Diabetes Association. *Diabetes Care* 31 Suppl 1:S61–S78.
Bergheim, I., S. Weber, M. Vos, et al. 2008. Antibiotics protect against fructose-induced hepatic lipid accumulation in mice: Role of endotoxin. *J Hepatol* 48:983–992.
Browning, J. D., L. S. Szczepaniak, R. Dobbins, et al. 2004. Prevalence of hepatic steatosis in an urban population in the United States: Impact of ethnicity. *Hepatology* 40:1387–1395.
Capanni, M., F. Calella, M. R. Biagini, et al. 2006. Prolonged n-3 polyunsaturated fatty acid supplementation ameliorates hepatic steatosis in patients with non-alcoholic fatty liver disease: A pilot study. *Aliment Pharmacol Ther* 23:1143–1151.
Cortez-Pinto, H., L. Jesus, H. Barros, et al. 2006. How different is the dietary pattern in non-alcoholic steatohepatitis patients? *Clin Nutr* 25:816–823.
Dansinger, M. L., J. A. Gleason, J. L. Griffith, H. P. Selker, and E. J. Schaefer. 2005. Comparison of the Atkins, Ornish, Weight Watchers and Zone diets for weight loss and heart disease risk reduction: A randomized trial. *JAMA* 293:43–53.
Day, C. P., and O. F. James. 1998. Steatohepatitis: A tale of two "hits"? *Gastroenterology* 114:842–845.

Diehl, A. M. 2004. Tumor necrosis factor and its potential role in insulin resistance and non-alcoholic fatty liver disease. *Clin Liver Dis* 8:619–638, x.

Esmaillzadeh, A., F. Tahbaz, I. Gaieni, H. Alavi-Majd, and L. Azadbakht. 2004. Concentrated pomegranate juice improves lipid profiles in diabetic patients with hyperlipidemia. *J Med Food* 7:305–308.

Esposito, K., R. Marfella, M. Ciotola, et al. 2004. Effect of a Mediterranean-style diet on endothelial dysfunction and markers of vascular inflammation in the metabolic syndrome: A randomized trial. *JAMA* 292:1440–1446.

Fujimoto, M., K. Tsuneyama, M. Kainuma, et al. 2008. Evidence-based efficacy of Kampo formulas in a model of nonalcoholic fatty liver. *Exp Biol Med (Maywood)* 233:328–337.

Fujioka, K., F. Greenway, J. Sheard, and Y. Ying. 2006. The effects of grapefruit on weight and insulin resistance: Relationship to the metabolic syndrome. *J Med Food* 9:49–54.

Harrison, S. A., S. Torgerson, P. Hayashi, J. Ward, and S. Schenker. 2003. Vitamin E and vitamin C treatment improves fibrosis in patients with nonalcoholic steatohepatitis. *Am J Gastroenterol* 98:2485–2490.

Kris-Etherton, P. M., T. A. Pearson, Y. Wan, et al. 1999. High-monounsaturated fatty acid diets lower both plasma cholesterol and triacylglycerol concentrations. *Am J Clin Nutr* 70:1009–1015.

Kugelmas, M., D. B. Hill, B. Vivian, L. Marsano, and C. J. McClain. 2003. Cytokines and NASH: A pilot study of the effects of lifestyle modification and vitamin E. *Hepatology* 38:413–419.

Laaksonen, D. E., K. Nyyssonen, L. Niskanen, T. H. Rissanen, and J. T. Salonen. 2005. Prediction of cardiovascular mortality in middle-aged men by dietary and serum linoleic and polyunsaturated fatty acids. *Arch Intern Med* 165:193–199.

Li, Z., S. Yang, H. Lin, et al. 2003. Probiotics and antibodies to TNF inhibit inflammatory activity and improve nonalcoholic fatty liver disease. *Hepatology* 37:343–350.

Lichtenstein, A. H. 2006. Thematic review series: Patient-oriented research. Dietary fat carbohydrate and protein: Effects on plasma lipoprotein patterns. *J Lipid Res* 47:1661–1667.

Lirussi, F., E. Mastropasqua, S. Orando, and R. Orlando. 2007. Probiotics for non-alcoholic fatty liver disease and/or steatohepatitis. *Cochrane Database Syst Rev* CD005165.

Marchesini, G., E. Bugianesi, G. Forlani, et al. 2003. Nonalcoholic fatty liver, steatohepatitis, and the metabolic syndrome. *Hepatology* 37:917–923.

McAuley, K. A., C. M. Hopkins, K. J. Smith, et al. 2005. Comparison of high-fat and high-protein diets with a high-carbohydrate diet in insulin-resistant obese women. *Diabetologia* 48:8–16.

Mozaffarian, D. 2006. *trans* Fatty acids—effects on systemic inflammation and endothelial function. *Atheroscler Suppl* 7:29–32.

Ornish, D., L. W. Scherwitz, J. H. Billings, et al. 1998. Intensive lifestyle changes for reversal of coronary heart disease. *JAMA* 280:2001–2007.

Porikos, K. P. and T. B. Van Itallie. 1983. Diet-induced changes in serum transaminase and triglyceride levels in healthy adult men. Role of sucrose and excess calories. *Am J Med* 75:624–630.

Ros, E., I. Nunez, A. Perez-Heras, et al. 2004. A walnut diet improves endothelial function in hypercholesterolemic subjects: A randomized crossover trial. *Circulation* 109:1609–1614.

Salen, G., S. Patel, and A. K. Batta. 2002. Sitosterolemia. *Cardiovasc Drug Rev* 20:255–270.

Samuels, R., U. V. Mani, U. M. Iyer, and U. S. Nayak. 2002. Hypocholesterolemic effect of spirulina in patients with hyperlipidemic nephrotic syndrome. *J Med Food* 5:91–96.

Sandhya, V. G., and T. Rajamohan. 2006. Beneficial effects of coconut water feeding on lipid metabolism in cholesterol-fed rats. *J Med Food* 9:400–407.

Schulze, M. B., J. E. Manson, D. S. Ludwig, et al. 2004. Sugar-sweetened beverages, weight gain, and incidence of type 2 diabetes in young and middle-aged women. *JAMA* 292:927–934.

Selmi, C., T. K. Mao, C. L. Keen, H. H. Schmitz, and M. Eric Gershwin. 2006. The anti-inflammatory properties of cocoa flavanols. *J Cardiovasc Pharmacol* 47 Suppl 2:S163–S171; discussion S172–S176.

Tapsell, L. C., L. J. Gillen, C. S. Patch, et al. 2004. Including walnuts in a low-fat/modified-fat diet improves HDL cholesterol-to-total cholesterol ratios in patients with type 2 diabetes. *Diabetes Care* 27:2777–2783.

Trichopoulou, A., T. Costacou, C. Bamia, and D. Trichopoulos. 2003. Adherence to a Mediterranean diet and survival in a Greek population. *N Engl J Med* 348:2599–2608.

Trinidad, T. P., A. S. Loyola, A. C. Mallillin, et al. 2004. The cholesterol-lowering effect of coconut flakes in humans with moderately raised serum cholesterol. *J Med Food* 7:136–140.

Wang, D., Y. Wei, and M. J. Pagliassotti. 2006. Saturated fatty acids promote endoplasmic reticulum stress and liver injury in rats with hepatic steatosis. *Endocrinology* 147:943–951.

Werner, A., R. Havinga, T. Bos, et al. 2005. Essential fatty acid deficiency in mice is associated with hepatic steatosis and secretion of large VLDL particles. *Am J Physiol Gastrointest Liver Physiol* 288:G1150–G1158.

Wolfram, S., Y. Wang, and F. Thielecke. 2006. Anti-obesity effects of green tea: From bedside to bench. *Mol Nutr Food Res* 50:176–187.

10 Dietary Fatty Acids and the Pathogenesis of Liver Disease in Alcoholism

Amin A. Nanji

CONTENTS

10.1 FATTY ACIDS: INTRODUCTION

The purpose of this review is to bring together information on the role of fatty acids in alcoholic liver disease (ALD). Quite apart from the effects of fatty acids on liver disease, fatty acids are important precursors of prostaglandins (PGs), leukotrienes (LTs), and hydroxyl fatty acids. There is considerable evidence that the amount of fat in the diet is a key determinant of lesions in ALD (Nanji, 2003). Furthermore, dietary lipids are a key source of lipids accumulating in livers of ethanol-fed animals (Nanji and French, 1986). Findings of initial studies on the Lieber-DeCarli model showed a steatogenic effect of dietary fat in ALD (Nanji, 2003). Results of studies on the intragastric feeding rat model revealed that when fat constituted 5% of calories, focal necrosis and steatosis were induced in the centrilobular areas of ethanol-fed rats. When experiments on intragastrically fed rats were conducted again with 25% and 35% of calories as fat, centrilobular fibrosis, resembling that seen in baboons and humans, developed in more than half of the rats (Nanji, 2003).

The role of different types of dietary fat in ALD is supported by epidemiological correlations indicating that the susceptibility to alcohol is related to different types of fatty acids in the diet (Nanji and French, 1986). In one study, deviation from expected mortality from cirrhosis was correlated with intake of saturated and unsaturated fatty acids (Nanji, 2004). The findings supported the notion that saturated fatty acids (SFAs) were protective against ALD. In contrast, unsaturated fatty acids promoted ALD. As a follow-up to these epidemiological correlations, studies were carried out by using the intragastric feeding rat model for ALD. In rats fed ethanol and tallow (beef fat, SFAs), none of the features of ALD developed, minimal to moderate pathological changes occurred in animals fed ethanol and lard (2.5% linoleic acid), and the most severe changes were seen in rats fed ethanol with corn oil (55–60% linoleic acid). The importance of polyunsaturated fatty acids (PUFAs), rather than linoleic acid alone, has also been evaluated in rats fed fish oil. Compared with findings for rats fed corn oil with ethanol, more severe liver injury, particularly necrosis and inflammation, is seen in rats fed fish oil with ethanol (Nanji, 2004).

10.2 EFFECT OF FATTY ACIDS ON PATHOLOGICAL AND PATHOPHYSIOLOGICAL CHANGES IN ETHANOL-FED RATS

10.2.1 ARACHIDONIC ACID AND EICOSANOIDS

The key link between fatty acids and inflammation is the eicosanoid family of inflammatory mediators generated from 20 carbon PUFAs liberated from cell membrane phospholipids. The membrane phospholipids of inflammatory cells taken from humans consuming Western-type diets typically contain approximately 20% of fatty acids as the n-6 PUFA arachidonic acid (AA). In contrast, the proportions of 20 other carbon PUFAs, such as n-6 PUFA di-homo-y-linolenic acid and n-3 PUFA eicosa-pentaenoic acid (EPA), are typically about 2%. Thus, AA is usually the dominant substrate for eicosanoid synthesis. Eicosanoids include PGs, thromboxanes, LTs, and hydroxyeicosatetraenoic acids (HETEs). AA in cell membrane phospholipids can be mobilized by various phospolipase enzymes, most notably phospholipase A1, and the free acid can subsequently act as a substrate for the enzymes that synthesize eicosanoids.

Under inflammatory conditions, increased production rates of AA-derived eico-sanoids are noted and elevated levels of these eicosanoids are observed in blood and tissues of patients with acute and chronic inflammatory conditions.

10.2.2 PROTECTIVE EFFECTS OF SFA IN ALD: ROLE OF ADIPONECTIN

Adiponectin may be one link between the consumption of SFAs and protection against alcoholic liver injury (You et al., 2005). As mentioned above, diets enriched in SFAs or medium-chain triglycerides (MCTs) protect against alcoholic liver injury.

Protection against alcoholic liver injury, particularly steatosis, may be due to increased levels of adipose-derived adiponectin (You et al., 2005).

Chronic ethanol intake is associated with inhibition of AMP-activated kinase (AMPK) and peroxisome proliferators activated receptor α (PPAR-α). Both mol-ecules are key regulatory factors in fatty acid oxidation. Comparing results obtained in mice fed ethanol with PUFAs versus SFAs, the study demonstrated that ethanol with SFAs, but not PUFAs, led to AMPK phosphorylation. AMPK is a key "meta-bolic switch" controlling lipid metabolism, and its activation by adiponectin leads to increased hepatic fatty acid oxidation and reduced lipid accumulation in liver (Anania, 2005).

10.2.3 ROLE OF SIRTUIN 1

Accumulation of fat in the liver is a crucial initial step in ALD. Evidence has accu-mulated that chronic ethanol administration increases levels of nuclear hepatic levels of sterol regulatory element–binding protein 1 (SREBP-1) and its targeted transcripts, which include acetyl-CoA carboxylase, fatty acid synthase, stearoyl-CoA desatu-rase 1, ATP citrate lyase, and mitochondrial glycerol 3-phosphate acyltransferase. Activation of these transcripts increases fatty acid synthesis and accumulation of tri-glycerides in liver. Post-transcriptional modification of SREBP-1 by reversible acyla-tion regulates proteosome-mediated degradation of SREBP-1. An additional regulator of liver lipid storage is sirtuin 1 (SIRT-1), a nicotinamide adenine dinucleotide-dependent histone deaclyase that regulates the activity of several transcription fac-tors including SREBP-1 (You et al., 2008). The regulation of SIRT-1 by SFAs may be important in regulating lipogenic enzymes.

10.2.4 MITOCHONDRIA

Mitochondria are emerging as the key target of ethanol toxicity, and mitochon-drial dysfunction is considered the major event in the pathogenesis of liver injury secondary to chronic alcohol consumption. Cytochrome P450 2 E1 (CYP2E1) is also localized in these organelles, and its induction after a variety of endogenous or exogenous molecules is responsible for the excessive local generation of reactive oxygen species (ROS) and associated lipid peroxidation damaging important components of the respiratory chain and mitochondrial DNA. Possible attenuation of these alcohol-induced injuries through diet manipulation has been proposed. Replacement of long-chain triglycerides (LCT; 42% of total dietary calories) with MCTs attenuates hepatic steatosis in alcohol-fed rats (Lieber et al., 2007). One reason for this difference is the propensity of MCTs for oxidation rather than esterification, whereas the converse is true for LCT. Recently, MCTs have been shown to play a beneficial role in experimental nonalcoholic fatty liver disease in the absence of dietary LCTs.

One mechanism for the beneficial effect of MCT possibly results from their rapid absorption and transport into the mitochondrial membrane with prevention of the alcohol-induced block of fatty acid β oxidation and associated lipid peroxidations.

There was an almost complete elimination of alcohol-induced liver pathology, including marked reduction of steatosis, as the saturated fat fraction of total dietary fat increased from 0% to 30% (Ronis et al., 2004). However, this study showed that the protective effects of saturated fat on the development of ALD was dose responsive and occurred even when substantial concentrations of unsaturated fat remain in the diet. The reduction in liver pathology was accompanied by significant reductions in indexes of oxidative stress, such as the glutathione/glutathione disulfide ratio and markers of lipid peroxidation (thiobarbituric acid reactive substances). However, there were no changes in induction of CYP2E1, because neither CYP2E1 apoprotein expression nor a direct measure of CYP2E1-dependent activity (p-nitrophenol hydroxylation) differed in any of the ethanol-treated groups.

10.3 EFFECT OF FATTY ACIDS ON ENDOTOXIN LEVELS AND ENDOTOXIN SIGNALING

10.3.1 Effect of Dietary Fatty Acids on Endotoxin-Mediated Signaling Pathways, Nuclear Factor κB, and Cytokines in Experimental ALD

Endotoxins are lipopolysaccharide components of the outer wall of most gram-negative bacteria. Considerable evidence supports the hypothesis that endotoxins are involved in alcohol-dependent liver injury. Endotoxin levels are within normal limits in rats fed SFAs and ethanol intragastrically. In rats fed corn oil and fish oil with ethanol, endotoxin levels begin to increase within 2 weeks of ethanol administration and increase sixfold by 9 weeks (Nanji et al., 1993). The mechanism (or mechanisms) by which ethanol causes endotoxemia is unknown, but it is probably related to increased mucosal permeability of the colon and reduction in the capacity of Kupffer cells to detoxify endotoxin (Purohit et al., 2008). Further support for the hypothesis that endotoxin is a contributory factor to alcoholic liver injury is derived from studies in which gut sterilization, with either lactobacilli or broad-spectrum antibiotics, leads to a marked decrease in endotoxin levels and absence of pathological changes in the liver (Nanji et al., 1994). Multiple mammalian receptors for endotoxins have been identified. Of these receptors, two glycoproteins are implicated in the interaction between endotoxin and macrophages. These two glycoproteins, lipopolysaccharide-binding protein (LBP) and membrane-bound CD 14 (mCD14), were evaluated in rats fed ethanol and different dietary fatty acids. The highest levels of mCD14 and LBP were found in rats exhibiting necrosis and inflammation. Expression of mCD14 was restricted to Kupffer cells, and LBP expression was restricted to hepatocytes (Su et al., 1998).

10.3.2 NUCLEAR FACTOR κB

Work has shown that both endotoxin and oxidative stress lead to the activation of nuclear factor κB (NF-κB), a ubiquitous transcription factor implicated in the activation of many genes, several of which are involved in alcoholic liver injury. Activation of NF-κB in experimental alcoholic liver injury is seen only in rats fed corn oil and fish oil, and these animals have increased levels of endotoxin and oxidative stress, as well as necroinflammatory changes on histological evaluation (Nanji et al., 1999). Activation of NF-κB in these animals occurs as a result of proteolytic degradation of inhibitor κB α. Several of the genes that show increased expression in association with activation of NF-κB also show increased expression in alcoholic liver injury. These genes include tumor necrosis factor α (TNF-α) interleukin 1α and chemokines. It is important to point out relevant findings showing that the increase in levels of oxidant stress and NF-κB activation precedes the development of pathological liver injury in intragastrically fed rats (Jokelainen et al., 2001). In addition, oxidant stress can directly injure liver cells by triggering apoptosis or predisposing them to TNF-induced apoptosis. It is likely that the major cell type in liver responsible for activation of NF-κB is the Kupffer cell, although contributions from endothelial cells and hepatic stellate cells (HSCs) cannot be ruled out. Although inhibition of NF-κB by reduction of oxidant stress is a potential therapeutic strategy, consideration should be given to the fact that NF-κB plays a protective role in hepatocyte survival.

10.3.3 TUMOR NECROSIS FACTOR

In ALD, several lines of evidence support the involvement of TNF-α. In the intragastric alcohol feeding model, liver injury was reduced in TNF-R1 knockout mice by neutralizing antibodies against TNF-α or antibiotic treatment to remove bacteria. TNF-α levels increase in a chronic alcohol feeding model in which gut permeability to bacterial-derived LPS is enhanced.

TNF-α is a proinflammatory cytokine that regulates cell proliferation, differentiation, and apoptosis and induces production of other cytokines and immune responses. TNF-α is mainly produced by macrophages and also by a broad variety of other tissues including lymphoid cells, mast cells, endothelial cells, fibroblasts, and neuronal tissues. Dysregulated TNF-α function is implicated in pathological processes of many diseases including ALD (Li and Lin, 2008). Like other signaling ligands, TNF-α exerts its cellular effect through two distinct surface receptors: 55 kDa receptor 1 (TNF-R1) and 75 kDa receptor (TNF-R2). TNF-R1 is ubiquitously expressed, whereas TNF-R2 is primarily found on cells of the immune system and is highly regulated.

10.4 EFFECT OF FATTY ACIDS ON NF-κB AND INFLAMMATORY SIGNALING PATHWAYS

10.4.1 CYCLOOXYGENASE 2

There are two major isoforms of cyclooxygenase: cyclooxygenase 1 (COX-1) and cyclooxygenase 2 (COX-2) (Shu and Klotz, 2008). They differ in several respects. COX-1 exists constitutively in several tissues and is responsible for normal physiologic functions, such as maintenance of gastric mucosal function and regulation of renal blood flow. In contrast, COX-2, which is not detected in most normal tissues, is induced by lipid peroxidation and inflammatory stimuli, such as cytokines and endotoxins, all of which are important contributors to alcohol-induced liver injury. Moreover, compared with control mice, COX-2–deficient (COX-2$^{-/-}$) mice are less sensitive to endotoxin-mediated liver injury. These observations, taken together with the known proinflammatory effects of the products of COX-2–catalyzed reactions, have led to a proposal that induction of COX-2 is an important final common pathway for mediation of alcohol-induced liver injury (Nanji, 2004). Of the inflammatory mediators that induce COX-2, endotoxin and TNF-α are most relevant to alcoholic liver injury. Reactive oxygen intermediates and lipid hydroperoxides also regulate the expression of COX-2. Also of note is that oxidant tone regulates the response of COX-2 to endotoxin. Compared with COX-1, initiation of COX-2 activity requires considerably lower levels of hydroperoxides. In intragastrically fed rats, increased levels of COX-2 are seen in rats fed ethanol with corn oil and fish oil, which indicate evidence of pathological liver injury, as well as increased levels of TNF-α, endotoxin, and lipid peroxides. It is interesting that TNF-α and COX-2 are coexpressed in the Kupffer cells of ethanol-fed rats with evidence of necroinflammatory changes. Decreased expression of COX-1 is also seen in Kupffer cells of ethanol-fed rats exhibiting necroinflammatory changes. This lower degree of activity can account for the decreased production of prostacylin and prostaglandin E_2 (PGE2) in rats exhibiting pathological liver injury (Nanji et al., 1994).

10.4.2 LONG-CHAIN N-3 PUFAS AND EICOSANOID PRODUCTION

Increased consumption of long-chain n-3 PUFAs, EPA, and docosahexaenoic acid (DHA) results in increased proportions of those fatty acids in inflammatory cell membrane phospholipids, partly at the expense of AA. Thus, because there is less substrate available for synthesis of eicosanoids from AA, fish oil supplementation of the human diet has been shown to result in decreased production of PGE_2, TXB_2, LTB_4, 5-HETE, and LTE_4 by inflammatory cells. EPA also acts as a substrate for COX and lipoxygenase (LOX) enzymes, thus giving rise to a different family of eicosanoids: the 3-series PGs and thromboxane (TXs) and the 5-series LTs and hydroxyeicosapentaenoic acids. Thus, the reason for the increased severity of ALD in fish oil ethanol-fed rats is intriguing (Pawlosky and Salem, 2004).

In addition to long-chain n-3 PUFAs modulating the generation of eicosanoids from AA and to EPA acting as substrate for the generation of alternative eicosanoids, recent studies have identified a novel group of mediators, called E-series resolvins, formed from EPA by COX-2/LOX that appear to exert anti-inflammatory actions. In addition, DHA-derived mediators termed D-series resolvins, docosatrienes, and neuroprotectins, also produced by COX-2/LOX under some conditions, have been identified, and these too appear to be anti-inflammatory and inflammation-resolving.

10.5 EFFECT OF FATTY ACIDS ON OXIDATIVE AND NITROSATIVE STRESS

A significant body of evidence supports a role for reactive oxygen intermediates in alcohol-induced liver injury (Day and Cederbaum, 2006). The main oxidant sources are cytochrome P4502E1 and iron. Levels of antioxidant enzymes and antioxidants such as glutathione are decreased in the livers of alcohol-fed animals.

The oxidation of n-3 PUFAs in the endoplasmic reticulum involves the initial formation of ω-hydroxy or (ω-1)-hydroxy fatty acids catalyzed by microsomal cytochrome P450 (CYP4A1 and CYP2E1). Dicarboxylic fatty acids, derived from ω-hydroxy and (ω-1)-hydroxy fatty acids, are increased in states of impaired mitochondrial fatty acid β oxidation. Microsomal ω hydroxylation via CYP2E1 and CYP4A1 is increased in alcohol-fed rats. Evidence in the literature suggests that fatty acids and their ω oxidation products activate PPARs. PPARs are actively involved in regulating genes involved in fatty acid metabolism, such as enzymes of the extramitochondrial fatty acid oxidation pathways (e.g., peroxysomal fatty acyl CoA oxidase, CYP4A1, liver fatty acid–binding protein). The induction of hepatic extramitochondrial pathways of fatty acid oxidation by means of PPAR-α serves to provide the liver cell with alternative means for the catabolism of fatty acids under conditions of markedly increased fatty acids flux and fatty acid overload. PPAR-α appears to act as a cellular transducer that senses the presence of fatty acid overload states and directs the appropriate adaptive hepatocellular gene response.

Alcohol is one of the many known causes of impaired mitochondrial long-chain fatty acid oxidation, resulting in fatty acid overload, by which fatty acids accumulating in the cell are diverted into esterification (triglyceride synthesis) and extramitochondrial fatty acid oxidation (Bailey and Cunningham, 2002). The latter involves ω-1 oxidation by CYP2E1 and CYP3A4 in the endoplasmic reticulum and β oxidation in the peroxisomes. The fatty acid overload hypothesis indicates a role for PUFAs in the hepatotoxic sequelae associated with alcohol, that is, impaired fatty oxidation.

Whereas many studies have been carried out with n-6 series PUFAs, less is known about the role of n-3 series PUFAs in the development of ALD.

The intragastric infusion model of ethanol feeding is associated with the induction of high levels of CYP2E1 and greatly increased lipid peroxidation, which appear to contribute to the liver injury. AA induces toxicity in HepG2 E47 cells, a cell line that expresses CYP2E1, but not control, HepG2 cells, which do not express CYP2E1. AA also induces toxicity in pyrazole-induced rat heptatocytes with high levels of CYP2E1 but not in saline control hepatocytes. This CYP2E1-dependent AA toxicity is prevented by inhibitors of CYP2E1 and antioxidants.

A key feature of liver fibrosis is the increase in collagen I protein. Collagen is a heterotrimeric protein composed of two $\alpha1$ chains and one $\alpha2$ chain encoded by collagen 1A (*COL1A1*) and *COL1A2* genes. Both *COL1A1* and *COL1A2* genes are highly sensitive to ROS and acetaldehyde, a product from alcohol metabolism. It has been reported that the *COL1A2* promoter contains at least two putative NF-κB binding sites. Oxidant stress is a major factor inducing NF-κB. In view of the potential link between oxidative stress and the activation of the *COL1A1* and *COL1A2* genes in HSCs, it was speculated that feeding fish oil plus alcohol can lead to the activation of collagen 1 and subsequent fibrosis (Nieto, 2007).

The intragastric feeding rat model for ALD was used to assess the relation among pathological liver injury, oxidant stress, and levels of hepatic antioxidant enzymes. Male Wistar rats were fed ethanol with MCTs, palm oil, corn oil, or fish oil. Control animals were fed isocaloric amounts of dextrose. Activity and protein concentrations were evaluated by using immunoblot analysis in each group for manganese-SOD, copper-zinc SOD, catalase, and glutathione peroxidase. Among ethanol-fed rats, fish oil showed the most severe pathological changes and the highest levels of lipid peroxidation; rats fed corn oil showed less severe pathological changes and lower levels of lipid peroxidation compared to fish oil–fed rats. Palm oil–fed rats showed fatty liver only, and rats fed MCTs had normal livers. Levels of lipid peroxidation correlated closely in groups with severity of pathological changes in the liver. Among the antioxidant enzymes, the lowest levels of catalase, glutathione peroxidase, and copper-zinc SOD were seen in fish oil–fed rats. An inverse correlation was observed among the severity of pathological changes (especially necrosis and inflammation), lipid peroxidation, and the antioxidant enzyme levels and activity (Polavarapu et al., 1998).

10.5.1 Nitric Oxide

Nitric oxide (NO) has earned the reputation of being a signaling mediator with many diverse and often opposing biological activities. The diversity in response to this simple diatomic molecule comes from the enormous variety of chemical reactions and biological properties associated with it. In the past few years, the importance of steady-state NO concentration has emerged as a key determinant of its biological function. Precise cellular responses are differentially regulated by a specific NO concentration. In general, lower NO concentrations promote cell survival and proliferation, whereas higher levels favor cell cycle arrest and apoptosis. Free radical interactions also influence NO signaling. The resulting reactive nitrogen species generated from these reactions can also have biological effects and increase oxidative and nitrosative stress responses (Thomas et al., 2008).

NO is thought to play a pivotal role in the development of various types of liver disease. Despite extensive evidence that NO has critical roles in various processes in liver disease, it remains controversial whether NO is protective or injurious.

10.5.2 Nitrotyrosine

10.5.2.1 Tyrosine Nitration Yields and Relationship with Disease

Low levels of free and protein-bound 3-nitrotyrosine (3-NT) are normally detected and reflect the low steady state of oxidizing and nitrating species produced under basal conditions. In disease states associated with nitroxidative stress, there is a significant increase of 3-NT (Thomas et al., 2008).

In livers of animals and patients with ALD, increased expression of COX-2, inducible nitric oxide synthase (iNOS), and nitrotyrosine are observed. Nitric oxide synthase (NOS) catalyzes the conversion of L-arginine to NO, whereas COX-2 uses AA as substrate-forming vasoactive metabolites such as thromboxane and prostacyclin via specific synthases. The involvement of NOS and COX in altering vascular function has been implicated in conditions characterized by oxidative stress. Peroxynitrate-induced nuclear translocation of NF-κB leads to increased expression of iNOS and COX-2. Peroxinitrate formed by iNOS induction also reduces protacyclin synthase activity by increasing the proteolytic degradation of protacyclin synthase protein.

10.5.3 ROLE OF ISOPROSTANES IN LIVER ENDOTHELIAL DYSFUNCTION

F_2 isoprostanes are PG isomers derived from free radical–catalyzed peroxidation of AA. As products of lipid peroxidation, they are considered reliable markers of enhanced systemic oxidative stress *in vivo*.

Potential mechanisms for the hepatic dysfunction may be a direct vasoconstrictive effect of isoprostanes. Isoprostanes have been shown to enhance vasoconstriction *in vitro* and *in vivo*. The potential role of isoprostanes as participants in alcohol liver disease is further supported by their presence in human and experimental alcohol liver disease.

The measurement of F_2 isoprostanes is considered a reliable method in assessing lipid peroxidation and oxidative stress *in vivo*. Both systemic and urinary isoprostane levels may represent total lipid peroxidation, but not necessarily local isoprostanes production, because of the large variability between peripheral and local levels of isoprostanes in different organs.

10.6 EFFECT OF FATTY ACIDS ON THE PROTEOSOME AND PROTEIN TRAFFICKING

10.6.1 PROTEASOME: INTRACELLULAR PROTEOLYSIS

Protein turnover, defined here as the breakdown and replenishment of cellular proteins, is a continuous process. Although eukaryotic cells have three prominent protein catabolic pathways (lysosomes, calpains, and the proteasome), an estimated 75–90% of intracellular proteins are degraded by the proteasome. This enzyme and its protein marker, ubiquitin protein that is covalently attached to protein substrates, were at first largely unrecognized until it became apparent that the ubiquitin-proteasome pathway is involved in all the aforementioned cellular processes.

10.6.2 ETHANOL CONSUMPTION AND THE UBIQUITIN-PROTEASOME SYSTEM

In ethanol-fed experimental animals, the intracellular level of ubiquitin (representing both the free and conjugated forms) is elevated in hepatoytces of rats orally administered with ethanol. However, oral ethanol feeding has variable effects on the peptidase activities of the proteasome. When high blood ethanol levels are achieved, proteasome activity is significantly inhibited. In fact, both published and unpublished data from a number of oral feeding studies with rats and mice have indicated an inverse correlation between serum ethanol levels and hepatic proteasome chymotrypsin-like activity, indicating that hepatic proteasome activity is inhibited by high blood ethanol levels. Conversely, slight elevations in proteasome activity after oral ethanol feeding have been reported in animals with low to moderate serum ethanol levels (i.e., 25–40 mM). The latter results indicate that milder forms of oxidative stress actually activate the proteasome, and related work reported elsewhere supports this notion. In contrast to oral ethanol feeding, when ethanol is administered to animals via continuous intragastric feeding, it produces higher blood ethanol levels (i.e., $\geq$ 40 mM or 186 mg/dL), markedly more liver damage than after oral feeding, and a 35–40% reduction of the proteasome activity (Radi, 2004).

Furthermore, other studies with livers of intragastrically fed rats have shown that serum ethanol concentration alone is not sufficient to bring about a decline in proteasome activity. The level of oxidative stress derived from consumption of PUFAs combined with ethanol causes a significant decline in proteasome activity, whereas diets containing ethanol and SFAs do not. Rats given ethanol and MCT exhibited no significant liver pathology, whereas cumulative pathology scores in ethanol-fed rats given palm oil, corn oil, or fish oil were 2.5, 5.4, and 7.0, respectively, indicating that ethanol and fish oil caused the greatest liver damage. The severity of liver pathology in the last three groups of animals correlated with levels of lipid peroxides and serum F isoprostanes. Alpha smooth muscle actin, an indicator of stellate cell activation, was increased relative to controls in the livers of all ethanol-fed rats. In livers of corn oil and fish oil ethanol-fed rats, proteasome chymotrypsin-like activity was decreased by 55–60%, but there was no quantitative alteration in 20S proteasome subunit content. In contrast, ethanol affected neither proteasome activity nor its content in MCT- and palm oil–treated animals.

10.6.3   CYP2E1-PROTEASOME INTERACTIONS

The proteasome complex plays a major role in CYP2E1 turnover and therefore in regulation of CYP2E1 levels in liver cells. Ethanol and other low molecular weight ligands prevent proteasome-mediated CYP2E1 turnover. This is a major mechanism by which ethanol "induces" CYP2E1. Lowering of proteasome activity potentiates CYP2E1-dependent toxicity. This is associated with accumulation of oxidized and nitrated protein adducts and increases in CYP2E1 levels. During CYP2E1-dependent oxidant stress, there is an increase in ubiquitylated protein levels and protein aggregates. This is associated with a decline in proteasome trypsinlike proteolytic activity. The proteasome itself becomes oxidized and is a target of CYP2E1-generated oxidant stress. These CYP2E1-proteasome interactions may play a role in the decline in proteasome activity, the formation of oxidized protein adducts, and the accumulation of protein after chronic ethanol treatment. These interactions may also be important in CYP2E1-catalyzed toxicity of hepatotoxins and procarcinogens.

10.6.4 RECEPTOR-MEDIATED ENDOCYTOSIS MEDIATED BY THE ASIALOGLYCOPROTEIN RECEPTOR AND A ROLE FOR THIS RECEPTOR DURING ALCOHOLIC LIVER INJURY

The asialoglycoprotein receptor (ASGP-R) is a hepatocyte-specific receptor responsible for the uptake of serum glycoproteins with terminal galactosyl/N-acetylgalactosamine residues. Potential physiological roles for the ASGP-R include general glycoprotein clearance, immunoglobulin (Ig)A uptake, clearance of antigen-antibody complexes, cell adhesion, clearance of apoptotic bodies, and clearance of related molecules such as desialylated forms of apoptotic bodies. ASGP-R–mediated uptake of apoptotic cells is altered after ethanol administration (Casey et al., 2007). Consequences of the altered ASGP-R clearance of apoptotic cells include the activation of other cells through the interaction of accumulating apoptotic bodies with specific cell receptors. This activation process then stimulates the release of proinflammatory and profibrogenic substances providing enhanced signaling and the production of molecular factors that could be involved in the promotion of adverse liver pathology.

REFERENCES

Anania, F. A. 2005. Adiponectin and alcoholic fatty liver: Is it, after all, what you eat? *Hepatology* 42:530–532.

Bailey, S. M., and C. C. Cunningham. 2002. Contribution of mitochondria to oxidative stress associated with alcoholic liver disease. *Free Radic Biol Med* 32:11–16.

Casey, C. A., S. M. L. Lee, R. Aziz-Sieble, and B. L. McVicker. 2007. Impaired receptor-mediated endocytosis: Its role in alcohol-induced apoptosis. *J Gastroenterol Hepatol* 23 Suppl 1:S46–S49.

Day, A., and A. I. Cederbaum. 2006. Alcohol and oxidative liver injury. *Hepatology* S63–S74.

Jokelainen, K., L. A. Reinke, and A. A. Nanji. 2001. NF-kappaB activation is associated with free radical generation and endotoxemia and precedes pathological liver injury in experimental alcoholic liver disease. *Cytokine* 16:36–39.

Li, H., and X. Lin. 2008. Positive and negative signaling components involved in TNFα-induced NF-κB activation. *Cytokine* 41:1–8.

Lieber, C. S., Q. Cao, L. M. DeCarli, M. A. Leo, et al. 2007. Role of medium-chain triglycerides in the alcohol-mediated cytochrome P450 2E1 Induction of mitochondria. *Alcohol Clin Exp Res* 31:1660–1668.

Nanji, A. A. 2003. Alcoholic Liver Disease, in *Hepatology: A Textbook of Liver Disease*, ed. E. Zakim and T. Boyer. Philadelphia, PA: W. B. Saunders.

Nanji, A. A. 2004. Role of dietary fatty acids in the pathogenesis of experimental alcoholic liver disease. *Alcohol* 34:21–25.

Nanji, A. A., and S. W. French. 1986. Dietary factors and alcoholic cirrhosis. *Alcohol Clin Exp Res* 10:271–273.

Nanji, A. A., K. Jokelainen, A. Rahemtulla, et al. 1999. Activation of nuclear factor kappa B and cytokine imbalance in experimental alcoholic liver disease in the rat. *Hepatology* 30:934–943.

Nanji, A. A., U. Khettry, S. M. H. Sadrzadeh, and T. Yamanaka. 1993. Severity of liver injury in experimental alcoholic liver disease. Correlation with plasma endotoxin, prostaglandin E$_2$, leukotriene B$_4$ and thromboxane B$_2$. *Am J Pathol* 142:367–373.

Nanji, A. A., U. Khettry, and S. M. H. Sadrzadeh. 1994. Lactobacillus feeding reduces endotoxemia and severity of experimental alcoholic liver (disease). *Proc Soc Exp Biol Med* 205:243–247.

Nanji, A. A., S. Khwaja, and S. M. H. Sadrzadeh. 1994. Decreased prostacyclin production by liver non-parenchymal cells precedes liver injury in experimental alcoholic liver disease. *Life Sci* 54:455–461.

Nieto, N. 2007. Ethanol and fish oil induce NF-κB transactivation of the collagen α2(1) promoter through lipid peroxidation-driven activation of the PKC-P13K-Akt Pathway. *Hepatology* 45:1433–1445.

Pawlosky, R. J., and N. Salem Jr. 2004. Perspectives on alcohol consumption: Liver polyunsaturated fatty acids and essential fatty acid metabolism. *Alcohol* 34:27–33.

Polavarapu, R., D. R. Spitz, J. E. Sim, et al. 1998. Increased lipid peroxidation and impaired antioxidant enzyme function is associated with pathological liver injury in experimental alcoholic liver disease in rats fed diets high in corn oil and fish oil. *Hepatology* 27:1317–1323.

Purohit, V., J. C. Bode, C. Bode, et al. 2008. Alcohol, intestinal bacterial growth, intestinal permeability to endotoxin, and medical consequences: Summary of a symposium. *Alcohol* 42:349–361.

Radi, R. 2004. Nitric oxide, oxidants, and protein tyrosine nitration. *Proc Natl Acad Sci U S A* 101:4003–4008.

Ronis, M. J. J., S. Korourian, M. Zipperman, R. Hakkak, and T. M. Badger. 2004. Dietary saturated fat reduces alcoholic hepatoxicity in rats by altering fatty acid metabolism and membrane composition. *J Nutr* 134:904–912.

Shu, S., and U. Klotz. 2008. Clinical use and pharmacological properties of selective COX-2 inhibitors. *Eur J Clin Pharmacol* 64:233–252.

Su, G. L., A. Rahemtulla, P. Thomas, R. D. Klein, S. C. Wang, and A. A. Nanji. 1998. CD14 and lipopolysaccharide binding protein expression in a rat model of alcoholic liver disease. *Am J Pathol* 152:841–849.

Thomas, D. D., L. A. Ridnour, J. S. Isenberg, et al. 2008. The chemical biology of nitric oxide: Implications in cellular signaling. *Free Radic Biol Med* 45:18–31.

You, M., Q. Cao, X. Liang, J. M. Ajmo, and G. C. Ness. 2008. Mammalian sirtuin 1 is involved in the protective action of dietary saturated fat against alcoholic fatty liver in mice. *J Nutr* 138:497–501.

You, M., R. V. Considine, T. C. Leone, D. P. Kelly, and D. W. Crabb. 2005. Role of Adiponectin in the protective action of dietary saturated fats against alcoholic fatty liver in mice. *Hepatology* 42:568–577.

11 Long-Term Management of Alcoholic Liver Disease

*Zhanxiang Zhou, Zhenyuan Song,
Danielle Pigneri, Marion McClain,
Charles L. Mendenhall,
Luis S. Marsano, and Craig J. McClain*

CONTENTS

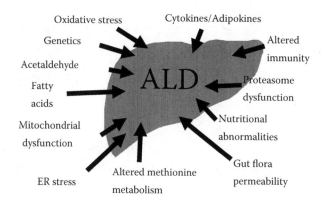

FIGURE 11.1 Mechanisms of liver injury. Nutritional abnormalities/deficiencies play a mechanistic role in the development of ALD, and interact with other mechanisms such as oxidative stress and cytokines.

11.1   INTRODUCTION

Malnutrition is common in most forms of cirrhosis including alcohol-induced cirrhosis. Moreover, virtually all patients with alcoholic hepatitis have some evidence of malnutrition. Patients may have global protein calorie malnutrition and/or isolated nutrient deficiencies, such as zinc deficiency. Nutritional deficiencies in alcoholic liver disease (ALD) may be caused by inadequate intake/anorexia, malabsorption, decreased nutrient storage, increased nutrient need, increased excretion, or decreased ability to metabolize nutrients into their active forms. Malnutrition may play a mechanistic role in the development of ALD, either directly or indirectly by modifying factors such as gut permeability, oxidative stress, or cytokine production (Figure 11.1). This chapter will review (1) two major nutritional abnormalities (alterations in zinc and methionine metabolism) of major research interest to our research group and of major importance in the pathogenesis and treatment of ALD; (2) selected other nutrient abnormalities; and (3) overall nutritional therapy in ALD. Because the role of lipids/fatty acids and iron is covered in other chapters, it will not be discussed here.

11.2   ZINC

11.2.1   Occurrence of Zinc Deficiency in ALD

Zinc deficiency is one of the most consistently observed nutritional/biochemical abnormalities in ALD. Decreases in serum zinc levels (hypozincemia) in patients with ALD are well documented. In a representative study, the serum zinc concentration in alcoholic patients was 7.52 μmol/L, which is significantly lower than 12.69 μmol/L in control subjects.[1] The decrease in serum zinc correlates with progression of liver damage. Patients with alcoholic cirrhosis showed a lower serum zinc level (80 μg/dL) than noncirrhotic patients (97 μg/dL), decreased by −37% and −24%, respectively, in comparison to normal subjects (127 μg/dL).[2] Furthermore, serum zinc levels in patients with hepatic encephalopathy were significantly lower than in cirrhotic patients without hepatic encephalopathy (0.54 vs. 0.96 mmol/L).[3] Zinc in the serum is mainly bound to albumin (83.7%) and macroglobulin (16.30%),[4] and a decrease in serum albumin in association with zinc decrease was also found in alcoholic patients.[5] Serum zinc also decreases with stress/inflammation, which regularly occurs in ALD.

11.2.2   Mechanisms for Altered Zinc Metabolism in ALD

A balance between intestinal absorption and urinary excretion has been suggested as a major mechanism underlying body zinc homeostasis.[6] To understand the mechanisms by which ethanol induces zinc deficiency, the effects of ethanol consumption on zinc metabolism have been investigated by measuring intestinal zinc absorption and urinary zinc excretion. Using a dual isotope absorption technique, the intestinal absorption rate of ^{65}Zn was 56% in normal subjects, whereas the intestinal ^{65}Zn absorption was 37% (a −34% decrease) in alcoholic patients.[7,8] On the other hand, an increase in urinary zinc excretion (hyperzincuria) has been well documented in alcoholic cirrhosis. In comparison to urinary zinc excretion of 734 µg/day in controls, urinary zinc excretion was 1777 µg/day in patients with alcoholic cirrhosis. Zinc intake is another factor affecting zinc homeostasis, with 90% of alcoholics having inadequate dietary zinc intake.[9] Therefore, multiple factors including inadequate zinc intake, impaired zinc absorption, and increased urinary zinc excretion have been implicated in the development of zinc deficiency in ALD.

To determine the link between ethanol consumption and zinc imbalance, prolonged ethanol administration was performed in five alcoholic subjects who were admitted to a metabolic ward for 34 days.[10] Ethanol was administered orally for 17 days, every 2 hours for 18 hours each day, to maintain a blood ethanol level of 100 mg/dL, followed by 17 days of abstinence. Urinary zinc excretion during the drinking period was nearly twice as high as that during the nondrinking period. With ethanol administration, the serum zinc level was decreased but normalized after ethanol was discontinued. This study clearly demonstrated a direct effect of ethanol on zinc metabolism, with a negative correlation between urinary and serum zinc levels.

11.2.3   Zinc Deficiency and Liver Function

Zinc is the second most abundant trace element in the body next to iron. Zinc is involved in all major aspects of cell functions such as metabolism, detoxification, antioxidant defenses, signal transduction, and gene regulation. Thus, zinc deficiency can cause physiological defects and, ultimately, cell injury. Manifestations of zinc deficiency include anorexia, skin lesions, growth retardation, neurosensory defects, and immune dysfunction in humans[11] (Table 11.1). Zinc deficiency has been documented in multiple types of liver diseases.[12] Experimental zinc deficiency increased the susceptibility to lipopolysaccharide (LPS)-induced liver injury.[13] In patients with ALD, hepatic zinc deficiency has been found to be correlated with liver dysfunction as indicated by decreased serum albumin, increased serum bilirubin, and decreased galactose elimination capacity and antipyrine clearance.[5,14,15]

TABLE 11.1

Selected Functional Consequences of Zinc Deficiency of Relevance to ALD

1. Skin lesions
2. Anorexia (with possible alterations in taste and smell acuity)
3. Growth retardation
4. Depressed wound healing
5. Hypogonadism
6. Altered immune function
7. Impaired night vision, altered vitamin A metabolism
8. Diarrhea
9. Depressed mental function
10. Susceptibility to alcohol-induced liver injury

Zinc participates in cell functions mainly by binding to thousands of zinc proteins including metalloenzymes. Zinc coordination has catalytic, structural, or regulatory roles in zinc proteins, and removal of zinc can exert deleterious effects on cell function.[16] Alcohol dehydrogenase is one of the major enzymes involved in ethanol metabolism. Alcohol dehydrogenase is a zinc-binding enzyme, and loss of zinc binding under conditions of oxidative and nitrosative stress resulted in the total loss of the activities of alcohol dehydrogenase.[17] In alcoholic patients, the activity of alcohol dehydrogenase has been found to be decreased in association with zinc deficiency in the liver.[18] One of the most important cellular antioxidants in the liver is Cu/Zn-SOD, a zinc-dependent enzyme. Measurements of Cu/Zn-SOD and Mn-SOD in hepatocytes from biopsies of patients with ALD demonstrated that the overall amount of Cu/Zn-SOD is significantly lower than in control biopsies, whereas no difference was found for Mn-SOD.[19] Hepatocyte apoptosis is a feature of alcoholic hepatitis, and active caspase 3 was significantly elevated in the livers of steatohepatitis patients.[20,21] In contrast to alcohol dehydrogenase and Cu/Zn-SOD, zinc release from caspase 3 will lead to enzymatic activation.[22] Thus, caspase 3 activation and apoptosis in the liver may be related to zinc deficiency.

The direct link between zinc status and zinc protein function has been determined in animals and cell culture studies. In a mouse model of ALD, chronic ethanol exposure caused a decrease in the protein level and DNA binding function of hepatocyte nuclear factor 4α (HNF-4α) association with hepatic zinc reduction.[23] A HepG2 cell culture study further demonstrated that zinc deprivation directly causes a decrease in DNA binding function of HNF-4α without affecting the protein level, indicating the requirement of zinc for proper zinc protein function. Dysfunction of HNF-4α induced by zinc deprivation resulted in repression of proteins involved in cell growth such as insulin-like growth factor 1 (IGF-1), insulin-like growth factor binding protein, and metallothionein (MT). Therefore, zinc mobilization from zinc proteins may be an important molecular mechanism by which zinc deficiency impairs liver function and contributes to the development of ALD.

11.2.4 ROLE OF MT IN ZINC HOMEOSTASIS AND ALD

Metallothioneins are low molecular weight, thiol-rich proteins.[24] MTs are composed of 61–68 amino acids with a highly conserved sequence of 20 cysteine residues. Under physiological conditions, MT primarily binds to zinc, and one MT molecule can bind up to seven zinc ions. There are four MT isoforms in mammals, MT-I– MT-IV; MT-I and MT-II are found in the liver. MT primarily serves as a cellular zinc reservoir, and zinc levels in the liver correlate with MT levels.[25] MT overexpression in the livers of MT transgenic mice is associated with a twofold increase in hepatic zinc concentration, whereas MT knockout (MT-KO) KO mice showed a decrease in hepatic zinc levels.[26,27] In a mouse model of ALD, the MT and zinc levels in the liver are not affected by acute ethanol exposure.[28] However, hepatic MT significantly decreased along with zinc decreases in the liver after chronic ethanol exposure.[29] MT depletion in the liver of an MT-KO mouse model intensified zinc deficiency and liver damage.[29] These studies indicate that a decrease in MT contributes to the disturbance in hepatic zinc homeostasis after chronic ethanol exposure.

MT also participates in intracellular zinc trafficking. MT locates in cytoplasm and nuclei, and translocation of MT from cytoplasm to nucleus has been demonstrated in the liver during times of high requirement for zinc.[30] In response to reactive oxygen species (ROS) exposure, induction of gene expression and nuclear translocation of MT has been detected in association with zinc trafficking from the cytoplasm into the nucleus.[31,32] *In vitro* studies with exogenous MT incubation have shown that MT can be imported into the membrane space of liver mitochondria and release zinc, which in turn inhibits respiration of coupled or uncoupled mitochondria.[33,34] However, hepatic MT concentration was decreased after chronic ethanol exposure in mice, although ROS accumulation were detected in the liver.[29] This may explain why alcoholic patients had lower zinc levels in both total zinc and subcellular fractions.

11.2.5 ZINC SUPPLEMENTATION IN ALD

The beneficial effects of zinc supplementation on the incidence or severity of diseases including ALD has received some attention from investigators. To assess the duration of zinc intake necessary to normalize serum and hepatic zinc concentrations, zinc supplementation in patients with ALD has been performed in a time-dependent manner.[35] Alcoholic patients without cirrhosis received zinc sulfate at 600 mg/day for 10 days and alcoholic patients with cirrhosis for 10, 30, and 60 days. Serum zinc concentrations were increased to normal values in all groups of patients during 10 days to 2 months of zinc supplementation. Zinc concentrations in the liver biopsies were significantly increased in patients with cirrhosis after zinc supplementation for 10 and 60 days, but some patients remained under normal values, particularly those with cirrhosis. No adverse reactions of zinc supplementation were observed in this study.

A long-term oral zinc supplementation (200 mg t.i.d. for 2–3 months) to cirrhotic patients including alcoholics produced beneficial effects on both liver metabolic function and nutritional parameters.[15] Quantitative liver function tests, including galactose elimination capacity and antipyrine clearance, demonstrated that oral zinc supplementation significantly improved liver metabolic function. Similarly, the Child-Pugh score, an overall estimation of hepatocellular failure, was improved by zinc supplementation on average by more than 1 point. Zinc supplementation also significantly improved nutritional parameters, including urinary excretion of creatinine, serum prealbumin, retinol-binding protein, and IGF-1. In particular, the serum IGF-1 was increased on average by 30% after zinc therapy. However, all nutritional parameters remained on average below the lower limit of the normal range. Glucose disappearance was improved by more than 30% in response to zinc therapy. There were no changes in pancreatic insulin secretion and systemic delivery or in the hepatic extraction of insulin. Insulin sensitivity, which was reduced by 80% before treatment, did not change. Glucose effectiveness was nearly halved in cirrhosis before treatment, and significantly increased after zinc therapy. The data suggest that zinc treatment in advanced cirrhosis improves glucose tolerance via an increasing the effects of glucose per se on glucose metabolism.

In a recent study, the effects of a zinc compound (polaprezinc) on liver fibrosis in patients with chronic liver disease, including ALD, were determined.[36] Patients received 34 mg zinc/day for 24 weeks. Oral polaprezinc supplementation increased serum zinc concentrations by 16.6% and 31.6% at 12 and 24 weeks, respectively. Serum type IV collagen levels, which reflect liver fibrosis, were decreased significantly at 24 weeks in comparison to baseline level in the patients showing increased serum zinc level after polaprezinc supplementation. The tissue inhibitors of metalloproteinase 1 (TIMP-1) levels were reduced significantly in these patients. However, no significant changes were detected in the levels of other enzyme markers of fibrogenesis and fibrolysis such as MMP-1, MMP-2, MMP-3, and TIMP-2. The results suggest that zinc may have an inhibitory effect on liver fibrosis through down-regulation of TIMP-1.

Several recent mechanistic studies in animal models have shown that zinc functions as a hepatoprotective agent through regulation of antioxidant defense, cell proliferation, and cell death. Zinc supplementation attenuates ethanol-induced hepatic zinc depletion and suppresses ethanol-induced oxidative stress, in part through enhancing glutathione (GSH)-related antioxidant capacity in the liver.[29] At the cellular level, zinc supplementation inhibits alcohol-induced hepatocyte apoptosis partially through suppression of death receptor–mediated pathway.[37] Zinc supplementation also stimulates hepatocyte proliferation through preservation of HNF-4α.[23] There are also extrahepatic actions of zinc in the prevention of alcoholic liver injury. Zinc supplementation preserves intestinal integrity and prevents endotoxemia, leading to inhibition of endotoxin-induced tumor necrosis factor α (TNF-α) production in the liver.[38] Induction of MT in the liver and intestine was associated with zinc supplementation, suggesting a link between MT with zinc action. Indeed, MT has been shown to have protective action against alcoholic hepatotoxicity in MT-TG mice.[28] Although the hepatic and extrahepatic effects of zinc could be independent of MT,[28,39] MT is critical to maintain high levels of zinc in the liver. Low levels of MT in the liver reduce endogenous zinc reservoir and sensitize the organ to alcohol-induced injury.[29] The coordination between zinc and MT is that MT maintains high levels of zinc in the liver, and releases zinc under oxidative stress conditions, leading to hepatoprotective action. Therefore, developing methods to maintain a high level of MT in the liver is an attractive strategy to improve zinc homeostasis under ethanol exposure.

In summary, it is clear from animal studies that zinc attenuates the development/progression of experimental ALD. Data in humans demonstrate reversal of certain zinc deficiency signs and symptoms with zinc supplementation. Major randomized long-term trials of zinc therapy in human ALD are unfortunately limited. Because of its excellent safety profile and because of the regular occurrence of zinc deficiency in ALD, we currently regularly supplement patients with ALD with 220 mg of zinc sulfate (50 mg elemental zinc) once a day with meals. Potential side effects are nausea (which is reduced with food intake) and copper deficiency with high doses (usually more than 220 mg of zinc sulfate three times a day).

11.3 METHIONINE

11.3.1 Intracellular Methionine Metabolism

In mammals, the liver plays a central role in methionine metabolism (Figure 11.2), as nearly half of the daily intake of methionine is metabolized there. The intracellular methionine metabolism is initiated by the formation of S-adenosylmethionine (SAM) in a reaction catalyzed by methionine adenosyltransferase (MAT). SAM is the principal biological methyl donor via the transmethylation pathway, the precursor of aminopropyl groups used in polyamine biosynthesis, and in the liver, a precursor of GSH through its conversion to cysteine via the transsulfuration pathway. A healthy human adult produces 6–8 g of SAM per day, most of it in the liver where

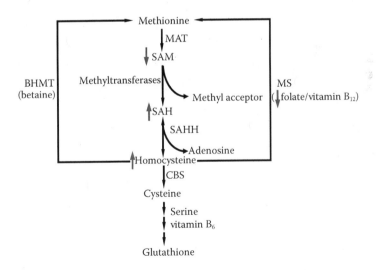

FIGURE 11.2 Altered methionine metabolism in ALD. MAT, methionine adenosyltransferase; SAM, S-adenosylmethionine; SAH, S-adenosylhomocysteine; SAHH, SAH hydrolase; CBS, cystathionine β-synthase; BHMT, betaine-homocysteine methyltransferase; MS, methionine synthase.

it is also utilized in a variety of reactions. Under normal conditions, most of the SAM generated per day is used in transmethylation reactions in which methyl groups are added to a vast number of molecules including both high- and low-molecular weight compounds, via specific methyltransferases. These compounds include DNA, RNA, biogenic amines, phospholipids, histones, and other proteins; their methylation may modulate cellular functions and integrity. In this process, SAM is converted to S-adenosylhomocysteine (SAH), which is a potent competitive inhibitor of most methyltransferases studied; both an increase in SAH level as well as a decrease in the SAM/SAH ratio are known to inhibit transmethylation reactions.[40-45] Therefore, the removal of SAH is essential.

The reaction that converts SAH to homocysteine and adenosine is reversible and catalyzed by SAH hydrolase. Because the thermodynamics favor the synthesis of SAH, the reaction proceeds in the direction of hydrolysis only if the products, adenosine and homocysteine, are rapidly removed. In the liver, homocysteine is metabolized by transsulfuration and methionine resynthesis pathways. In the transsulfuration pathway, homocysteine condenses with serine to form cystathionine in a reaction catalyzed by cystathionine β-synthase, which requires vitamin B6 as a cofactor. The activity of cystathionine β-synthase is allosterically regulated by SAM. Cystathionine is then cleaved by another vitamin B_6-dependent enzyme, β-cystathionase, which results in the release of free cysteine, the rate-limiting precursor for reduced GSH synthesis. In the methionine resynthesis pathway, homocysteine can be converted to methionine by two alternate reactions. One is catalyzed by methionine synthase (MS), which requires normal levels of folate and vitamin B_{12}. A methyl group is transferred from N^5-methyltetrahydrofolate (MTHF) to vitamin B_{12} to form methylcobalamine, which in turn transfers the methyl group to homocysteine to produce methionine. Another pathway is catalyzed by betaine-homocysteine methyltransferase (BHMT), which requires betaine, a metabolite of choline.[46-50]

11.3.2 ABNORMAL METABOLISM OF METHIONINE AND ITS IMPLICATION IN THE DEVELOPMENT OF ALD

Abnormal hepatic methionine metabolism is well documented in ALD, generally characterized by decreased hepatic SAM and folate levels, and increased hepatic SAH and homocysteine accumulation. A link between ethanol consumption and hepatic SAM depletion has been well established in both animal and human studies. Chronic ethanol administration depleted the hepatic concentrations of SAM in a variety of animal models of ALD including rats, mice, baboons, and micropigs.[51-54] Reduced hepatic SAM concentrations have also been reported in alcoholic hepatitis patients. Hepatic SAM depletion by chronic ethanol administration is associated with liver injury of variable magnitude including fatty liver, inflammation, and hepatitis in humans.[55] Several mechanisms have been proposed for SAM depletion, those including inactivation of MAT, excessive consumption of SAM by the liver, and inhibition of endogenous methionine synthesis due to impaired homocysteine methylation.

MAT is a critical cellular enzyme because it catalyzes the only reaction that generates SAM from methionine. In mammals, two different genes, *MAT1A* and *MAT2A*, encode for two homologous MAT catalytic subunits, $\alpha1$ and $\alpha2$. *MAT1A* is expressed only in the liver, whereas *MAT2A* is expressed in extrahepatic tissues and induced during liver growth and dedifferentiation.[56,57] The decreased MAT activity in ALD occurs primarily by posttranslational mechanisms through either a change in the oligomeric equilibrium of the liver-specific MAT (decrease in ratio of tetramer to dimer) or covalent modification of the enzyme without a change in the oligomeric equilibrium.[58] Since the liver-specific MAT contains several critical cysteine residues, its activity is sensitive to oxidative stress. Modifications of these critical cysteine residues can inactivate the enzyme by direct interference with the substrate binding site(s) or by causing dissociation of the oligomers.[59] Moreover, LPS administration results in liver-specific MAT inactivation via nitrosylation of its certain cysteine residues both *in vitro* and *in vivo* in animals.[60] Since both oxidative stress and endotoxemia occur in ALD and contribute to the liver injury, these may represent critical mechanisms underlying the inactivation of the liver-specific MAT. Moreover, chronic alcohol exposure may deplete hepatic SAM concentrations by increasing SAM consumption. This was observed in a rat study in which chronic alcohol administration decreased hepatic SAM and GSH concentrations without affecting MAT activity,[61] suggesting that the utilization of SAM is increased as a precursor for the synthesis of GSH to counteract alcohol-induced oxidative stress. Chronic ethanol administration has also been shown to decrease the hepatic activity of MS and reduce hepatic concentrations of folate and betaine,[54,62–64] the factors known to participate in the resynthesis of endogenous methionine from homocysteine. Thus, alcohol may deplete hepatic SAM by inhibiting the synthesis of its endogenous precursor methionine.

Folate deficiency is another well-characterized metabolic abnormality in ALD. Folate is a water-soluble vitamin that plays an integral role in methionine metabolism and DNA synthesis. Folate in its 5-methyltetrahydrofolate (5-MTHF) form can transfer a methyl group to homocysteine via an MS-catalyzed reaction to form endogenous methionine, which is a precursor of SAM. Thus, folate helps maintain normal concentrations of homocysteine, methionine, and SAM. Folate deficiency can impair methionine metabolism, leading to hyperhomocysteinemia as well as depletion of methionine and SAM, the important features of ALD.[65] Decreased serum or red blood cell folate concentrations in alcoholic patients who consume >80 g ethanol/day have been reported both in the United States and in several European countries. Several potential mechanisms may be involved in folate deficiency in chronic alcoholism: intestinal malabsorption that may be due to decreased transcription of the reduced folate carrier required for folate transport across intestinal membranes, decreased liver folate storage, decreased liver uptake, or increased urinary excretion.[66–68]

In contrast to its effects on SAM and folate, chronic alcohol exposure elevates hepatic levels of homocysteine and SAH, two other important metabolites in hepatic methionine metabolism. Homocysteine is formed from methionine after removal of the methyl group on SAM and hydrolysis of SAH. Results of recent studies support the suggestion that hyperhomocysteinemia may play an important role in the development of alcohol-induced fatty liver, liver injury, and hepatic fibrogenesis.[69] Elevated plasma homocysteine levels in patients with ALD is likely to be a consequence of deficiencies in vitamin B_{12}, folate, and vitamin B_6, as well as of decreased activities of enzymes that metabolize homocysteine, such as MS, BHMT, and cystathionine β-synthase.[70,71] Multiple cellular mechanisms are implicated in homocysteine-induced liver disease. Homocysteine-induced endoplasmic reticulum stress in hepatocytes[72,73] and suppressed adiponectin production in adipocytes[74] both contribute to the pathogenesis of ALD. Homocysteine enhances the production of several proinflammatory cytokines, including monocyte chemoattractant protein 1 and interleukin 8, a T-lymphocyte and neutrophil chemoattractant.[75,76] Moreover, in vascular smooth muscle cells, homocysteine promotes DNA synthesis and enhances collagen production, suggesting that homocysteine may serve as a direct fibrogenic mediator for vascular atherosclerosis.[77–79] Furthermore, Torres et al.[80] demonstrated induction of α1(I) procollagen and TIMP-1 mRNA expression by a human stellate cell line and TIMP-1 mRNA and activator protein 1 activation by cultured hepatocytes.

SAH, a direct product after SAM transfers its methyl groups to various compounds, is catalyzed by many different methyltransferases, and, in turn, is a potent endogenous inhibitor of most methyltransferases. SAH is further metabolized to homocysteine and adenosine through a reversible reaction catalyzed by SAH hydrolase. The generation of SAH from homocysteine is thermodynamically favored over the synthesis of homocysteine. The reaction proceeds toward homocysteine synthesis only when the products (homocysteine and adenosine) are removed by further metabolism. Chronic ethanol feeding has been shown to increase hepatic concentrations of SAH in different animal models of ALD. Furthermore, hepatocytes obtained from ethanol-fed rats showed a significant twofold increase in SAH concentrations, which were further elevated when the hepatocytes were incubated with methionine. Although it remains unclear mechanistically, homocysteine accumulation may be one of the main causes for increased hepatic SAH concentrations. Recent results from our studies provide strong evidence that SAH accumulation plays an etiologic role in the pathogenesis of ALD. Our studies demonstrated that chronic alcohol exposure not only caused hepatic SAM deficiency in mice but also increased SAH levels, leading to significantly decreased intracellular SAM/SAH ratio, a reliable indicator of inhibited transmethylation reactions. Also, we found that increased SAH accumulation sensitized hepatocytes to TNF-induced cell death.[81] Moreover, SAH accumulation inhibited mitochondrial SAM transporters and thereby decreased intramitochondrial SAM levels. Furthermore, we showed that mitochondrial SAM depletion sensitizes hepatocytes to TNF cytotoxicity.[82] Lastly, abnormal SAM metabolism may play a role in the emerging area of epigenetics in ALD.

11.3.3 Correction of Abnormal Methionine Metabolism as a Therapy

11.3.3.1 SAM Therapy

SAM therapy for ALD is based on the fact that SAM is essential for multiple metabolic reactions and that chronic ethanol administration depletes its hepatic concentration in association with liver injury in animals and humans. SAM administration attenuated alcohol-induced steatosis and restored hepatic GSH concentrations in rats, and it attenuated ethanol-induced depletion of mitochondrial GSH and restored mitochondrial function in hepatocytes.[83] In mice, SAM treatment significantly attenuated acute alcohol–induced liver injury characterized by attenuation of alcohol-induced steatosis, necrosis, and increased alanine transaminase activity, which was associated with restoration of hepatic SAM and mitochondrial GSH concentrations and attenuation of lipid peroxidation.[84] In baboons, SAM attenuated alcohol-induced liver injury by repairing mitochondrial injury, which restored plasma GSH concentrations and decreased plasma concentrations of AST.[51] Clinically, the therapeutic potential of SAM was tested in a 24-month randomized, placebo-controlled, double-blind, multicenter clinical trial in 123 patients with alcoholic cirrhosis.[85] SAM treatment improved survival or delayed the need for liver transplantation in patients with alcoholic liver cirrhosis, especially in those with less advanced liver disease. In this trial, increased hepatic concentrations of GSH may have contributed to the beneficial effect of SAM because, in another study, oral administration of 1.2 g SAM/day for 6 months significantly increased hepatic GSH concentrations in ALD patients.[86] Although this one large multicenter study showed some beneficial effect of SAM, other studies are needed to document this beneficial effect and define appropriate dosing schedules.

11.3.3.2   Folate Therapy

It is clear that folate deficiency in micropigs accelerates alcohol-induced liver injury through multiple pathways. However, with folic acid fortification in the current American diet, chronic alcohol exposure may not lead to major hepatic folate deficiency. Whether further folate administration will attenuate human ALD is unknown. Despite unclear indications, we frequently supplement with folate in patients with ALD.

11.3.3.3   Betaine Therapy

Betaine is highly effective in reducing homocysteine levels and removing fat from the liver in experimental models of alcohol-induced liver injury. Unfortunately, good randomized studies in human ALD are lacking, as are dose-finding studies in humans. This is unfortunate because betaine is much more stable than SAM, and its absorption is much better characterized. Human studies are clearly warranted, but we do not supplement with betaine at present.

11.4   SELECTED OTHER VITAMIN AND MINERAL DEFICIENCIES AS RELATED TO ALD

11.4.1   VITAMINS

11.4.1.1   Vitamin B$_1$/Thiamine

Thiamine deficiency is common in many forms of cirrhosis, including alcoholic cirrhosis. In a comparison study among patients with alcoholic cirrhosis, hepatitis C virus–induced cirrhosis, and hepatitis C without cirrhosis (no healthy controls were used), thiamine deficiency frequency was similar in cirrhotic patients regardless of cause. No patients with hepatitis C without cirrhosis were found to have thiamine deficiency, suggesting that hepatitis infection itself does not affect thiamine levels. No correlation was found between thiamine deficiency and severity of liver disease as measured by Child–Pugh score, serum albumin, Knodell activity index, or fibrosis score.[87] Thiamine deficiency can be caused by inadequate intake, decreased hepatic storage, and both acute and chronic impairment of intestinal absorption by ethanol.[88]

Wernicke–Korsakoff syndrome (WKS) is a severe mental disturbance caused by thiamine deficiency and is often associated with alcoholism (due to the high prevalence of thiamine deficiency among alcoholics). WKS can be described in two distinct stages. The first stage is Wernicke's encephalopathy, due to acute thiamine deficiency, which is generally reversible by treatment with large doses of thiamine. If this treatment is not given, long-term damage to brain tissue may occur, resulting in Korsakoff's psychosis. Supplementation with thiamine will not reverse the effects of Korsakoff's psychosis because of permanent brain damage. Signs/symptoms of WKS include acute confusion, nystagmus, ophthalmoplegia (paralysis of the ocular muscles), ataxia, short-term memory loss, and even death, although not all of these symptoms need to be present to diagnose WKS. Onset of WKS is often precipitated by illness, alcoholic seizures, or delirium tremens.[89]

Peripheral neuropathy has also been associated with deficiencies of vitamins such as thiamine, folate, pyridoxine, pantothenic acid, or nicotinic acid.[89] Alcoholic patients sometimes experience peripheral neuropathy, and 90% of these patients also had low serum thiamine levels in one study.[90]

11.4.1.2   Vitamin B$_2$/Riboflavin

Riboflavin deficiencies have been noted in both alcoholic and nonalcoholic cirrhotic patients. This may be explained by inadequate intake, increased utilization, deficient absorption and storage, or abnormal metabolism.[91] Low levels of riboflavin may be associated with glossitis, cheilitis, and lingual papillae atrophy in alcoholic patients.[90]

11.4.1.3   Vitamin B$_3$/Niacin

Niacin deficiency, or pellagra, may be associated with chronic alcoholism. Alcoholic pellagra encephalopathy (APE) is less common than WKS and is thought to be underdiagnosed. Symptoms include confusion, oppositional hypertonus, myoclonus, cogwheel rigidity, hallucinations, insomnia, tremor, ataxia, peripheral neuropathy, seizures, anxiety, depression, excitement, neurasthenia, grasping and suckling reflexes, and fecal or urinary incontinence. Because APE often occurs concomitantly with other alcoholic encephalopathies, it is often difficult to diagnose. Vitamin supplementation (e.g., thiamine, pyridoxine) for other diagnosed encephalopathies without treatment of APE (via niacin supplementation) has often intensified or induced APE symptoms.[89]

11.4.1.4   Vitamin B$_6$/Pyridoxine

Chronic alcohol abuse has been shown to lower hepatic stores of pyridoxine.[92] Low pyridoxine levels may contribute to hypochromic anemia in alcoholic patients with normal iron levels. Vitamin B$_6$ is required for the production of GSH from homocysteine (see previous sections). GSH is an important antioxidant, and free radical damage contributes to the development of ALD. B$_6$ deficiency in alcoholics may contribute to the liver damage caused by alcohol and other toxic agents.[93]

11.4.1.5 Vitamin D

Decreased serum vitamin D among alcoholics may be attributable to inadequate intake, malabsorption resulting from cholestasis and pancreatic insufficiency, or low sunlight exposure. Decreased vitamin D may contribute to lowered bone density and mass as well as increased susceptibility to osteonecrosis and bone fractures.[92]

In a study of 181 alcoholic men and 43 healthy male controls, vitamin D, osteocalcin, parathyroid hormone, IGF-1, and bone mass were all found to be decreased among alcoholics. No correlation was found between bone loss and amount of alcohol consumed or severity of liver disease. Rather, a correlation was found between malnutrition and bone loss. Alcoholic patients tended to have significantly lower body mass index (BMI), but for patients with a similar BMI to healthy controls, bone loss was more severe in alcoholics. Alcoholics with very irregular food intake habits drink more ethanol and present greater impairment of nutritional status, indicating that periods of malnutrition may intensify bone loss.[94] Indeed, in a study in rats, serum vitamin D levels decreased with a protein-deficient diet, and this effect was compounded when ethanol was also administered. Vitamin D levels were found to be directly related to final weight, serum albumin, and serum osteocalcin.[95]

The vitamin D receptor is a nuclear hormone receptor, and its activation is increasingly recognized as important in functions unrelated to bone, especially immune function. Potential anti-inflammatory and antifibrotic effects are under active investigation.[96]

11.4.1.6 Vitamin A/Retinol

The liver is the major storehouse for vitamin A, with high levels in hepatic stellate cells. When quiescent stellate cells become activated, they lose their vitamin A stores and are then capable of producing collagen and subsequent fibrosis. Vitamin A deficiency (low serum levels and abnormal dark adaptation) is present in approximately 50% of alcoholic cirrhotic patients,[10] and alcoholics have been shown to have very low concentrations of hepatic vitamin A at all stages of their disease.[97] Thus, hepatic stores of vitamin A may become severely depleted in ALD, even if liver damage is moderate, and serum vitamin A and retinol-binding protein levels are still within normal limits. This occurs both via a migration of vitamin A from the liver to extrahepatic tissues and by an increased rate of retinoid catabolism. This effect is amplified when drugs and other xenobiotics are combined with ethanol.

The retinoic acid receptor, retinoid X receptor α (RXRα), is a nuclear hormone receptor highly expressed in the liver. Knockout RXRα mice were used to study the role of RXRα in ethanol metabolism, in part because vitamin A and ethanol are metabolized through overlapping pathways and that vitamin A deficiency and ethanol toxicity cause similar birth defects.[98] RXRα-KO mice were found to have increased alcohol dehydrogenase 1 (ADH-1) protein and activity levels, whereas mRNA levels remained unchanged. Ethanol clearance from the blood and livers of knockout mice was also enhanced, which was attributed to the increased ADH-1 activity. Activity of acetaldehyde dehydrogenase (ALDH) and glutathione S-transferase (GST) were decreased in knockout mice. The decreased ALDH activity contributed to the slower clearance of acetaldehyde. Faster production of acetaldehyde by ADH-1 combined with slower clearance by ALDH contributed to an observed rise in circulating acetaldehyde. RXRa-KO mice had a greater susceptibility to ALD, which was likely caused by the increased levels of circulating acetaldehyde. Moreover, Dai et al.[99] found that a deficiency in the expression of the RXRα led to a reduction of SAM and GSH levels and resulted in a more severe liver injury in mice fed ethanol intragastrically for 25 days. These cumulative data suggest that activation of the RXRα by vitamin A may have a hepatoprotective effect against ALD,[98] and this activation may be inadequate in vitamin A–deficient alcoholics.

11.4.2 Minerals

11.4.2.1 Magnesium

Magnesium deficiency is common among alcoholics. Indeed, serum magnesium has been reported to be decreased in both alcoholic and nonalcoholic steatosis. Depleted intracellular magnesium stores in alcoholics can occur for multiple reasons including decreased intake and/or accumulation of saturated fatty acids on cell membranes.[100] Urinary excretion of magnesium and calcium was found to be increased in a dose-dependent manner following even moderate amounts of alcohol intake,[101] and this can contribute to the magnesium deficiency in alcoholics.

Magnesium deficiency has frequently been associated with peripheral insulin resistance. Indeed, nondiabetic patients with insulin resistance have been treated with magnesium with improvement of peripheral insulin resistance.[102] Magnesium deficiency also has been reported to significantly improve AST levels in some studies.[103] Lastly, magnesium is often associated with muscle cramps, and magnesium supplementation has been shown to significantly improve muscle cramps during pregnancy.[104] We frequently use magnesium supplements in our patients with alcoholic cirrhosis who experience muscle cramps (magnesium oxide, one tablet, p.o. daily).

11.4.2.2 Selenium

Selenium is incorporated as selenocysteine at the active sites of multiple selenoproteins.[105,106] The best recognized of these are the GSH peroxidase enzymes, which play a critical role in antioxidant defense systems. Thioredoxin reductase is also a selenocysteine-containing enzyme. Selenoproteins are also important for thyroid function, muscle metabolism, and sperm function, as well as immune function. Selenium status is usually determined by the serum selenium concentration, or by determining a marker of selenium status, such as erythrocyte GSH peroxidase activity.

Several studies have shown that subjects with ALD have decreased serum, whole blood, and hepatic selenium.[107–111] Dworkin et al.[110] noted that hepatic selenium deficiency correlated with prothrombin time, but not bilirubin, albumin, or AST. Gonzalez-Reimers and colleagues[109] also found that selenium levels were related to prothrombin activity and nutritional status, and more closely related to nutritional status. A German study including mild to moderate ALD found that even in males consuming a normal diet (with alcohol as added calories), selenium status was depressed.[111] We could not find trials of isolated selenium supplementation in ALD patients, but selenium and multiple other antioxidants did not significantly improve alcoholic hepatitis.[112]

11.5 OVERALL NUTRITIONAL INTERVENTION

Interest in the role of nutritional support as therapy for ALD was first stimulated by early studies by Patek and Post[113] demonstrating that a "nutritious diet" improved 5-year outcome in patients with alcoholic cirrhosis, compared with historical controls. Two large Veterans Administration Cooperative Studies[114–116] highlight the regular occurrence of malnutrition in hospitalized patients with alcoholic hepatitis. The first demonstrated that every patient with alcoholic hepatitis had some degree of malnutrition, and severity of malnutrition correlated with mortality (Table 11.2).[117] An inverse relation was noted between energy intake and mortality rate (Figure 11.3). Before hospitalization, patients with alcoholic hepatitis were consuming more than 3000 calories a day, but almost 50% of those calories were in the form of alcohol, which represents "empty calories" with virtually no nutritional benefit. Although caloric intake was high, protein consumption was low, with less than 8% of calories being consumed as protein. Moreover, when patients were stratified according to severity of their alcoholic hepatitis, patients with more severe disease consumed fewer nonalcohol calories. Once these patients were hospitalized, many tended to have severe anorexia. Indeed, despite the fact that these patients had aggressive dietary and nursing support, only 67% of patients consumed recommended calories in the hospital. These studies highlighted the high frequency of malnutrition in patients with alcoholic hepatitis and the potential need for tube feeding in subjects unable to voluntarily consume enough food.

Several more recent studies support a role for nutritional support in patients hospitalized for ALD. In one trial, liver function, as assessed by serum bilirubin levels and antipyrine clearance, improved significantly in patients who received enteral nutritional supplementation through a feeding tube, compared with that in patients who ate a hospital diet.[118] Patients who received nutritional supplementation also

TABLE 11.2
Acute and Long-term Mortality in Alcoholic Hepatitis Associated with Varying Degrees of Protein–Calorie Malnutrition (PCM)

Duration of Follow-Up (months)	Severity of PCM (%)			p
	Mild (110)	Moderate (209)	Severe (33)	
1	2	15	52	< .001
6	7	31	67	< .001
12	14	43	76	< .001

Source: Data from Mendenhall, C. L., Tosch, T., Weesner, R. E., Garcia-Pont, P., et al., *Am J Clin Nutr* 43, 213–218, 1986.

Note: n, number of patients; p value at each period is determined by χ^2 test.

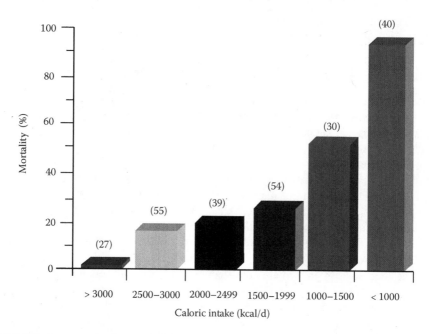

FIGURE 11.3   Voluntary food intake correlated in a dose response fashion with mortality from alcoholic hepatitis. (From Mendenhall, C., Roselle, G. A., Gartside, P., and Moritz, T., *Alcohol Clin Exp Res* 19, 635–641, 1995.)

had significantly greater protein and caloric intake. In a pivotal multicenter study by Cabré and coworkers,[119] patients were randomized to receive prednisone, 40 mg daily, or a liver-specific formula containing 2000 calories per day, through a feeding tube. The 1-month mortality rates were similar in both groups, but the 1-year mortality rate was significantly lower in the patients who received the enteral nutrition, in great part because of reduced infectious complications, in comparison with patients who received glucocorticoids. This study clearly demonstrates the important role of enteral nutrition in hospitalized patients with severe ALD. Tube feeding in patients with ALD is probably underutilized in most hospitals because of concerns about precipitating hepatic encephalopathy or stimulating bleeding from esophageal varices, neither of which has been documented. Most patients can probably tolerate standard enteral products. Only selected patients with overt hepatic encephalopathy require liver-specific products rich in branched-chain amino acids in our opinion, although there remains debate in this area.[120,121] A well-defined approach is required to achieve appropriate nutritional support in the hospitalized patient with ALD, and our overall approach is outlined in Table 11.3.

Studies of nutritional support in outpatients are limited, but Hirsch and colleagues[122] demonstrated that patients from an outpatient liver clinic who took an enteral nutrition support product containing 1000 kcal and 34 g of protein had significantly improved protein intake and fewer hospitalizations in comparison with those not receiving the supplement. This group also showed that an enteral supplement

TABLE 11.3

Nutritional Recommendations for Patients with Liver Disease

- Early nutrition assessment and regular follow-ups
- Total energy: 1.2–1.4 × resting energy expenditure
- Protein: 1.0–1.5 g/kg/day
- Fat: 30–40% of nonprotein energy
- Formulate water and electrolyte intake to individual needs, renal function, diuretic sensitivity
- Replace vitamins and minerals (avoid excessive iron and copper intake)
- Complement daily requirements with enteral feedings (parenteral if enteral route otherwise contraindicated)

improved nutritional status and immune function in outpatients with alcoholic cirrhosis.[123] It is well documented that patients with alcoholic cirrhosis metabolically enter a starvation mode more rapidly than normal volunteers because of decreased glycogen stores in their livers. This is the rationale for nocturnal supplements to patients with cirrhosis. In probably the most comprehensive and recent outpatient study to date, daytime versus evening enteral supplements were evaluated in patients with cirrhosis.[124] Nighttime enteral supplements were shown to be superior by many nutritional indices and patients' improved nutritional status over a 1-year period as assessed by studies such as fat-free mass.

11.6   SUMMARY

We have described in detail the complex interactions of two nutritional alterations (zinc, methionine) in the development and progression of ALD and have highlighted other individual nutritional deficiencies in ALD. Nutritional support can improve nutritional status and, in some patients, may enhance liver function and decrease the risk of death in ALD. Assessment of nutritional status and nutritional supplementation should be pursued aggressively in both inpatients and outpatients with ALD, especially those with more severe alcoholic hepatitis and cirrhosis.

REFERENCES

1. Goode, H. F., J. Kelleher, and B. E. Walker. 1990. Relation between zinc status and hepatic functional reserve in patients with liver disease. *Gut* 31:694–697.
2. Rodríguez-Moreno, F., E. González-Reimers, F. Santolaria-Fernández, L. Galindo-Martín, O. Hernandez-Torres, N. Batista-López, and M. Molina-Perez. 1997. Zinc, copper, manganese, and iron in chronic alcoholic liver disease. *Alcohol* 14:39–44.
3. Rahelić, D., M. Kujundzić, Z. Romić, K. Brkić, and M. Petrovecki. 2006. Serum concentration of zinc, copper, manganese, and magnesium in patients with liver cirrhosis. *Coll Antropol* 30:523–528.
4. Foote, J. W., and H. T. Delves. 1984. Albumin bound and alpha 2-macroglobulin bound zinc concentrations in the sera of healthy adults. *J Clin Pathol* 37:1050–1054.

5. Wu, C. T., J. N. Lee, W. W. Shen, and S. L. Lee. 1984. Serum zinc, copper, and ceruloplasmin levels in male alcoholics. *Biol Psychiatry* 19:1333–1338.
6. King, J. C., D. M. Shames, and L. R. Woodhouse. 2000. Zinc homeostasis in humans. *J Nutr* 130:1360S–1366S.
7. Dinsmore, W. W., M. E. Callender, and D. McMaster. 1985. The absorption of zinc from a standardized meal in alcoholics and in normal volunteers. *Am J Clin Nutr* 42:688–693.
8. Valberg, L. S., P. R. Flanagan, C. N. Ghent, and M. J. Chamberlain. 1985. Zinc absorption and leukocyte zinc in alcoholic and nonalcoholic cirrhosis. *Dig Dis Sci* 30:329–333.
9. Watson, R. R., and T. K. Leonard-Green. 1990. Alcohol-induced malnutrition and immunosuppression. In: *Drugs of Abuse and Immune Function*, ed. R. R. Watson. Boca Raton: CRC Press, pp. 125–138.
10. Russell, R. M. 1980. Vitamin A and zinc metabolism in alcoholism. *Am J Clin Nutr* 33:2741–2749.
11. McClain, C. J., L. Adams, and S. Shedlofsky. 1988. Zinc and the gastrointestinal system. In: *Essential and Toxic Trace Elements in Human Health and Disease*. New York: Alan R. Liss Inc., pp. 55–73.
12. Stamoulis, I., G. Kouraklis, and S. Theocharis. 2007. Zinc and the liver: An active interaction. *Dig Dis Sci* 52:1595–1612.
13. Shea-Budgell, M., M. Dojka, M. Nimmo, D. Lee, and Z. Xu. 2006. Marginal zinc deficiency increased the susceptibility to acute lipopolysaccharide-induced liver injury in rats. *Exp Biol Med* 231:553–558.
14. Atukorala, T. M., C. A. Herath, and S. Ramachandran. 1986. Zinc and vitamin A status of alcoholics in a medical unit in Sri Lanka. *Alcohol Alcohol* 21:269–275.
15. Bianchi, G. P., G. Marchesini, M. Brizi, B. Rossi, G. Forlani, P. Boni, N. Melchionda, K. Thomaseth, and G. Pacini. 2000. Nutritional effects of oral zinc supplementation in cirrhosis. *Nutr Res* 20:1079–1089.
16. Giles, N. M., A. B. Watts, G. I. Giles, F. H. Fry, J. A. Littlechild, and C. Jacob. 2003. Metal and redox modulation of cysteine protein function. *Chem Biol* 10:677–693.
17. Daiber, A., D. Frein, D. Namgaladze, and V. Ullrich. 2002. Oxidation and nitrosation in the nitrogen monoxide/superoxide system. *J Biol Chem* 277:11882–11888.
18. Mills, P. R., G. S. Fell, R. G. Bessent, L. M. Nelson, and R. I. Russell. 1983. A study of zinc metabolism in alcoholic cirrhosis. *Clin Sci (Lond)* 64:527–535.
19. Zhao, M., K. Matter, J. A. Laissue, and A. Zimmermann. 1996. Copper/zinc and manganese superoxide dismutases in alcoholic liver disease: Immunohistochemical quantitation. *Histol Histopathol* 11:899–907.
20. Natori, S., C. Rust, L. M. Stadheim, A. Srinivasan, L. J. Burgart, and G. J. Gores. 2001. Hepatocyte apoptosis is a pathologic feature of human alcoholic hepatitis. *J Hepatol* 34:248–253.
21. Ramalho, R. M., H. Cortez-Pinto, R. E. Castro, S. Solá, A. Costa, M. C. Moura, M. E. Camilo, and C. M. Rodrigues. 2006. Apoptosis and Bcl-2 expression in the livers of patients with steatohepatitis. *Eur J Gastroenterol Hepatol* 18:21–29.
22. Chimienti, F., M. Seve, S. Richard, J. Mathieu, and A. Favier. 2001. Role of cellular zinc in programmed cell death: Temporal relationship between zinc depletion, activation of caspases, and cleavage of Sp family transcription factors. *Biochem Pharmacol* 62:51–62.
23. Kang, X., Z. Song, C. J. McClain, Y. J. Kang, and Z. Zhou. 2008. Zinc supplementation enhances hepatic regeneration by preserving hepatocyte nuclear factor–α in mice subjected to a long-term ethanol administration. *Am J Pathol* 172:916–925.
24. Vallee, B. L. 1995. The function of metallothionein. *Neurochem Int* 27:23–33.
25. Davis, S. R., and R. J. Cousins. 2000. Metallothionein expression in animals: A physiological perspective on function. *J Nutr* 130:1085–1088.

26. Iszard, M. B., J. Liu, Y. Liu, T. Dalton, G. K. Andrews, R. D. Palmiter, and C. D. Klaassen. 1995. Characterization of metallothionein-I-transgenic mice. *Toxicol Appl Pharmacol* 133:305–312.
27. Masters, B. A., E. J. Kelly, C. J. Quaife, R. L. Brinster, and R. Palmiter. 1994. Targeted disruption of metallothionein I and II genes increases sensitivity to cadmium. *Proc Natl Acad Sci U S A* 91:584–588.
28. Zhou, Z., X. Sun, J. C. Lambert, J. T. Saari, and Y. J. Kang. 2002. Metallothionein-independent zinc protection from alcoholic liver injury. *Am J Pathol* 160:2267–2274.
29. Zhou, Z., L. Wang, Z. Song, J. T. Saari, C. J. McClain, and Y. J. Kang. 2005. Zinc supplementation prevents alcoholic liver injury in mice through attenuation of oxidative stress. *Am J Pathol* 166:1681–1690.
30. Tohyama, C., J. S. Suzuki, J. Hemelraad, N. Nishimura, and H. Nishimura. 1993. Induction of metallothionein and its localization in the nucleus of rat hepatocytes after partial hepatectomy. *Hepatology* 18:1193–1201.
31. Spahl, D. U., D. Berendji-Grün, C. V. Suschek, V. Kolb-Bachofen, and K. D. Kröncke. 2003. Regulation of zinc homeostasis by inducible NO synthase-derived NO: Nuclear metallothionein translocation and intranuclear Zn^{2+} release. *Proc Natl Acad Sci U S A* 100:13952–13957.
32. Takahashi, Y., Y. Ogra, and K. T. Suzuki. 2005. Nuclear trafficking of metallothionein requires oxidation of a cytosolic partner. *J Cell Physiol* 202:563–569.
33. Ye, B., W. Maret, and B. L. Vallee. 2001. Zinc metallothionein imported into liver mitochondria modulates respiration. *Proc Natl Acad Sci U S A* 98:2317–2322.
34. Costello, L. C., Z. Guan, R. B. Franklin, and P. Feng. 2004. Metallothionein can function as a chaperone for zinc uptake transport into prostate and liver mitochondria. *J Inorg Biochem* 98:664–666.
35. Zarski, J. P., J. Arnaud, H. Labadie, M. Beaugrand, A. Favier, and M. Rachail. 1987. Serum and tissue concentrations of zinc after oral supplementation in chronic alcoholics with or without cirrhosis. *Gastroenterol Clin Biol* 11:856–860.
36. Takahashi, M., H. Saito, M. Higashimoto, and T. Hibi. 2007. Possible inhibitory effect of oral zinc supplementation on hepatic fibrosis through downregulation of TIMP-1: A pilot study. *Hepatol Res* 37:405–409.
37. Zhou, Z., J. Liu, Z. Song, C. J. McClain, and Y. J. Kang. 2008. Zinc supplementation inhibits hepatic apoptosis in mice subjected to a long-term ethanol exposure. *Exp Biol Med* 233:540–548.
38. Lambert, J. C., Z. Zhou, and Y. J. Kang. 2003. Suppression of Fas-mediated signaling pathway is involved in zinc inhibition of ethanol-induced liver apoptosis. *Exp Biol Med* 228:406–412.
39. Lambert, J. C., Z. Zhou, L. Wang, Z. Song, C. J. McClain, and Y. J. Kang. 2004. Prevention of intestinal integrity by zinc is independent of metallothionein in alcohol-intoxicated mice. *Am J Pathol* 164:1959–1966.
40. Lu, S. C., Z. Z. Huang, H. Yang, J. M. Mato, M. A. Avila, and H. Tsukamoto. 2000. Changes in methionine adenosyltransferase and *S*-adenosylmethionine homeostasis in alcoholic rat liver. *Am J Physiol Gastrointest Liver Physiol* 279:G178–G185.
41. Avila, M. A., E. R. Garcia-Trevijano, M. L. Martinez-Chantar, M. U. Latasa, I. Perez-Mato, L. A. Martinez-Cruz, M. M. del Pino, F. J. Corrales, and J. M. Mato. 2002. *S*-Adenosylmethionine revisited: Its essential role in the regulation of liver function. *Alcohol* 27:163–167.
42. McClain, C. J., D. B. Hill, Z. Song, R. Chawla, W. Watson, T. Chen, and S. Barve. 2002. *S*-Adenosylmethionine, cytokines, and alcoholic liver disease. *Alcohol* 27:185–192.
43. Mato, J. M., L. Alvarez, P. Ortiz, and M. A. Pajares. 1997. *S*-Adenosylmethionine synthesis: Molecular mechanisms and clinical implications. *Pharmacol Ther* 73:265–280.

44. Chiang, P. K., R. K. Gordon, J. Tal, G. C. Zeng, B. P. Doctor, K. Pardhasaradhi, and P. P. McCann. 1996. *S*-Adenosylmethionine and methylation. *FASEB J* 10:471–480.
45. Hoffman, D. R., S. W. Marion, W. E. Cornatzer, and J. A. Duerre. 1980. *S*-Adenosylmethionine and *S*-adenosylhomocysteine metabolism in isolated rat liver. Effects of L-methionine, L-homocysteine, and adenosine. *J Biol Chem* 255: 10822–10827.
46. Finkelstein, J. D. 1990. Methionine metabolism in mammals. *J Nutr Biochem* 1: 228–237.
47. Mato, J. M., F. J. Corrales, S. C. Lu, and M. A. Avila. 2002. *S*-Adenosylmethionine: A control switch that regulates liver function. *FASEB J* 16:15–26.
48. Finkelstein, J. D., W. E. Kyle, J. L. Martin, and A. M. Pick. 1975. Activation of cystathionine synthase by adenosylmethionine and adenosylethionine. *Biochem Biophys Res Commun* 66:81–87.
49. Taoka, S., L. Widjaja, and R. Banerjee. 1999. Assignment of enzymatic functions to specific regions of the PLP-dependent heme protein cystathionine beta-synthase. *Biochemistry* 38:13155–13161.
50. Lu, S. C. 1999. Regulation of hepatic glutathione synthesis: Current concept and controversies. *FASEB J* 13:1169–1183.
51. Lieber, C. S., A. Casini, L. M. DeCarli, C. I Kim., N. Lowe, R. Sasaki, and M. A. Leo. 1990. *S*-Adenosyl-L-methionine attenuates alcohol-induced liver injury in the baboon. *Hepatology* 11:165–172.
52. Barak, A. J., H. C. Beckenhauer, and D. J. Tuma. 1994. *S*-Adenosylmethionine generation and prevention of alcoholic fatty liver by betaine. *Alcohol* 11:501–503.
53. Song, Z., Z. Zhou, T. Chen, D. Hill, J. Kang, S. Barve, and C. McClain. 2003. *S*-Adenosylmethionine (SAMe) protects against acute alcohol induced hepatotoxicity in mice. *J Nutr Biochem* 14:591–597.
54. Halsted, C. H., J. Villanueva, C. J. Chandler, S. P. Stabler, R. H. Allen, L. Muskhelishvili, S. J. James, and L. Poirier. 1996. Ethanol feeding of micropigs alters methionine metabolism and increases hepatocellular apoptosis and proliferation. *Hepatology* 23:497–505.
55. Lee, T. D., M. R. Sadda, M. H. Mendler, T. Bottiglieri, G. Kanel, J. M. Mato, and S. C. Lu. 2004. Abnormal hepatic methionine and glutathione metabolism in patients with alcoholic hepatitis. *Alcohol Clin Exp Res* 28:173–181.
56. Kotb, M., and N. M. Kredich. 1985. *S*-Adenosylmethionine synthetase from human lymphocytes. Purification and characterization. *J Biol Chem* 260:3923–3930.
57. Kotb, M., S. H. Mudd, J. M. Mato, A. M. Geller, N. M. Kredich, J. Y. Chou, and G. L. Cantoni. 1997. Consensus nomenclature for the mammalian methionine adenosyltransferase genes and gene products. *Trends Genet* 13:51–52.
58. Alvarez, L., F. Corrales, A. Martín-Duce, and J. M. Mato. 1993. Characterization of a full-length cDNA encoding human liver *S*-adenosylmethionine synthetase: Tissuespecific gene expression and mRNA levels in hepatopathies. *Biochem J* 293:481–486.
59. Avila, M. A., J. Mingorance, M. L. Martínez-Chantar, M. Casado, P. Martin-Sanz, L. Boscá, and J. M. Mato. 1997. Regulation of rat liver *S*-adenosylmethionine synthetase during septic shock: Role of nitric oxide. *Hepatology* 25:391–396.
60. Ruiz, F., F. J. Corrales, C. Miqueo, and J. M. Mato. 1998. Nitric oxide inactivates rat hepatic methionine adenosyltransferase in vivo by *S*-nitrosylation. *Hepatology* 28:1051–1057.
61. Aleynik, S. I., and C. S. Lieber. 2003. Polyenylphosphatidylcholine corrects the alcoholinduced hepatic oxidative stress by restoring *S*-adenosylmethionine. *Alcohol Alcohol* 38:208–213.
62. Barak, A. J., H. C. Beckenhauer, M. Junnila, and D. J. Tuma. 1993. Dietary betaine promotes generation of hepatic *S*-adenosylmethionine and protects the liver from ethanolinduced fatty infiltration. *Alcohol Clin Exp Res* 17:552–555.

63. Villanueva, J. A., and C. H. Halsted. 2004. Hepatic transmethylation reactions in micropigs with alcoholic liver disease. *Hepatology* 39:1303–1310.
64. Kharbanda, K. K., and A. J. Barak. 2005. Defects in methionine metabolism: Its role in ethanol-induced liver injury. In: *Comprehensive Handbook of Alcohol-Related Pathology*, Vol 2, ed. V. R. Preedy and R. R. Watson. New York, NY: Academic Press, Elsevier Sciences, pp. 735–747.
65. Halsted, C. H. 2004. Nutrition and alcoholic liver disease. *Semin Liver Dis* 24:289–304.
66. Herbert, V., R. Zalusky, and C. S. Davidson. 1963. Correlation of folate deficiency with alcoholism and associated macrocytosis, anemia, and liver disease. *Ann Intern Med* 58:977–988.
67. Gloria, L., M. Cravo, M. E. Camilo, M. Resende, J. N. Cardoso, A. G. Oliveira, C. N. Leitão, and F. C. Mira. 1993. Nutritional deficiencies in chronic alcoholics: Relation to dietary intake and alcohol consumption. *Am J Gastroenterol* 92:485–489.
68. Leevy, C. M., L. Cardi, O. Frank, R. Gellene, and H. Baker. 1965. Incidence and significance of hypovitaminemia in a randomly selected municipal hospital population. *Am J Clin Nutr* 17:259–271.
69. Refsum, H., P. M. Ueland, O. Nygård, and S. E. Vollset. 1998. Homocysteine and cardiovascular disease. *Annu Rev Med* 49:31–62.
70. Cravo, M. L., L. M. Glória, J. Selhub, M. R. Nadeau, M. E. Camilo, M. P. Resende, J. N. Cardoso, C. N. Leitão, and F. C. Mira. 1996. Hyperhomocysteinemia in chronic alcoholism: Correlation with folate, vitamin B-12, and vitamin B-6 status. *Am J Clin Nutr* 63:220–224.
71. Selhub, J., and J. W. Miller. 1992. The pathogenesis of homocysteinemia: Interruption of the coordinate regulation by *S*-adenosylmethionine of the remethylation and transsulfuration of homocysteine. *Am J Clin Nutr* 55:131–138.
72. Ji, C., and N. Kaplowitz. 2004. Hyperhomocysteinemia, endoplasmic reticulum stress, and alcoholic liver injury. *World J Gastroenterol* 10:1699–1708.
73. Ji, C., and N. Kaplowitz. 2003. Betaine decreases hyperhomocysteinemia, endoplasmic reticulum stress, and liver injury in alcohol-fed mice. *Gastroenterology* 124:1488–1499.
74. Song, Z., Z. Zhou, I. Deaciuc, T. Chen, and C. J. McClain. 2008. Inhibition of adiponectin production by homocysteine: A potential mechanism for alcoholic liver disease. *Hepatology* 47:867–879.
75. Poddar, R., N. Sivasubramanian, P. M. DiBello, K. Robinson, and D. W. Jacobsen. 2001. Homocysteine induces expression and secretion of monocyte chemoattractant protein–1 and interleukin-8 in human aortic endothelial cells: Implications for vascular disease. *Circulation* 103:2717–2723.
76. Zeng, X., J. Dai, D. G. Remick, and X. Wang. 2003. Homocysteine mediated expression and secretion of monocyte chemoattractant protein-1 and interleukin-8 in human monocytes. *Circ Res* 93:311–320.
77. Majors, A., L. A. Ehrhart, and E. H. Pezacka. 1997. Homocysteine as a risk factor for vascular disease. Enhanced collagen production and accumulation by smooth muscle cells. *Arterioscler Thromb Vasc Biol* 17:2074–2081.
78. Tsai, J. C., H. Wang, M. A. Perrella, M. Yoshizumi, N. E. Sibinga, L. C. Tan, E. Haber, T. H. Chang, R. Schlegel, and M. E. Lee. 1996. Induction of cyclin A gene expression by homocysteine in vascular smooth muscle cells. *J Clin Invest* 97:146–153.
79. Tsai, J. C., M. A. Perrella, M. Yoshizumi, C. M. Hsieh, E. Haber, R. Schlegel, and M. E. Lee. 1994. Promotion of vascular smooth muscle cell growth by homocysteine: A link to atherosclerosis. *Proc Natl Acad Sci U S A* 91:6369–6373.
80. Torres, L., E. R. García-Trevijano, J. A. Rodríguez, M. V. Carretero, E. Bustos, E. Fernández, E. Eguinoa, J. M. Mato, and M. A. Avila. 1999. Induction of TIMP-1 expression in rat hepatic stellate cells and hepatocytes: A new role for homocysteine in liver fibrosis. *Biochim Biophys Acta* 1455:12–22.

81. Song, Z., Z. Zhou, S. Uriarte, L. Wang, Y. J. Kang, T. Chen, S. Barve, and C. J. McClain. 2004. S-Adenosylhomocysteine sensitizes to TNF-alpha hepatotoxicity in mice and liver cells: A possible etiological factor in alcoholic liver disease. *Hepatology* 40:989–997.

82. Song, Z., Z. Zhou, M. Song, S. Uriarte, T. Chen, I. Deaciuc, and C. J. McClain. 2007. Alcohol-induced S-adenosylhomocysteine accumulation in the liver sensitizes to TNF hepatotoxicity: Possible involvement of mitochondrial S-adenosylmethionine transport. *Biochem Pharmacol* 74:521–531.

83. Feo, F., R. Pascale, R. Garcea, L. Daino, L. Pirisi, S. Frassetto, M. E. Ruggiu, C. Di Padova, and G. Stramentinoli. 1984. Effect of the variations of S-adenosyl-L-methionine liver content on fat accumulation and ethanol metabolism in ethanol-intoxicated rats. *Toxicol Appl Pharmacol* 83:331–341.

84. Song, Z., Z. Zhou, T. Chen, D. Hill, J. Kang, S. Barve, and C. McClain. 2003. S-Adenosylmethionine (SAMe) protects against acute alcohol induced hepatotoxicity in mice. *J Nutr Biochem* 14:591–597.

85. Mato, J. M., J. Cámara, P. Ortiz, J. Rodés, and the Spanish Collaborative Group for the Study of Alcoholic Liver Cirrhosis. 1999. S-Adenosylmethionine in the treatment of alcoholic liver cirrhosis: A randomized, placebo-controlled, double-blind multicentre clinical trial. *J Hepatol* 30:1081–1089.

86. Vendemiale, G., E. Altomare, T. Trizio, C. Le Grazie, C. Di Padova, M. T. Salerno, V. Carrieri, and O. Albano. 1989. Effects of oral S-adenosyl-L-methionine on hepatic glutathione in patients with liver disease. *Scand J Gastroenterol* 24:407–415.

87. Levy, S., C. Herve, E. Delacoux, and S. Erlinger. 2002. Thiamine deficiency in Hepatitis C virus and alcohol-related liver diseases. *Dig Dis Sci* 47:543–548.

88. Hoyumpa, A. M. 1980. Mechanisms of thiamin deficiency in chronic alcoholism. *Am J Clin Nutr* 33:2750–2761.

89. Cook, C. C. H., P. M. Hallwood, and A. D. Thomson. 1998. B vitamin deficiency and neuropsychiatric syndromes in alcohol misuse. *Alcohol Alcohol* 33:317–336.

90. Leevy, C. M., J. Baker, W. TenHove, O. Frank, and G. R. Cherrick. 1965. B-complex vitamins in liver disease of the alcoholic. *Am J Clin Nutr* 16:339–346.

91. Roongpisuthipong, C., A. Sobhonslidsuk, K. Nantiruj, and S. Songchitsomboon. 2001. Nutritional assessment in various stages of liver cirrhosis. *Nutrition* 17:761–765.

92. Leevy, C. M., and S. A. Moroianu. 2005. Nutritional aspects of alcoholic liver disease. *Clin Liver Dis* 9:67–81.

93. Purohit, V., M. F. Abdelmalek, S. Barve, N. J. Benevenga, C. H. Halsted, N. Kaplowitz, K. K. Kharbanda, Q. Liu, S. C. Lu, C. J. McClain, C. Swanson, and S. Zakhari. 2007. Role of S-adenosylmethionine, folate, and betaine in the treatment of alcoholic liver disease: Summary of a symposium. *Am J Clin Nutr* 86:14–24.

94. Santolaria, F., E. Gonzalez-Reimers, J. L. Perez-Manzano, A. Milena, M. A. Gomez-Rodriguez, A. Gonzalez-Diaz, M. J. de la Vega, and A. Martinez-Riera. 2000. Osteopenia assessed by body composition analysis is related to malnutrition in alcoholic patients. *Alcohol* 22:147–157.

95. Gonzalez-Reimers, E., M. C. Duran-Castellon, R. Martin-Olivera, A. Lopez-Lirola, F. Santolaria-Fernandez, M. J. De La Vega-Prieto, A. Perez-Ramirez, and E. Garcia-Valdecasas Campelo. 2005. Effect of zinc supplementation on ethanol-mediated bone alterations. *Food Chem Toxicol* 43:1497–1505.

96. Szatmari, I., and L. Nagy. 2008. Nuclear receptor signaling in dendritic cells connects lipids, the genome and immune function. *EMBO J* 27:2353–2362.

97. Leo, M. A., and C. S. Lieber. 1999. Alcohol, vitamin A, and beta-carotene: Adverse interactions, including hepatotoxicity and carcinogenicity. *Am J Clin Nutr* 69:1071–1085.

98. Gyamfi, M. A., M. G. Kocsis, L. He, G. Dai, A. J. Mendy, and Y. Y. Wan. 2006. The role of retinoid X receptor alpha in regulating alcohol metabolism. *J Pharmacol Exp Ther* 319:360–368.

99. Dai, T., Y. Wu, A. S. Leng, Y. Ao, R. C. Robel, S. C. Lu, S. W. French, and Y. J. Wan. 2003. RXRalpha-regulated liver SAMe and GSH levels influence susceptibility to alcohol-induced hepatotoxicity. *Exp Mol Pathol* 75:194–200.

100. Wells, I. C. 2008. Evidence that the etiology of the syndrome containing type 2 diabetes mellitus results from abnormal magnesium metabolism. *Can J Physiol Pharmacol* 86:16–24.

101. Rylander, R., Y. Megevand, B. Lasserre, W. Amstutz, and S. Granbom. 2001. Moderate alcohol consumption and urinary excretion of magnesium and calcium. *Scand J Clin Invest* 61:401–405.

102. Guerrero-Romero, F., H. E. Tamez-Perez, G. Gonzalez-Gonzalez, A. M. Salinas-Martinez, J. Montes-Villarreal, J. H. Trevino-Ortiz, and M. Rodriguez-Moran. 2004. Oral magnesium supplementation improves insulin sensitivity in non-diabetic subjects with insulin resistance. A double-blind placebo-controlled randomized trial. *Diabetes Metab* 30:253–258.

103. Poikolainen, K., and H. Alho. 2008. Magnesium treatment in alcoholics: A randomized clinical trial. *Subst Abuse Treat Prev Policy* 3:1.

104. Dahle, L. O., G. Berg, M. Hammar, M. Hurtig, and L. Larsson. 1995. The effect of oral magnesium substitution on pregnancy-induced leg cramps. *Am J Obstet Gynecol* 173:175–180.

105. Brown, K. M., and J. R. Arthur. 2001. Selenium, selenoproteins and human health: As review. *Public Health Nutr* 4:593–599.

106. Neve, J. 2000. New approaches to assess selenium status and requirement. *Nutr Rev* 58:363–369.

107. Czuczejko, J., B. A. Zachara, E. Stubach-Topczewska, W. Halota, and J. Kedziora. 2003. Selenium, glutathione and glutathione peroxidases in blood of patients with chronic liver diseases. *Acta Biochim Pol* 50:1147–1154.

108. Jablonska-Kaszewska, I., R. Swiatkowska-Stodulska, J. Lukasiak, W. Dejneka, A. Dorosz, E. Dabrowska, and B. Falkeiwicz. 2003. Serum selenium levels in alcoholic liver disease. *Med Sci Monit* 9 Suppl 3:15–18.

109. Gonzalez-Reimers, E., L. Galindo-Martin, F. Santorlaria-Fernandez, M. J. Sanchez-Perez, J. Alvisa-Negrin, E. Garcia-Valdecasas-Campelo, J. M. Gonzalez-Perez, and M. C. Martin-Gonzalez. 2008. Prognostic value of serum selenium levels in alcoholics. *Biol Trace Elem Res* 125:22–29.

110. Dworkin, B. M., W. S. Rosenthal, R. E. Stahl, and N. K. Panesar. 1988. Decreased hepatic selenium content in alcoholic cirrhosis. *Dig Dis Sci* 33:1213–1217.

111. Bergheim, I., A. Parlesak, C. Dierks, J. C. Bode, and C. Bode. 2003. Nutritional deficiencies in German middle-class male alcohol consumers: Relation to dietary intake and severity of liver disease. *Eur J Clin Nutr* 57:421–438.

112. Steward, S., M. Prince, M. Bassendine, M. Hudson, O. James, D. Jones, C. Record, and C. P. Day. 2007. A randomized trial of antioxidant therapy alone or with corticosteroids in acute alcoholic hepatitis. *J Hepatol* 47:277–283.

113. Patek, A. J., Jr., and J. Post. 1948. Dietary treatment of cirrhosis of the liver; results in 124 patients observed during a 10 year period. *J Am Med Assoc* 138:543–549.

114. Mendenhall, C. L., S. Anderson, R. E. Weesner, S. J. Goldberg, and K. A. Crolic. 1984. Protein-calorie malnutrition associated with alcoholic hepatitis. Veterans Administration Cooperative Study Group on Alcoholic Hepatitis. *Am J Med* 76:211–222.

115. Mendenhall, C. L., T. E. Moritz, G. A. Roselle, T. R. Morgan, B. A. Nemchausky, C. H. Tamburro, E. R. Schiff, C. J. McClain, L. S. Marsano, J. I. Allen, et al. 1993. A study of oral nutritional support with oxandrolone in malnourished patients with alcoholic hepatitis: Results of a Department of Veterans Affairs cooperative study. *Hepatology* 17:564–576.

116. Mendenhall, C., G. A. Roselle, P. Gartside, and T. Moritz. 1995. Relationship of protein calorie malnutrition to alcoholic liver disease: A reexamination of data from two Veterans Administration Cooperative Studies. *Alcohol Clin Exp Res* 19:635–641.

117. Mendenhall, C. L., T. Tosch, R. E. Weesner, P. Garcia-Pont, S. J. Goldberg, T. Kiernan, L. B. Seeff, M. Sorell, C. Tamburro, R. Zetterman, et al. 1986. VA cooperative study on alcoholic hepatitis. II: Prognostic significance of protein-calorie malnutrition. *Am J Clin Nutr* 43:213–218.

118. Kearns, P. J., H. Young, G. Garcia, T. Blaschke, G. O'Hanlon, M. Rinki, K. Sucher, and P. Gregory. 1992. Accelerated improvement of alcoholic liver disease with enteral nutrition. *Gastroenterology* 102:200–205.

119. Cabré, E., P. Rodríguez-Iglesias, J. Caballería, J. C. Quer, J. L. Sánchez-Lombraña, A. Parés, M. Papo, R. Planas, and M. A. Gassull. 2000. Short- and long-term outcome of severe alcohol-induced hepatitis treated with steroids or enteral nutrition: A multicenter randomized trial. *Hepatology* 32:36–42.

120. Charlton, M. 2003. Branched-chain amino acid–enriched supplements as therapy for liver disease: Rasputin lives. *Gastroenterology* 124:1980–1982.

121. Marchesini, G., G. Bianchi, M. Merli, P. Amodio, C. Panella, C. Loguercio, F. Rossi Fanelli, R. Abbiati, and Italian BCAA Study Group. 2003. Nutritional supplementation with branched-chain amino acids in advanced cirrhosis: A double-blind, randomized trial. *Gastroenterology* 124:1792–1801.

122. Hirsch, S., D. Bunout, P. de la Maza, H. Iturriaga, M. Petermann, G. Icazar, V. Gattas, and G. Ugarte. 1993. Controlled trial on nutrition supplementation in outpatients with symptomatic alcoholic cirrhosis. *JPEN J Parenter Enteral Nutr* 17:119–124.

123. Hirsch, S., M. P. de la Maza, V. Gattás, G. Barrera, M. Petermann, M. Gotteland, C. Muñoz, M. Lopez, and D. Bunout. 1999. Nutritional support in alcoholic cirrhotic patients improves host defenses. *J Am Coll Nutr* 18:434–441.

124. Plank, L. D., E. J. Gane, S. Peng, C. Muthu, S. Mathur, L. Gillanders, K. McIlroy, A. J. Donaghy, and J. L. McCall. 2008. Nocturnal nutritional supplementation improves total body protein status of patients with liver cirrhosis: A randomized 12-month trial. *Hepatology* 48:557–566.

12 Nutritional Therapy for Inherited Metabolic Liver Disease

Robin H. Lachmann and Helen Mundy

CONTENTS

12.1 INTRODUCTION

A number of inborn errors of metabolism lead to liver disease. In some of these errors, the functional metabolic defect is located in the liver. For some of these diseases, dietetic therapy is central to their management. In this chapter we discuss the nutritional management of aminoacidopathies, glycogen storage disease (GSD), and disorders of fatty acid oxidation.

12.2 DISORDERS OF AMINO ACID CATABOLISM

There are many disorders of amino acid catabolism. Some disorders, such as PKU, are specific to individual amino acids. In others, the deficient enzyme is involved in the breakdown of a group of amino acids [e.g., branched-chain ketoacid dehydrogenase (BCKD) in maple syrup urine disease (MSUD)]. In urea cycle disorders (UCDs), the detoxification of ammonia, common to the breakdown of all amino acids, is affected. Although these disorders are metabolic intoxications that predominantly affect the nervous system and do not cause liver disease per se, the involved enzymes are expressed in hepatocytes and the metabolic defect is present in the liver. Indeed, liver transplantation can be curative in these disorders (Meyburg and Hoffmann, 2005).

In the following sections, we will briefly describe some of the more common aminoacidopathies, discuss the general principles involved in their dietary management, and give some specific examples of how they are applied in practice (Table 12.1).

12.2.1 PHENYLKETONURIA

Phenylketonuria (PKU) is one of the most common inherited metabolic disorders, with an incidence of about 1 in 10,000 (Scriver and Kaufman, 2001). The majority of cases result from a deficiency in phenylalanine hydroxylase (PAH), which converts phenylalanine into tyrosine. In rare cases, deficiency of tetrahydrobiopterin (a cofactor of PAH) is the culprit. Key concepts of inborn errors and their dietary management are summarized in Table 12.1.

TABLE 12.1

Summary of the Key Concepts Underlying Inherited Metabolic Diseases and Their Dietary Management

1. Inherited metabolic diseases are genetic diseases involving the pathways of intermediary metabolism.
2. Many of these metabolic pathways are expressed in the liver.
3. Disease can be caused by buildup of toxic molecules that can no longer be degraded or by deficiency of essential products that are no longer made.
4. Severity of disease depends on the residual flux through the affected pathway.
5. Patients commonly present in an acute crisis, often triggered by intercurrent infection or by fasting.
6. Dietary treatments are aimed at restoring metabolic balance either by minimizing flux through the affected pathway, and hence preventing the accumulation of toxic metabolites, and/or by replacing missing products of metabolism.

The infant brain is sensitive to high phenylalanine levels and, if left untreated, PKU can lead to severe mental retardation. Microcephaly is common and about 25% of patients have epilepsy. Many older patients have behavioral problems and some suffer from psychotic illnesses. A few patients develop movement disorders with pyramidal and extrapyramidal signs (Brenton and Pietz, 2000). Although most of the pathology is related to brain damage, eczema is also common.

The evidence suggests that high levels of phenylalanine are directly toxic to the developing brain, but the mechanism by which phenylalanine causes damage has not been elucidated. It has been suggested that abnormalities in neurotransmitters, particularly dopamine, which is derived from tyrosine, the levels of which can be low in PKU, might be involved (Surtees and Blau, 2000).

12.2.2 MAPLE SYRUP URINE DISEASE

MSUD is a defect of catabolism of the branched-chain amino acids (BCAAs) valine, leucine, and isoleucine, due to deficiency of BCKD (Chuang and Shih, 2001). MSUD derives its name from the aroma of the accumulated ketoacids excreted in urine. Classical untreated MSUD, with complete deficiency of BCKD, usually presents in the first week of life with nonspecific symptoms that rapidly progress to encephalopathy and death. Partial enzyme activity can result in an intermediate phenotype with variable developmental delay and sometimes intermittent, acute encephalopathic episodes.

Neurotoxicity is directly related to the degree and duration of elevation of the plasma leucine concentration. Acute MSUD is characterized by confusion, hyperactivity, hallucinations, dystonia, and ataxia, which eventually lead to coma. With timely treatment, death and neurodisability can be avoided, even in severe classical forms of MSUD.

12.2.3 METHYLMALONIC ACIDURIA AND PROPIONIC ACIDEMIA

Propionic and methylmalonic acid are biochemical intermediates of BCAA degradation (Fenton et al., 2001). These organic acids have many roles in intermediary metabolism; they participate in the degradation of other amino acids, fatty acid metabolism, the Krebs cycle, gluconeogenesis, and detoxification of ammonia. The most severe forms result in neonatal encephalopathy, which is often fatal. Milder phenotypes may present later in life with acute encephalopathy, developmental delay, movement disorder, or behavioral disturbance. Survivors can suffer from a number of long-term problems; acute pancreatitis, cardiomyopathy and osteopenia occur in both diseases, whereas progressive renal tubular disease is a specific feature of methylmalonic aciduria.

12.2.4 UREA CYCLE DISORDERS

The breakdown of dietary and endogenous protein leads to the production of nitrogen, which must be excreted from the body. The urea cycle is the metabolic pathway that achieves this by incorporating excess nitrogen into urea to be excreted in

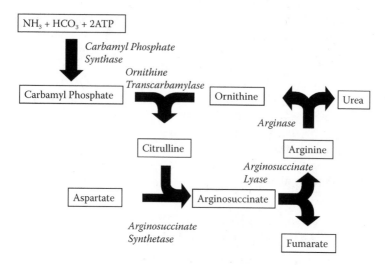

FIGURE 12.1 The urea cycle. Reactions of the urea cycle are shown. Urea cycle disorders can be caused by deficiency of any of these enzymes (shown in italics).

the urine (Figure 12.1). Enzyme defects interrupting this pathway lead to hyperammonemia (Brusilow and Horwich, 2001). In its most severe form, this presents in the neonatal period and results in encephalopathy, cerebral edema, and death. In patients presenting later in life, and particularly adult patients, hyperammonemia can present subacutely, often with psychiatric features. Metabolic decompensation is often triggered by intercurrent illness, or fasting, which can lead to a catabolic state and breakdown of endogenous protein; excessive dietary protein intake can also be a precipitant.

12.2.5 Practical Applications

12.2.5.1 Principles of Dietary Management

In disorders of amino acid metabolism, toxic metabolites are produced when there is excessive breakdown of protein. The protein entering the degradative pathway can either be exogenous in origin (e.g., dietary protein) or endogenous (e.g., in generalized catabolic states such as starvation or intercurrent infection). The amount of protein turnover that can be tolerated varies from patient to patient and depends on the residual activity of the affected metabolic pathway.

The basic aim of dietary management is to reduce the flux through the affected metabolic pathway to a point where the accumulation of toxic metabolites is prevented or controlled at levels that do not give rise to significant clinical manifestations. Management can be split into two phases: long-term treatment, which is aimed at maintaining health by preventing acute episodes, and long-term complications and control of acute metabolic decompensations.

12.2.5.2   Long-Term Management

Diet is a major element in the management of all these disorders. We will use PKU as an example to illustrate the principles involved in the dietary management of amino acid disorders and discuss some specific issues relating to other disorders.

12.2.5.3   Phenylketonuria

Newborn screening for PKU was introduced in the UK in 1969. Diagnosis is now made in the first week of life, and it is possible to institute dietary therapy before the infant sustains any irreversible brain damage. This has completely transformed the prognosis of this disorder.

There are four elements in the dietary management of PKU: restriction of natural protein, use of synthetic supplements to provide adequate essential amino acids and micronutrients, use of special protein-free foods to provide adequate calorie intake, and regular monitoring of blood phenylalanine concentrations.

Natural protein intake, traditionally measured in the UK as phenylalanine exchanges (one exchange containing 50 mg of phenylalanine) is titrated to maintain blood phenylalanine concentrations lower than set target levels, which vary with age and country (Table 12.2). Synthetic, phenylalanine-free amino acid supplements are given (Macdonald et al., 2004). In childhood, the dose is adjusted to maintain normal growth. In adults, a fixed dose (equivalent to 60 g of natural protein in our clinic) is given. Modern supplements often include micronutrients as well, but if necessary these can be given separately. If protein-restricted diet and supplements do not supply enough calories to maintain growth in children or weight in adults, then special low-protein and protein-free dietary products (bread, pasta, rice, flour, etc.) can be added to the diet to meet energy requirements.

Strict control of phenylalanine levels in infancy and early childhood allows normal intellectual development, and patients with PKU now lead normal lives with intellectual and physical achievements similar to their peers. Their diet, however, is quite demanding and although compliance is normally good in infants and young children, it is not uncommon for older children and young adults to want to be able to eat the same things as their friends and family. Although there was initially much concern about what would happen to adolescent patients if they stopped their

TABLE 12.2
Target Blood Phenylalanine Concentrations for UK Patients with PKU on Dietary Treatment

Age (years)	Target Blood Phenylalanine Concentrations (µmol/L)
0–4	120–360
5–10	120–480
11–12	120–700
Adolescents/Adults	120–700

Note: Normal adult reference range is 33–81 µmol/L.

low-protein diets and their phenylalanine levels went up, experience has on the whole been good, and it now seems that after the age of 10 years, the brain is no longer susceptible to the sort of irreversible injury seen in infant brains exposed to high phenylalanine levels (Brenton and Pietz, 2000).

There continue to be concerns about the possible effects of long-term exposure to high phenylalanine levels on the adult brain. There have been case reports of the development of complications such as spastic paraplegia, but these seem to relate to the micronutrient deficiencies these patients can develop when they stop taking their supplements (due to the poor quality of their diets) rather than to phenylalanine exposure per se. Magnetic resonance imaging studies have shown areas of high signal intensity in some patients with high phenylalanine levels, but these are reversible with the reinstitution of diet and do not appear to be clinically significant (Cleary et al., 1995). Neuropsychological studies have shown that performance on certain tests of executive function can be related to phenylalanine levels, but these effects are not consistent and their significance to everyday life is unclear (Channon et al., 2007). Some patients choose to remain on diet because they feel they function better when phenylalanine levels are controlled, often citing improved energy levels and concentration.

In the UK, however, up to 75% of adult patients are on unrestricted diets, and most of them do not feel that this has a significant impact on their lives and are clinically well. However, these patients, who initiated diet in infancy, are still relatively young and it is important to continue to monitor them closely, both to check their micronutrient status and to carefully document their neurological progress as they continue to age.

12.2.6 OTHER DISORDERS

The management of disorders in which the degradation of specific amino acids is impaired (MSUD, tyrosinemia) is basically the same as that of PKU with different, specific amino acid supplements being available for each disorder.

In UCDs, the aim is to restrict protein intake to a level where the residual urea cycle activity is sufficient to prevent ammonia levels from rising excessively. The problem here is that, as ammonia can be generated from all amino acids, it is not possible to use a synthetic supplement to make up the protein requirements (Singh, 2007). Fortunately, there are available drugs that can detoxify ammonia through alternative metabolic pathways (e.g., sodium benzoate, sodium phenylbutyrate) (Enns et al., 2007). In more severely affected patients, these can be used to increase protein tolerance and allow the introduction of essential amino acid supplements.

12.2.7 MANAGEMENT OF ACUTE DECOMPENSATION

Acute metabolic decompensations can occur in MSUD, the organic acidemias, and UCDs. These can be triggered by excessive dietary protein intake, but are more often related to catabolism triggered by an intercurrent illness, by fasting, often before surgery or, particularly in UCDs, in the puerperium, when involution of the uterus involves considerable protein breakdown.

In acute decompensation, medical treatment is often required to reduce the levels of toxic metabolites. Hemodialysis can be used to remove ammonia and toxic amino acids (e.g., leucine in MSUD) from the circulation. Intravenous drugs such as sodium benzoate, sodium phenylbutyrate, and arginine are used in hyperammonemia. The aim of dietary management is to reduce protein breakdown by removing all dietary sources of exogenous protein while providing enough calories to prevent catabolism of endogenous protein.

Initially, calories are given in the form of carbohydrate. If the patient is capable of taking them orally, glucose polymers such as Maxijul can be used. They can also be given to the unconscious patient via a feeding tube. Otherwise, an intravenous infusion of 10% dextrose is given at a rate of 2 mL/kg/h, in adults. Sometimes this will be successful in switching off catabolism, and metabolite levels will decrease and the patient's condition will start to improve after several hours.

If the patient's condition does not improve within 24–48 hours, then more complex nutrition will be required. By this stage, continuing absolute protein restriction will enhance endogenous protein breakdown to sustain obligatory *de novo* protein synthesis and, therefore, becomes counterproductive. If the patient is eating, then (s)he should be given amino acid supplements and it may be possible to introduce some natural protein into the diet. If the patient is unconscious, supplements should be given enterally by tube feeding if possible. Occasionally, TPN may be required; in these cases, it is important to use products with suitable amino acid contents.

12.2.8 PREGNANCY

Pregnancy in women with aminoacidopathies offers a new set of challenges because it is necessary to consider the well-being of the fetus as well as the mother.

Maternal PKU syndrome, consisting of a combination of cardiac and skeletal defects, microcephaly, developmental delay, and low birth weight, is well recognized in babies exposed to high levels of phenylalanine *in utero* (Levy and Ghavami, 1996). It was thought that the teratogenicity of phenylalanine would limit the reproductive options of women with diet-treated PKU: phenylalanine levels in the target ranges used for adults did not prevent the maternal PKU syndrome. Further research has shown, however, that with very strict dietary control, maintaining plasma phenylalanine levels between 100 and 250 μmol/L throughout pregnancy, birth defects can be prevented and the developmental outcome appears to be good. Ideally, mothers are commenced on a preconception diet, with the aim of getting phenylalanine levels into this target range before they conceive (Maillot et al., 2008). If women do conceive when phenylalanine levels are higher than this, then the evidence suggests that, provided that the levels can be brought into the target range before 8 weeks of gestation, the outcome can be good.

Maintaining these phenylalanine levels can be challenging, particularly during early pregnancy. Morning sickness poses special problems: low calorie intake can lead to a catabolic state, which pushes phenylalanine levels up. In these conditions, it may be necessary to omit all natural protein from the diet and it is important to make sure that women are taking sufficient amino acid supplements and calories to suppress catabolism and support fetal growth. Fortunately, as pregnancy progresses and fetal growth accelerates, the mother's protein tolerance tends to increase markedly and their diet becomes less restricted. Once the baby is born, the mother may return to a normal, unrestricted diet, if she wishes.

Although the clinical experience of pregnancy in the other aminoacidopathies is limited, concerns for fetal health are less and raised maternal levels of amino acids such as leucine do not appear to be teratogenic. Careful monitoring is recommended throughout to ensure that the nutritional needs of both mother and fetus are met. In UCDs and MSUD, mothers are at risk for metabolic decompensation in the puerperium, as the uterus involutes, and it is important to remember that the mothers' protein tolerance may decline sharply after birth (although the demands of breastfeeding should be taken into account).

12.3   GLYCOGEN STORAGE DISEASES

GSDs are a heterogeneous group of inherited disorders of carbohydrate metabolism. They are individually rare, with an incidence of 1 in 100,000 to 1 in 300,000 (Chen, 2001). With intensive therapy, their childhood mortality has improved but has brought a burden of chronic adult morbidity.

Most GSDs are single enzyme defects within the glycogenolytic or gluconeogenic pathways (Table 12.3). Enzymes may be required for hepatic or muscular glycogenolysis or both. The pivotal role of the liver in providing energy to the muscle during exercise means that isolated hepatic defects will still have secondary muscle effects. GSD type II and type IV are not defects in energy metabolism and thus have little in common with the others and will not be considered here further.

TABLE 12.3
Classification of GSDs

Type	Enzyme Deficiency	Eponym
Ia	Glucose-6-phosphatase	Von Gierke
Ib	Glucose-6-phosphate transporters	
II	Lysosomal acid maltase	Pompe
III	Debrancher enzyme	Cori/Forbe
IV	Brancher enzyme	Andersen
V	Myophosphorylase	McArdle
VI	Hepatic phosphorylase	Hers
VII	Phosphofructokinase	Tarui
IX	Phosphorylase b kinase	
XI	GLUT 2	Fanconi-Bickel
0	Glycogen synthase	

Note: Classification of GSDs according to the historical numbering system, the enzyme defect, and the eponym.

12.3.1 HEPATIC GLYCOGENOSES

Hepatic glycogenoses present with fasting hypoglycemia, hepatomegaly, central and facial adiposity, short stature, and poor musculature.

GSD I is the most severe disorder as there is not only an abnormality of glycogenolysis, but also of gluconeogenesis. Glucose-6-phosphate cannot cross cell membranes and is metabolized within the liver leading to hyperlactatemia, hypercholesterolemia, hypertriglyceridemia, and hyperuricemia (Figure 12.2).

In GSD 0, III, VI, and IX, gluconeogenesis is preserved. Fasting induces intense ketosis. Some individuals have chronic lipid abnormalities, but milder than in GSD I.

12.3.2 PRACTICAL APPLICATIONS

The aim of therapy is to mimic the role of the liver in providing a continuous and responsive delivery of glucose to the body on fasting. Hypoglycemia is prevented as are the secondary metabolic abnormalities, which result from the hormonal responses to hypoglycemia.

Dietary therapy aims to provide a continuous supply of glucose based on basal glucose production rates in normal children. The method of administration varies with age of the child and between centers. Babies are commenced on continuous overnight nasogastric feeding with milk and frequent, usually 2-hourly, milk feeds during the day to give the calculated glucose requirement. At weaning, some milk feeds are exchanged for measured carbohydrate meals. To prevent excess supply of other nutrients and decrease of appetite in older infants, overnight milk is replaced with a glucose polymer solution.

In children, uncooked cornstarch (UCCS) is given as a slurry made with milk or water. UCCS is not easily absorbed and needs to be introduced slowly to avoid bloating and diarrhea. UCCS is slowly digested to release glucose. The aim is to allow a normal eating pattern with three meals per day. There is variable practice with regard to UCCS at night. Some feel the risk of sudden devastating hypoglycemia with discontinuation of continuous feed contraindicates this approach unless there is no alternative (Wolfsdorf and Crigler, 1997). In some individuals, normoglycemia is only maintained for a very short time after UCCS and they would require multiple doses at night with disruption of sleep and growth (Lee et al., 1996). In practice, the dose and frequency of UCCS is assessed by measuring the glucose and metabolite profile after a single dose. This allows the development of a tailored diet plan, which is updated throughout childhood.

The European Study on GSD I recommended that lactose, fructose, and sucrose be restricted because the inability to metabolize these sugars to glucose may worsen hyperlactatemia (Rake et al., 2002). However, in individuals with poor appetite, this further restricts choice. A modest increase in lactate may also provide an alternative fuel source for the brain in the event of sudden hypoglycemia.

These simple nutritional approaches have revolutionized the outcome for GSD patients but there are many unsolved issues. Growth of most treated patients has improved but the nutritional content of the diet, particularly for adults, is very poor (Mundy et al., 2003). Body composition studies report reduced bone mineral density

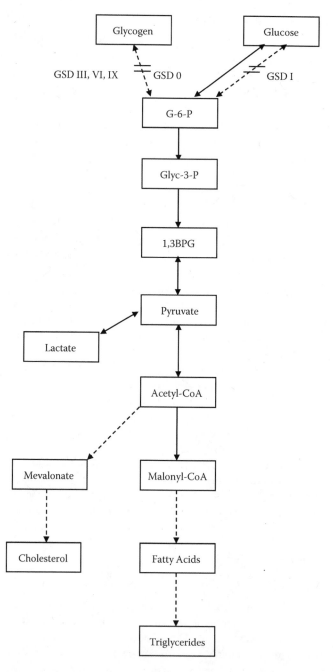

FIGURE 12.2   Abnormal glucose metabolism in GSD I. In GSD I, G-6-P cannot be transported out of the hepatocyte and is metabolized within the liver leading to hyperlactatemia, hypercholesterolemia, and hypertriglyceridemia. Glyc-3-P, glyceraldehyde 3 phosphate; 1,3BPG, 1,3-bisphospheroglycerate; G-6-P, glucose 6-phosphate. Dashed lines indicate multiple reactions.

and body protein with substantially increased body fat, particularly centrally (Mundy et al., 2008).

Glucose requirements differ between patients and, for any individual, also vary depending on activity. Tailored regimens, aided by continuous indwelling glucose monitors, are needed. Recently, a physically modified form of waxy maize starch has been approved that, in some patients, appears able to either increase the length of normoglycemia or reduce the total daily starch dose (Bhattacharya et al., 2007).

Patients with GSD I have hypertriglyceridemia secondary to overproduction of malonyl-CoA, which inhibits carnitine palmitoyltransferase I (Figure 12.2). This is required for long-chain fats to enter the mitochondrion for beta oxidation. A novel approach tested in a few patients has taken advantage of the ability of medium-chain triglycerides (MCT) to enter the mitochondrion without the carnitine system. Further work is needed to validate this approach (Nagasaka et al., 2007).

A subgroup of patients with milder disease found that as the basal metabolic rate reduces with age, they no longer require overnight feeding to maintain normoglycemia. However, other metabolites and counterregulatory hormones remain abnormal. This may manifest as faltering growth and pubertal delay. Some GSD IX adults who ceased treatment in childhood develop marked reduction in bone mineral density.

Alcohol is a potent inhibitor of gluconeogenesis and adults are advised to drink only very moderately and always combined with food.

GSD patients need an emergency regime to be used during illness, when normal diet is not tolerated. This consists of glucose polymer solution given either 2-hourly or continuously via a pump. For diarrhea, an oral rehydration salt can be added but must not be given alone, as the glucose content is insufficient. Failure to tolerate oral fluids requires emergency admission for administration of intravenous dextrose.

Pregnancy in adults with mild disease frequently requires reintroduction of UCCS to maintain normoglycemia. Monitoring of glucose profiles particularly in the second and third trimesters is recommended. The physical demands of labor combined with the usual avoidance of eating necessitate supplementation with intravenous dextrose. Pregnancies are not common but with these measures, outcomes appear good.

12.3.3 Muscle Glycogenoses

Fuel utilization within muscle depends on the duration, type, and intensity of exercise along with intrinsic factors such as conditioning and genetic variation in muscle fiber type. Disorders of glycogenolysis are imposed upon this variance. Symptoms tend to fall into two types: acute exercise intolerance with cramps and even rhabdomyolysis, and chronic progressive muscle dysfunction causing weakness.

Dietary therapy focuses on providing alternative fuels to compensate for the lack of glucose from glycogenolysis. Although therapies such as BCAAs or creatine supplements aimed at improving acute symptoms have appeared effective in a few patients, the results in larger studies are conflicting.

It has been postulated in GSD III that as gluconeogenesis from alanine is possible, then progressive myopathy may be due to degradation of muscle protein to supplement liver gluconeogenesis. Some recommend a very high protein diet for these patients (Slonim et al., 1984). However, this diet is difficult and may have no more benefit than supplementation with carbohydrate.

12.4   FATTY ACID OXIDATION DISORDERS

Fatty acids contribute significantly to energy requirements of the heart at rest and of skeletal muscle during exercise. They supply energy to all tissues during fasting and are a source of ketone bodies, which are the only energy forms, other than glucose, accessible to the brain.

During exercise or fasting, hormonal signals trigger lipolysis in the adipocyte, causing release of free fatty acids from triacylglycerol, which are transported to muscle or liver. Most fatty acids are initially long chain, that is, they have 16–18 carbons attached to a carboxylic acid group. To enter the mitochondrion, they must be first bound by carnitine (Figure 12.3). In the mitochondrion, acetyl-CoA molecules are sequentially released in a spiral of four reactions. The enzyme performing each step depends on the number of remaining carbon atoms and defects can therefore be divided according to whether they affect long-, medium-, or short-chain fatty acid oxidation. With each turn of the spiral, dehydrogenation reactions release electrons to the mitochondrial respiratory chain for production of adenosine triphosphate (ATP). The acetyl-CoA units either enter the tricarboxylic acid cycle or are converted to ketones.

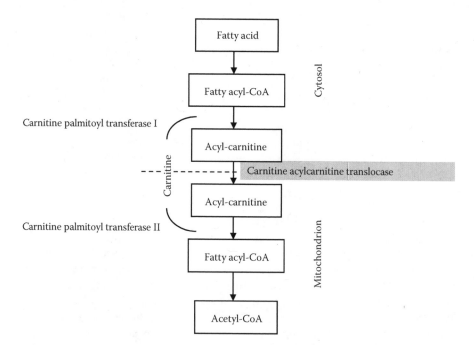

FIGURE 12.3   The carnitine long-chain fatty acid shuttle. To enter the mitochondrion, LCFAs must first be bound by carnitine. Once within the mitochondrion, the carnitine is recycled and acetyl-CoA molecules are sequentially released from the fatty acid, resulting in the generation of ATP by the mitochondrial respiratory chain.

12.4.1   MEDIUM-CHAIN ACYL-COA DEHYDROGENASE DEFICIENCY

Historically, this condition was often only diagnosed postmortem, after cot death, or after presentation with severe hypoketotic, hypoglycemic encephalopathy precipitated by intercurrent illness, resulting in severe morbidity in survivors. In most circumstances, the small baseline requirement for oxidation of medium-chain fats is probably covered by overlapping enzyme substrate specificity and, between episodes of decompensation, individuals with medium-chain acyl-CoA dehydrogenase deficiency (MCADD) appear well. Newborn screening is now available and has dramatically improved the outcome of this disorder.

12.4.2   PRACTICAL APPLICATIONS

Principles of therapy are simple: to avoid increased medium-chain fatty acid oxidation by limiting fasting and providing alternative energy sources during illness. Data on the maximum safe fasting period for individuals with MCADD are scanty. Guidelines for fasting tolerance have been established by the British Inherited Metabolic Disease Group (www.BIMDG.org.uk). These are cautious without being overrestrictive of normal life.

Treatment during intercurrent illness is similar to that already described for GSDs: 2-hourly provision of glucose polymer solution to meet energy requirements and admission for intravenous dextrose if this is not tolerated. The most potent precipitant of decompensation was shown in the prospective British Paediatric Surveillance Unit study of symptomatically presenting MCADD patients to be diarrhea. Therefore, although a regimen with additional salts from oral rehydration solutions is given, patients are recommended to seek additional help early if diarrhea is severe.

Theoretically, decompensation could be induced by hepatotoxic acyl-carnitine derivatives produced consequent to deficient metabolism of ingested MCT. In practice, the concentration of MCT in almost all foods is so low as to be inconsequential. The only products that must be avoided are MCT-enriched medicinal infant and pediatric formulas, and caution is advised in using large quantities of coconut oil.

Adults with MCADD rarely have difficulties unless they drink large quantities of alcohol particularly without eating or have fasted for long periods for medical procedures without adequate provision of dextrose.

Plasma carnitine levels in MCADD are frequently below those of the normal population, and there are rare reports of muscle carnitine deficiency. Treated patients do not appear to have muscle symptoms, and there is little information on exercise tolerance. Standard practice in the UK is not to supplement with carnitine, and outcome appears identical to those countries that do.

12.4.3   LONG-CHAIN FATTY ACID DISORDERS

Long-chain fats must be conjugated with carnitine before they can be transported into the mitochondrion (Figure 12.3). Deficiencies of the enzymes constituting the carnitine shuttle and the transporter for cellular uptake of carnitine cause problems with long-chain fatty acid metabolism. In addition, there are two defects of the fatty acid oxidative spiral: very long chain acyl-CoA dehydrogenase deficiency (VLCADD) and trifunctional protein deficiency, one part of which is long-chain 3-hydroxyacyl-CoA dehydrogenase (LCHAD).

Long-chain fatty acid oxidation disorders (FAODs) share similarities with MCADD in that presentation may be precipitated by metabolic stress and is often with a severe encephalopathy or sudden infant death. They have a more profound effect on muscle and, in particular, cardiac muscle. Long-chain FAODs are one of the few treatable causes of severe cardiomyopathy in childhood. Intercurrent infections are also associated with episodes of muscle breakdown and even rhabdomyolysis. In teenagers and adults, there are often troublesome cramping episodes unrelated to fasting or infections. LCHAD is also associated with peripheral neuropathy and pigmentary retinopathy (Saudubray et al., 1999).

12.4.4 PRACTICAL APPLICATIONS

Carnitine transporter defect can be treated very successfully with supplemental carnitine and use of a glucose polymer-based emergency regimen during illness. There is no need for dietary restriction.

For other disorders, therapy aims to minimize long-chain fatty acid oxidation. This is much more challenging than in MCADD because naturally occurring fats have chain lengths within this specificity. As adipose tissue is rich in long-chain fats, frequent feeds are required to minimize lipolysis.

In infants, overnight continuous nasogastric feeding is used. In adults and older children, multiple doses of UCCS are used. Dosing interval is assessed by profiling glucose, free fatty acids, and long-chain acylcarnitines after a UCCS load.

Dietary restriction of fat is severe. There is little experimental information to guide exact fat restrictions at differing ages. A recently presented European outcome census on long-chain disorders suggested that for patients with LCHAD severe restriction of fat is necessary throughout life, and even with these measures, prognosis is uncertain. The outcome for VLCADD is much better and relaxation of fat restriction may be possible during later life. This disorder shows variability even between siblings with asymptomatic elder siblings being discovered in late childhood after a severe presentation of a younger sibling.

Patients on severe fat-restricted diets require supplementation with essential fatty acids (EFAs) and fat-soluble vitamins. Walnut oil is commonly used in cooking to supplement EFA. Severely fat-restricted diets are energy poor, and this can be supplemented with dietary MCT. There may be an additional benefit in that dietary MCT is rapidly metabolized to ketone bodies, which may inhibit lipolysis.

The role of carnitine in all long-chain disorders is controversial. Untreated patients may be severely carnitine depleted even to the extent of making diagnosis by identification of accumulation of long-chain acylcarnitine species in blood difficult. There is a concern, however, that carnitine supplementation may generate toxic long-chain acylcarnitine derivatives, which may be arrhythmogenic (Corr et al., 1989). Our practice is to only use carnitine in the initial presentation and then only as a small oral dose (50 mg/kg/day).

A novel additional therapy has recently been proposed. Triheptanoate has been reported to have promising effects on cardiomyopathy and rhabdomyolysis in a number of long-chain FAODs (Roe et al., 2002). It is proposed that, in addition to providing acetyl-CoA units, as an odd-chain fat it provides propionyl-CoA, which can be anaplerotic for the tricarboxylic acid cycle. An increased rate of cataplerosis in long-chain fat disorders must be proposed for this theory to be plausible. Although this approach appears to be highly effective, it has been limited by the extreme difficulty in obtaining triheptanoate outside the centers pioneering its use.

For all long-chain FAODs, an emergency regimen, as previously described, for illness is required. Patients with long-chain FAODs are susceptible to decompensation and may require additional treatment with intravenous amino acids and insulin therapy if simple use of glucose polymer is insufficient to prevent catabolism.

12.5 SUMMARY POINTS

- The liver has important roles to play in intermediary metabolism, and many inborn errors of metabolism, even though they may not cause hepatic pathology per se, can be classified as liver diseases.
- The only effective treatment for the most severe forms of these disorders, where there is essentially no activity of the affected metabolic pathway, is liver transplantation.
- Where there is significant residual enzyme activity, nutritional management can be used to control the buildup of toxic metabolites and to replace missing products of metabolic pathways.
- Dietary treatment can be highly successful and, in PKU, has transformed prognosis, allowing patients to live normal lives.
- There is a growing need for physicians and dietitians with expertise in managing these complex disorders.

REFERENCES

Bhattacharya, K., R. C. Orton, X. Qi, H. Mundy, D. W. Morley, M. P. Champion, S. Eaton, R. F. Tester, and P. J. Lee. 2007. A novel starch for the treatment of glycogen storage diseases. *J Inherit Metab Dis* 30:350–357.

Brenton, D. P., and J. Pietz. 2000. Adult care in phenylketonuria and hyperphenylalaninaemia: The relevance of neurological abnormalities. *Eur J Pediatr* 159:S114–S120.

Brusilow, S. W., and A. L. Horwich. 2001. Urea cycle enzymes. In *The Metabolic and Molecular Bases of Inherited Disease*, ed. C. R. Scriver, A. L. Beaudet, W. S. Sly, and D. Valle. New York: McGraw-Hill.

Channon, S., G. Goodman, S. Zlotowitz, C. Mockler, and P. J. Lee. 2007. Effects of dietary management of phenylketonuria on long-term cognitive outcome. *Arch Dis Child* 92:213–218.

Chen, Y.-T. 2001. Glycogen storage disorders. In *The Metabolic and Molecular Bases of Inherited Disease*, ed. C. R. Scriver, A. L. Beaudet, W. S. Sly, and D. Valle. New York: McGraw-Hill.

Chuang, D. T., and V. E. Shih. 2001. Maple syrup urine disease (branched-chain ketoaciduria). In *The Metabolic and Molecular Bases of Inherited Disease*, ed. C. R. Scriver, A. L. Beaudet, W. S. Sly, and D. Valle. New York: McGraw-Hill.

Cleary, M. A., J. H. Walter, J. E. Wraith, F. White, K. Tyler, and J. P. Jenkins. 1995. Magnetic resonance imaging in phenylketonuria: Reversal of cerebral white matter change. *J Pediatr* 127:251–255.

Corr, P. B., M. H. Creer, K. A. Yamada, J. E. Saffitz, and B. E. Sobel. 1989. Prophylaxis of early ventricular fibrillation by inhibition of acylcarnitine accumulation. *J Clin Invest* 83:927–936.

Enns, G. M., S. A. Berry, G. T. Berry, W. J. Rhead, S. W. Brusilow, and A. Hamosh. 2007. Survival after treatment with phenylacetate and benzoate for urea-cycle disorders. *N Engl J Med* 356:2282–2292.

Fenton, W. A., R. A. Gravel, and D.S. Rosenblatt. 2001. Disorders of propionate and methylmalonate metabolism. In *The Metabolic and Molecular Bases of Inherited Disease*, ed. C. R. Scriver, A. L. Beaudet, W. S. Sly, and D. Valle. New York: McGraw-Hill.

Lee, P. J., M. A. Dixon, and J. V. Leonard. 1996. Uncooked cornstarch—efficacy in type I glycogenosis. *Arch Dis Child* 74:546–547.

Levy, H. L., and M. Ghavami. 1996. Maternal phenylketonuria: A metabolic teratogen. *Teratology* 53:176–184.

Macdonald, A., A. Daly, P. Davies, D. Asplin, S. K. Hall, G. Rylance, and A. Chakrapani. 2004. Protein substitutes for PKU: What's new? *J Inherit Metab Dis* 27:363–371.

Maillot, F., M. Lilburn, J. Baudin, D. W. Morley, and P. J. Lee. 2008. Factors influencing outcomes in the offspring of mothers with phenylketonuria during pregnancy: The importance of variation in maternal blood phenylalanine. *Am J Clin Nutr* 88:700–705.

Meyburg, J., and G. F. Hoffmann. 2005. Liver transplantation for inborn errors of metabolism. *Transplantation* 80:S135–S137.

Mundy, H. R., P. C. Hindmarsh, D. R. Matthews, J. V. Leonard, and P. J. Lee. 2003. The regulation of growth in glycogen storage disease type 1. *Clin Endocrinol (Oxf)* 58: 332–339.

Mundy, H. R., J. E. Williams, P. J. Lee, and M. S. Fewtrell. 2008. Reduction in bone mineral density in glycogenosis type III may be due to a mixed muscle and bone deficit. *J Inherit Metab Dis* 31:418–423.

Nagasaka, H., K. Hirano, A. Ohtake, T. Miida, T. Takatani, K. Murayama, T. Yorifuji, K. Kobayashi, M. Kanazawa, A. Ogawa, and M. Takayanagi. 2007. Improvements of hypertriglyceridemia and hyperlacticemia in Japanese children with glycogen storage disease type Ia by medium-chain triglyceride milk. *Eur J Pediatr* 166:1009–1016.

Rake, J. P., G. Visser, P. Labrune, J. V. Leonard, K. Ullrich, and G. P. Smit. 2002. Guidelines for management of glycogen storage disease type I—European Study on Glycogen Storage Disease Type I (ESGSD I). *Eur J Pediatr* 161:S112–S119.

Roe, C. R., L. Sweetman, D. S. Roe, F. David, and H. Brunengraber. 2002. Treatment of cardiomyopathy and rhabdomyolysis in long-chain fat oxidation disorders using an anaplerotic odd-chain triglyceride. *J Clin Invest* 110:259–269.

Saudubray, J. M., D. Martin, P. de Lonlay, G. Touati, F. Poggi-Travert, D. Bonnet, P. Jouvet, M. Boutron, A. Slama, C. Vianey-Saban, J. P. Bonnefont, D. Rabier, P. Kamoun, and M. Brivet. 1999. Recognition and management of fatty acid oxidation defects: A series of 107 patients. *J Inherit Metab Dis* 22:488–502.

Scriver, C. R., and S. Kaufman. 2001. Hyperphenylalaninaemia: Phenylalanine hydroxylase deficiency. In *The Metabolic and Molecular Bases of Inherited Disease*, ed. C. R. Scriver, A. L. Beaudet, W. S. Sly, and D. Valle. New York: McGraw-Hill.

Singh, R. H. 2007. Nutritional management of patients with urea cycle disorders. *J Inherit Metab Dis* 30:880–887.

Slonim, A. E., R. A. Coleman, and W. S. Moses. 1984. Myopathy and growth failure in debrancher enzyme deficiency: Improvement with high-protein nocturnal enteral therapy. *J Pediatr* 105:906–911.

Surtees, R., and N. Blau. 2000. The neurochemistry of phenylketonuria. *Eur J Pediatr* 159:S109–S113.

Wolfsdorf, J. I., and J. F. Crigler, Jr. 1997. Cornstarch regimens for nocturnal treatment of young adults with type I glycogen storage disease. *Am J Clin Nutr* 65:1507–1511.

Section III

Cancer, Viral, and
Immune Diseases

13 Biomarkers of Malnutrition in Liver Cirrhosis

Kazuyuki Suzuki and Yasuhiro Takikawa

CONTENTS

13.1 INTRODUCTION

The liver plays a central role in the metabolism of carbohydrate, protein, fat, vitamins, and minerals. Therefore, the metabolism of these nutritional elements is gradually disturbed with progressive chronic liver disease, resulting in undernourishment and/or malnutrition. Malnutrition is an established complication among patients with liver cirrhosis (LC) (Caregaro et al., 1996; Roongpisuthipong et al., 2001; Campillo et al., 2003; Riggio et al., 2003; Cabre and Gassull, 2005). It is characterized by protein-energy malnutrition (PEM) in LC, which is closely associated with the prognosis of LC, and many factors directly contribute to the pathogenesis of PEM in LC (Tajika et al., 2002; Guglielmi et al., 2005; Tsiaousi et al., 2008).

A flowchart to assess the nutritional status in patients with LC is shown in Figure 13.1. Indeed, statistical and dynamic nutritional assessments are generally recommended to assess the nutritional status of patients with LC (Table 13.1). Dietary assessment by a skilled dietitian, body composition analysis [height, body weight, body mass index (BMI), and anthropometric parameters], biochemical examinations (red blood cell count, hemoglobin, liver function tests, albumin, rapid turnover proteins, cholesterol, cholinesterase, prothrombin time activity, 3-methylhistidine

203

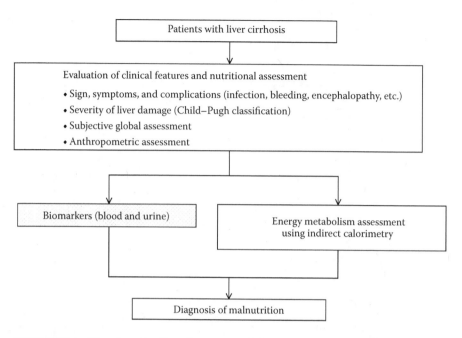

FIGURE 13.1 Flowchart detailing the process of diagnosing malnutrition in patients with LC. SGA and anthropometric parameters should be evaluated to assess the nutritional status in addition to the observation of clinical signs, symptoms, and complications in patients with LC. Because many biomarkers are synthesized by the liver and influenced by factors such as infections, burns, surgery, gastrointestinal disorders, chronic renal failure, and inadequate food intake, care is required to correctly interpret the biomarkers when evaluating PEM in LC. LC, liver cirrhosis; PEM, protein-energy malnutrition; SGA, subjective global assessment.

in urine, etc.), immune competence (total lymphocyte count, delayed cutaneous hypersensitivity, and reaction against purified protein derivative of tuberculin), and energy metabolism assessment [e.g., resting energy expenditure, nonprotein respiratory quotient (npRQ), and substrate oxidation rate for glucose, protein, and fat] using indirect calorimetry are needed to assess the complete nutritional status of patients with LC (Madden and Morgan, 1999; Peng et al., 2007). Although simple and easily applied methods such as the subjective global assessment and anthropometric parameters are recommended in the assessment of nutritional status (Atalay et al., 2008), an examination of biomarkers is essential for an accurate assessment of nutritional status in patients with LC. However, many biomarkers are synthesized by the liver and influenced by factors such as infections, burns, surgery, gastrointestinal disorders, chronic renal failure, and inadequate food intake (Johnson, 1999; Gabay and Kushner, 1999; Kalender et al., 2002). Care is required to correctly interpret the biomarkers when evaluating PEM in LC.

This chapter describes representative biomarkers with which to assess nutritional status in patients with LC.

TABLE 13.1
Recommended Nutritional Assessment in Patients with Liver Cirrhosis

1. Static nutritional status
   a. Daily food intake
   b. Body composition analyses
      Height, body weight, body mass index, anthropometric parameters
   c. Biomarkers
      Red blood cell count, hemoglobin, routine liver function tests, cholesterol, cholinesterase, albumin, rapid turnover protein, prothrombin time, etc. (adipocytokines, ghrelin, vitamins, minerals, etc.), creatinine height index in urine
   d. Immune competence
      Total lymphocyte count, delayed cutaneous hypersensitivity, purified protein derivate of tuberculin
2. Dynamic nutritional status
   a. Energy metabolism (indirect calorimetry)
   b. Nitrogen balance
   c. Urinary 3-methylhistidine excretion
   d. Biomarkers
      Plasma free amino acids (Fischer ratio, BTR)

Note: List of items in the assessment of nutritional status in patients with liver cirrhosis. Fischer ratio, total branched chain amino acids (BCAA)/aromatic amino acids (phenylalanine + tyrosine) molar ratio; BTR, BCAA/tyrosine ratio.

13.2 ALBUMIN, RAPID TURNOVER PROTEINS

Serum albumin is the main secretion protein synthesized by the liver and has multiple functions such as the maintenance of colloid osmotic pressure, ligand binding and transport, and enzymatic and antioxidative activities (Quinlan et al., 2005). The synthesis and degradation rate of serum albumin in patients with LC are decreased as compared with those in healthy individuals whose liver function is normal. The half-life of serum albumin is extended in patients with LC (Moriwaki et al., 2004). Albumin synthesis in the liver is influenced by the severity of liver damage, various hormones, and nutritional and catabolic status such as that conferred by infections and burns (Johnson, 1999; Gabay and Kushner, 1999). However, serum albumin is still frequently applied as a biomarker of malnutrition and/or the severity of liver damage in patients with LC (Child-Pugh classification) (Pugh et al., 1973). When serum albumin is used to assess malnutrition in patients with LC, physicians should confirm whether the daily food intake and pathophysiological conditions are properly and individually estimated.

Serum albumin assumes microheterogeneous, oxidized, and reduced forms (Kawakami et al., 2006). Serum total albumin decreases, whereas the ratio of oxidized albumin increases with LC progression (Watanabe et al., 2004). Furthermore, a recent study has also shown that the oxidation status of serum albumin changes in patients with LC after supplementation with branched-chain amino acids (BCAAs)

(Fukushima et al., 2007). Oxidative stress is an important factor in the progression of chronic liver disease (Moriya et al., 2001). These findings suggest that the oxidative state of serum albumin could be important as a novel marker of not only the severity of liver damage, but also of malnutrition in patients with LC. However, measurements of the oxidative states of serum albumin are time-consuming and rarely performed in the clinical setting.

Prealbumin (transthyretin), retinol-binding protein, and transferrin are markers of short-term nutritional status (Brose, 1990; Calamita et al., 1997; Devakonda et al., 2008) that are synthesized by the liver, and their half-lives are much shorter than that of albumin (Tables 13.2 and 13.3). These proteins are also influenced by baseline conditions such as surgery, infection, and anemia (Johnson, 1999; Gabay and Kushner, 1999).

Retinol-binding protein 4 (RBP-4) has been recently identified as an adipokine, which functions in the pathogenesis of insulin resistance associated with type 2 diabetes and obesity (Yang et al., 2005; Graham et al., 2006). Elevated serum RBP-4 level is an independent predictive marker of early insulin resistance and identifies individuals at risk of developing diabetes (Graham et al., 2006). Because hyperinsulinemia and glucose intolerance are frequently seen in patients with LC and because insulin resistance is an established risk factor for disease progression and survival in patients with chronic liver disease, serum RBP-4 might be a useful biomarker of malnutrition in patients with LC. Indeed, serum RBP-4 levels are decreased and closely correlated with the degree of liver damage according to the Child-Pugh classification (Yagmur et al., 2007). On the other hand, serum RBP-4 levels are impaired because of decreased hepatic production, but they are not associated with insulin resistance (Bahr et al., 2008). The features of serum RBP-4 in patients with LC are

---

TABLE 13.2
Biomarkers in Assessing the Nutritional State in Patients with Liver Cirrhosis

1. Biomarkers in the blood
   - Albumin
   - Rapid turnover proteins (prealbumin, retinol-binding protein, transferrin, etc.)
   - Fischer ratio (BTR)
   - Adipocytokines (leptin, adiponectin, resistin, etc.)
   - Ghrelin
   - Vitamins (A, D, E, K, thiamine, riboflavin, niacin, B_6, B_{12}, C, and folate)
   - Minerals (copper, zinc, iron, manganese, selenium, etc.)
   - Hormones (insulin-like growth factor, insulin-like growth factor–binding protein 3, reverse triiodothyronine, etc.)
2. Biomarkers in the urine
   - Nitrogen (nitrogen balance)
   - Creatinine (creatinine height index)
   - 3-Methylhistidine

Note: Biomarkers used in assessing the nutritional state of patients with liver cirrhosis. BTR, total branched chain amino acids/tyrosine ratio.

TABLE 13.3
Characteristics of Albumin and Rapid Turnover Proteins

	Albumin	Prealbumin	RBP	Transferrin
Half-life time	17–21 days	2 days	0.4–0.7 day	7–10 days
MW	67,000	55,000	21,000	76,500
Functions	Maintenance of colloid osmotic pressure, ligand, and transport of substances including hormones, and antioxidant action	Binding protein of thyroxin, vitamin A transport	Vitamin A transport	Carrier protein of iron, synthesis of hemoglobin
Baseline level Changes in serum level	3.5–5.5 g/dL	20–40 mg/dL	2.2–7.4 mg/dL	200–400 mg/dL
Increased	Dehydration, administration of hormones (steroid, insulin, thyroxin)	Chronic renal failure, hyperthyroidism, pregnancy	Chronic renal failure, fatty liver	Iron deficiency anemia, pregnancy, sex hormone administration
Decreased	Liver injury, nephrotic syndrome, protein-losing gastrointestinal diseases, acute inflammations, infections, burns	Protein malnutrition, liver injury, nephritic syndrome, gastrointestinal diseases, acute inflammations	Vitamin A deficiency, hyperthyroidism, liver injury, infections, burns	Protein malnutrition, liver injury, nephrotic syndrome, inflammations

Note: Characteristic features of albumin and rapid turnover proteins. RBP, retinol-binding protein; MW, molecular weight.

TABLE 13.4
Summary of Serum RBP-4 in Patients with LC

1. Serum RBP-4 levels are decreased in patients with LC and directly related with the severity of liver damage.
2. Serum RBP-4 levels do not correlate with insulin resistance in patients with LC.
3. Lowest RBP-4 levels are seen in cirrhotic patients with histological progression.
4. Hepatic RBP-4 expression is decreased in cirrhotic liver compared with normal liver.

Note: Indications of serum RBP-4 in patients with LC. LC, liver cirrhosis; RBP-4, retinol-binding protein 4.

summarized in Table 13.4. Further studies are required to elucidate how the serum RBP-4 contributes to the development of malnutrition in patients with LC.

13.3   PLASMA FREE AMINO ACIDS

The profile of plasma free amino acids shows characteristic changes in patients with LC (Fischer et al., 1976; Morgan et al., 1978). Levels of BCAAs (valine, leucine, and isoleucine) metabolized in the skeletal muscle are decreased, whereas those of aromatic amino acids (AAA; phenylalanine and tyrosine) metabolized in the liver are increased, resulting in a decreased BCAA/AAA molar ratio (Fischer ratio). These alterations are affected by the severity of liver damage and are closely associated with the development of hepatic encephalopathy (Fischer et al., 1976; Suzuki et al., 2004). However, analyzing amino acid profiles using high-performance liquid chromatography is expensive and time-consuming. Therefore, a straightforward and inexpensive enzymatic method of determining total BCAA and tyrosine levels in serum has been widely applied in Japan to measure the serum BCAA/tyrosine ratio (BTR) and to determine the amino acid balance and severity of liver damage (Azuma et al., 1989). Serum BTR is positively correlated with the plasma Fischer ratio and the serum albumin level in patients with LC (Figure 13.2A and B). A recent report has shown that BTR can help to predict a decrease in serum albumin levels associated with chronic liver disease (Suzuki et al., 2008). Thus, serum BTR might serve as a reliable biomarker of malnutrition in patients with LC.

13.4   ADIPOCYTOKINES

Leptin is a peptide hormone that is produced by adipose tissue affecting both food intake and energy metabolism via sympathetic nerves originating in the hypothalamus, and thus controls the ratio (%) of body fat (Zhang et al., 1994; Weigle et al., 1995). Leptin is involved in the pathogenesis of liver fibrosis (Din et al., 2005). Serum leptin levels are higher in females than males among patients with LC and healthy individuals, and levels positively correlate with BMI, but not with severity of liver damage (McCullough et al., 1998; Campillo et al., 2001). Moreover, serum leptin levels also correlate with arm muscle circumference (AMC) and triceps skinfold thickness (TSF) (Onodera et al., 2001). Because AMC and TSF are commonly decreased in LC patients with malnutrition, the serum leptin level might be useful in assessing malnutrition in such patients, although the gender difference should be considered.

Adiponectin, a peptide hormone produced by adipose tissue, is also an adipocytokine (Schere et al., 1995). Although its physiological role has not been fully elucidated, adiponectin critically influences several components of the metabolic syndrome such as diabetes mellitus and arteriosclerosis (Kadowaki and Yamauchi, 2005; Wang and Scherer, 2007). In particular, plasma adiponectin levels are invariably correlated negatively with BMI and body fat mass, fasting glucose and insulin levels, degree of insulin resistance, blood pressure, and serum total cholesterol and triglyceride levels (Hara et al., 2006). Several reports have described the relationship

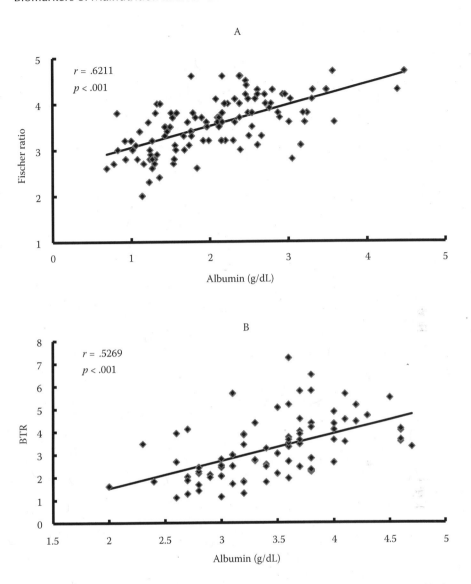

FIGURE 13.2 Correlation between levels of serum albumin and plasma amino acids in patients with LC. Eighty-five cirrhotic patients with or without hepatocellular carcinoma who were admitted at the Iwate Medical University Hospital were investigated. (A) Correlation between serum albumin levels and plasma Fischer ratio. (B) Correlation between serum albumin levels and serum BTR. Fischer ratio, valine + leucine + isoleucine/phenylalanine + tyrosine. BTR, valine + leucine + isoleucine/tyrosine.

between plasma adiponectin levels and steatosis in liver diseases including nonalcoholic steatohepatitis and hepatitis C virus–related chronic hepatitis (Jonsson et al., 2005; Petit et al., 2005). Tietge et al. (2004) and Sohara et al. (2004) have shown that circulating adiponectin levels are significantly increased in LC patients compared with healthy individuals and that they correlate with the severity of liver damage according to the Child-Pugh classification.

Serum adiponectin assumes three forms—low molecular weight, middle molecular weight, and high molecular weight (HMW)—and the latter is deeply involved in the pathogenesis of diabetes mellitus and metabolic syndrome (Kadowaki and Yamauchi, 2005; Hara et al., 2006). Figure 13.3 shows the relationship between plasma HMW adiponectin levels and malnutrition in LC patients. Plasma HMW adiponectin levels are elevated according to the severity of liver damage. Although the clinical significance of the HMW adiponectin remains somewhat obscure, it might be a promising biomarker of nutritional status in LC.

Resistin is a recently identified adipocytokine that might function in obesity and insulin resistance, although its role in humans is controversial (Bahr et al., 2006). However, circulating resistin levels correlate with the severity of liver damage in patients with LC (Kakizaki et al., 2008).

13.5 GHRELIN

Ghrelin was originally discovered as an orexigenic hormone that stimulates growth hormone release (Kojima et al., 1999). This hormone is mainly found in the gastric wall, and it plays a role in the hypothalamic centers to regulate feeding and caloric status (Nakazato et al., 2001). Recent reports have shown that ghrelin controls feeding

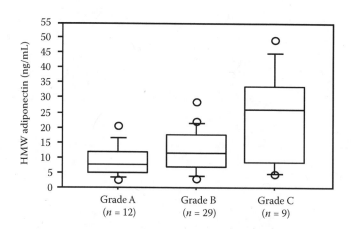

FIGURE 13.3 Relationship between plasma HMW adiponectin levels and severity of liver damage. Forty-seven cirrhotic patients (male 29, female 18) with or without hepatocellular carcinoma who were admitted at Iwate Medical University Hospital were investigated. Etiologies of these patients were HBV ($n = 3$), HCV ($n = 23$), HCV + alcohol ($n = 11$), alcohol ($n = 3$), primary biliary cirrhosis ($n = 3$), nonalcoholic steatohepatitis ($n = 1$), and unknown ($n = 3$). The severity of liver damage was classified into grade A, B, or C based on the Child-Pugh classification. Peripheral plasma samples were collected from all patients after overnight fasting and HMW adiponectin levels were measured using enzyme-linked immunosorbent assay (ELISA) (Fujirebio Co., Tokyo, Japan). LC, liver cirrhosis; HBV, hepatitis B virus; HCV, hepatitis C virus; HMW, high molecular weight.

behavior and the long-term regulation of body weight in association with leptin in the hypothalamic centers (Nakazato et al., 2001; Cummings et al., 2003). Circulating plasma ghrelin level has been considered a marker of pathological conditions such as obesity, insulin resistance, type 2 diabetes mellitus, hypertension, and *Helicobacter pylori* (HP) infection (Nwokolo et al., 2003; Kalaitzakis et al., 2007). Evaluation of plasma ghrelin levels in patients with LC has generated conflicting data (Tacke et al., 2003; Marchesini et al., 2004). However, we have recently shown that plasma ghrelin (desacyl form) levels in patients with LC are not higher than those in healthy controls, and that they do not correlate with the severity of liver damage; rather, the ghrelin level is closely associated with renal failure and inflammatory status (Takahashi et al., 2006). Figures 13.4 and 13.5 (reproduced with permission) show that the plasma ghrelin level significantly correlates with anthrometric parameters such as BMI, AMC, and TSF, and energy metabolic parameters such as npRQ, substrate oxidation rates for glucose (%CHO), and fat (%FAT) in patients with LC. Furthermore, plasma ghrelin level is negatively correlated with the level of serum leptin. Infection with HP did not influence the plasma ghrelin level in our study. Therefore, fasting plasma ghrelin level might be an interesting marker of malnutrition in patients with stable LC who do not have severe complications such as renal failure and infection.

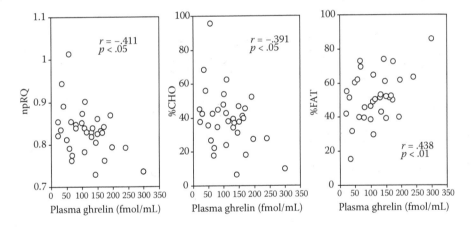

FIGURE 13.4 Relationship between plasma ghrelin levels and energy metabolism determined using indirect calorimetry. Thirty-four cirrhotic patients (male 20, female 14) with or without hepatocellular carcinoma who were admitted at Iwate Medical University Hospital were investigated. Etiologies of patients were HBV ($n = 1$), HCV ($n = 18$), HCV + alcohol ($n = 3$), alcohol ($n = 8$), primary biliary cirrhosis ($n = 1$), and unknown ($n = 3$). The severity of liver damage was classified into grade A, B, or C based on the Child-Pugh classification. Peripheral plasma samples were collected from all patients during the morning after overnight fasting and ghrelin levels were measured using ELISA (Mitsubishi Kagaku Iatoron Inc., Tokyo, Japan). Energy metabolism was measured using direct calorimeter (Deltatrac-II Metabolic Monitor, Datax Division Inst. Corp., Helsinki, Finland). npRQ, nonprotein respiratory quotients; %CHO, oxidation rate of glucose; %FAT, oxidation rate of fat; LC, liver cirrhosis; HBV, hepatitis B virus; HCV, hepatitis C virus. (From Takahashi, T., Kato, A., Onodera, K., and Suzuki, K., *Hepatol Res*, 24, 117–123, 2006. With permission.)

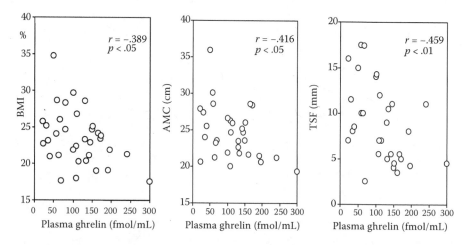

FIGURE 13.5 Relationship between plasma ghrelin levels and anthrometric parameters. AMC and TSF were measured using a commercial anthropometer. BMI, body mass index; AMC, arm muscle circumference; TSF, triceps skin-fold thickness. (From Takahashi, T., Kato, A., Onodera, K., and Suzuki, K., *Hepatol Res*, 24, 117–123, 2006. With permission.)

13.6   OTHER MARKERS

The nutritional status of patients with chronic liver diseases is often assessed using levels of vitamins (fat-soluble; A, D, E, K, and water-soluble; thiamine, riboflavin, niacin, B_6, B_{12}, C, and folate), minerals (mainly copper, zinc, iron, manganese, and selenium), and hormones (insulin-like growth factor 1, insulin-like growth factor–binding protein 3, reverse triiodothyronine, etc.) (Assy et al., 1998; Cabre and Gassull, 2005; Morgan and Heaton, 2008). However, because these biomarkers are also influenced by the severity of liver damage and baseline conditions such as food intake, alcohol abuse, cholestasis, and infection, the data must be carefully interpreted.

13.7   SUMMARY POINTS

- Subjective global assessment and measurement of anthrometric parameters are essential to accurately evaluate nutritional status in patients with LC.
- Malnutrition, in particular PEM type, is closely associated with the prognosis of patients with LC.
- Biomarkers, such as albumin, rapid turnover protein, amino acids, adipocytokines, ghrelin, vitamins, and minerals, are useful in assessing malnutrition.
- Data of biomarkers must be carefully interpreted, because they are often influenced by the severity of liver damage and other factors including diminished nutrient intake, alcohol, impaired digestion, absorption of nutrients, hypermetabolic, or catabolic state.

REFERENCES

Assy, N., Z. Hochberg, R. Enat, et al. 1998. Prognostic value of generation of growth hormone-stimulated insulin-like growth factor–1 (IGF-1) and its binding protein-3 in patients with compensated and decompensated liver cirrhosis. *Dig Dis Sci* 43:1317–1321.

Atalay, B. G., C. Yagmur, T. Z. Nursal, et al. 2008. Use of subjective global assessment and clinical outcomes in critically ill geriatric patients receiving nutrition support. *JPEN J Parenter Enteral Nutr* 32:454–459.

Azuma, Y., M. Maekawa, Y. Kuwabara, et al. 1989. Determination of branched-chain amino acid and tyrosine in serum of patients with various hepatic diseases and its clinical usefulness. *Clin Chem* 35:1399–1403.

Bahr, M. J., K. H. Boeker, M. P. Manns, et al. 2008. Decreased hepatic RBP4 secretion is correlated with reduced hepatic glucose production but not associated with insulin resistance in patients with liver cirrhosis. *Clin Endocrinol (Oxf)* 68:1–22. http://www.blackwell-synergy.com/loi/cen.pdf.

Bahr, M. J., J. Ockenga, K. H. W. Böker, et al. 2006. Elevated resistin levels in cirrhosis are associated but not with insulin resistance. *Am J Physiol Endocrinol Metab* 29:E199–E206.

Brose, L. 1990. Prealbumin as a marker of nutritional status. *J Burn Care Rehab* 11:372–375.

Cabre, E., and M. A. Gassull. 2005. Nutrition in liver cirrhosis. *Curr Opin Clin Nutr Metab Care* 8:545–551.

Calamita, A., I. Dichi, S. J. Papini-Berto, et al. 1997. Plasma levels of transthyretin and retinol-binding protein in Child-A cirrhotic patients in relation to protein-calorie status and plasma amino acids, zinc, vitamin A and plasma thyroid hormones. *Arq Gastroenterol* 34:139–147.

Campillo, B., J. P. Richardet, E. Scherman, et al. 2003. Evaluation of nutritional practice in hospitalized cirrhotic patients: Results of a prospective study. *Nutrition* 19:515–521.

Campillo, B., E. Sherman, J. P. Richardet, et al. 2001. Serum leptin levels in alcoholic liver cirrhosis: Relationship with gender, nutritional status, liver function and energy metabolism. *Eur J Clin Nutr* 55:980–988.

Caregaro, L., F. Alberino, P. Amodio, et al. 1996. Malnutrition in alcoholic and virus-related cirrhosis. *Am J Clin Nutr* 63:602–609.

Cummings, D. E., D. S. Weigle, S. Frayo, et al. 2003. Plasma ghrelin levels after diet-induced weight loss or gastric bypass surgery. *New Engl J Med* 346:1623–1630.

Devakonda, A., L. George, S. Raoof, et al. 2008. Transthyretin as a marker to predict outcome in critically ill patients. *Clin Biochem* 41:1126–1130.

Din, X., N. K. Saxena, S. Lin, et al. 2005. The role of leptin and adiponectin: A novel paradigm in adipocytokine regulation of liver fibrosis and stellate cell biology. *Am J Pathol* 166:1655–1699.

Fischer, J. E., H. M. Rosen, A. M. Ebeid, et al. 1976. The effect of normalization of plasma amino acids on hepatic encephalopathy. *Surgery* 80:77–91.

Fukushima, H., Y. Miwa, M. Shiraki, et al. 2007. Oral branched-chain amino acid supplementation improves the oxidized/reduced albumin ratio in patients with liver cirrhosis. *Hepatol Res* 37:765–70.

Gabay, C., and I. Kushner. 1999. Acute-phase proteins and other systemic responses to inflammation. *N Engl J Med* 340:448–454.

Graham, T. E., Q. Yang, M. Bluher, et al. 2006. Retinol-binding protein 4 and insulin resistance in lean, obese, and diabetic subjects. *N Engl J Med* 354:2552–2563.

Guglielmi, F. W., C. P. Panella, A. Buda, et al. 2005. Nutritional state and energy balance in cirrhotic patients with or without hypermetabolism. Multicenter prospective study by the 'Nutritional Problems in Gastroenterology' Section of the Italian Society of Gastroenterology (SIGE). *Dig Liver Dis* 37:681–688.

Hara, K., M. Horikoshi, T. Yamauchi, et al. 2006. Measurement of the high-molecular weight form of adiponectin in plasma is useful for the prediction of insulin resistance and metabolic syndrome. *Diabetes Care* 29:1357–1362.

Johnson, A. M. 1999. Low levels of plasma proteins malnutrition or inflammation? *Clin Chem Lab Med* 37:91–96.

Jonsson, J. R., A. R. Moschen, I. J. Hickman, et al. 2005. Adiponectin and its receptors in patients with chronic hepatitis C. *J Hepatol* 43:929–936.

Kadowaki, T., and T. Yamauchi. 2005. Adiponectin and adiponectin receptors. *Endocr Rev* 26:439–451.

Kakizaki, S., N. Sohara, Y. Yamazaki, et al. 2008. Elevated plasma resistin concentrations in patients with liver cirrhosis. *J Gastroenterol Hepatol* 23:73–77.

Kalaitzakis, E., I. Bosaeus, L. Ohman, et al. 2007. Altered postprandial glucose, insulin, leptin, and ghrelin in liver cirrhosis: Correlations with energy intake and resting energy expenditure. *Am J Clin Nutr* 85:808–815.

Kalender, B., B. Mutlu, M. Ersöz, et al. 2002. The effects of acute phase proteins on serum albumin, transferrin and haemoglobin in haemodyalysis patients. *Int J Clin Pract* 56:505–508.

Kawakami, A., K. Kubota, N. Yamada, et al. 2006. Identification and characterization of oxidized human serum albumin. A slight structural change impairs its ligand-binding and anti-oxidant functions. *FEBS J* 273:3346–3357.

Kojima, M., H. Hosoda, Y. Date, et al. 1999. Ghrelin is a growth-hormone–releasing acylated peptide from stomach. *Nature* 402:656–660.

Liu, C. J., P. J. Chen, Y. M. Jeng, et al. 2005. Serum adiponectin correlates with viral characteristics but not histological features in patients with chronic hepatitis C. *J Hepatol* 43:235–242.

Madden, A. M., and M. Y. Morgan. 1999. Resting energy expenditure should be measured in patients with cirrhosis, not predict. *Hepatology* 30:655–664.

Marchesini, G., N. Villanova, G. Bianchi, et al. 2004. Plasma ghrelin concentrations, food intake, and anorexia in liver disease. *J Clin Endocrinol Metab* 89:2136–2141.

McCullough, A. J., E. Bugianesi, G. Marchesini, et al. 1998. Gender-dependent alterations in serum leptin in alcoholic cirrhosis. *Gastroenterology* 115:947–953.

Morgan, M. Y., and K. W. Heaton. 2008. Nutrition, the liver, and gallstones. 2000. In *Human Nutrition and Dietetics*, ed. J. S. Garrow, W. P. T. Janes, and A. Ralph. London: Churchill Livingstone, pp. 575–603.

Morgan, M. Y., J. P. Milsom, and S. Sherlock. 1978. Plasma ratio of valine, leucine and isoleucine to phenylalanine and tyrosine in liver disease. *Gut* 19:1068–1073.

Moriwaki, H., Y. Miwa, M. Tajika, et al. 2004. Branched-chain amino acids as a protein- and energy-source in liver cirrhosis. *Biochem Biophys Res Commun* 313:405–409.

Moriya, K., K. Nakagawa, T. Santa, et al. 2001. Oxidative stress in the absence of inflammation in a mouse model for hepatitis C virus–associated hepatocarcinogenesis. *Cancer Res* 61:4365–4370.

Nakazato, M., N. Murakami, Y. Date, et al. 2001. A role of ghrelin in the central regulation of feeding. *Nature* 409:194–198.

Nwokolo, C. U., D. A. Freshwater, P. O'Hare, et al. 2003. Plasma ghrelin following cure of *Helicobacter pylori*. *Gut* 52:637–640.

Onodera, K., A. Kato, and K. Suzuki. 2001. Serum leptin concentrations in liver cirrhosis: Relationship to the severity of liver dysfunction and their characteristic diurnal profiles. *Hepatol Res* 21:205–212.

Peng, S., L. D. Plank, J. L. McCall, et al. 2007. Body composition, muscle function, and energy expenditure in patients with liver cirrhosis: A comprehensive study. *Am J Clin Nutr* 85:1257–1266.

Petit, J. M., A. Minello, V. Jooste, et al. 2005. Decreased plasma adiponectin concentrations are closely related to steatosis in hepatitis C virus–infected patients. *J Clin Endocrinol Metab* 90:2240–2243.

Pugh, R. N. H., I. M. Murray-Lyon, J. L. Dawson, et al. 1973. Transection of the oesophagus for bleeding oesophageal varices. *Br J Surg* 60:646–649.

Quinlan, G. J., G. S. Martin, and T. W. Evans. 2005. Albumin: Biochemical properties and therapeutic potential. *Hepatology* 41:1211–1219.

Riggio, O., S. Angeloni, L. Ciuffa, et al. 2003. Malnutrition is not related to alterations in energy balance in patients with stable liver cirrhosis. *Clin Nutr* 22:553–559.

Roongpisuthipong, C., A. Sobhonslidsuk, K. Nantiruj, et al. 2001. Nutritional assessment in various stages of liver cirrhosis. *Nutrition* 17:761–765.

Schere, P. E., S. Williams, M. Fogliano, et al. 1995. Novel serum protein similar to C1q produced exclusively in adipocytes. *J Biol Chem* 270:26746–26749.

Sohara, N., H. Takagi, S. Kakizaki, et al. 2004. Elevated plasma adiponectin concentrations in patients with liver cirrhosis correlate with plasma insulin levels. *Liver Int* 25:28–32.

Suzuki, K., A. Kato, and M. Iwai. 2004. Branched-chain amino acid treatment in patients with liver cirrhosis. *Hepatol Res* 30S:S25–S29.

Suzuki, T., K. Suzuki, K. Koizumi, et al. 2008. Measurement of serum branched-chain amino acid to tyrosine ratio level is useful in a prediction of a change of serum albumin level in chronic liver disease. *Hepatol Res* 38:267–272.

Tacke, F., G. Brabant, E. Kruck, et al. 2003. Ghrelin in chronic liver disease. *J Hepatol* 38:447–454.

Tajika, M., M. Kato, H. Mohri, et al. 2002. Prognostic value of energy metabolism in patients with viral liver cirrhosis. *Nutrition* 18:229–234.

Takahashi, T., A. Kato, K. Onodera, et al. 2006. Fasting plasma ghrelin levels reflect malnutrition state in patients with liver cirrhosis. *Hepatol Res* 24:117–123.

Tietge, U. J., K. H. Boker, M. P. Manns, et al. 2004. Elevated circulating adiponectin levels in liver cirrhosis are associated with reduced liver function and altered hepatic hemodynamics. *Am J Physiol Endocrinol Metab* 287:E82–E89.

Tsiaousi, I. E., A. I. Hatzitolios, S. K. Trygonis, et al. 2008. Malnutrition in end stage liver disease: Recommendations and nutritional support. *J Gastroenterol Hepatol* 23:527–533.

Wang, Z. V., and P. E. Scherer. 2007. Adiponectin, cardiovascular function, and hypertension. *Hypertension* 51:8–14.

Watanabe, A., S. Mastuzaki, H. Moriwaki, et al. 2004. Problem in serum albumin measurement and clinical significance of albumin microheterogeneity in cirrhosis. *Nutrition* 20:351–357.

Weigle, D. S., T. R. Bukowski, D. C. Foster, et al. 1995. Recombinant ob protein reduces feeding and body weight in the *ob/ob* mouse. *J Clin Invest* 96:2065–2070.

Yagmur, E., R. Weiskirchen, A. M. Gressner, et al. 2007. Insulin resistance in liver cirrhosis is not associated with circulating retinol-binding protein 4. *Diabetes Care* 30:1168–1172.

Yang, Q., T. E. Graham, N. Mody, et al. 2005. Serum retinol binding protein 4 contributes to insulin resistance in obesity and type 2 diabetes. *Nature* 436:356–362.

Zhang, Y., R. Procnca, M. Maffei, et al. 1994. Positional cloning of the mouse obese gene and its human homologue. *Nature* 372:425–432.

14 Malnutrition in Liver Cirrhosis: Effects of Nutritional Therapy

Kristina Norman and Matthias Pirlich

CONTENTS

14.1 PREVALENCE AND IMPACT OF MALNUTRITION IN LIVER CIRRHOSIS

Malnutrition with muscle wasting is a common complication in patients with liver cirrhosis (Tables 14.1 and 14.2). Reported prevalence from large cross-sectional studies ranges from approximately 30% to more than 50%, depending on the criteria used for the assessment of malnutrition (Norman et al., 2008a). There is evidence that malnutrition already occurs in the early stages of the disease but becomes more frequent with the progression of cirrhosis (Peng et al., 2007). Malnutrition in liver cirrhosis is mainly characterized by reduced visceral (lower plasma levels of albumin) as well as somatic protein deficiency, manifested by, for example, decreased muscle and body cell mass (Peng et al., 2007; Pirlich et al., 2000) and accompanied

217

TABLE 14.1

Key Features of Malnutrition and High Protein Intake in Liver Disease

1. Malnutrition is common in liver cirrhosis and impairs outcome.
2. Nutritional intake is frequently inadequate but can be enhanced by individualized nutritional counseling and oral supplements.
3. High protein intake is beneficial and recommended.
4. Hepatic encephalopathy is rarely attributable to high protein intake.
5. Energy and protein (with, e.g., BCAA) supplementation in the late evening reduces fat and protein oxidation and thus improves nitrogen retention and protein synthesis.

Note: Summary of key features concerning malnutrition and the nutritional therapy with high-protein intake and branched-chain amino acids (BCAA).

by muscle weakness (Peng et al., 2007) as well as impaired quality of life (Norman et al., 2006) (Table 14.3).

Nutritional intake is often reduced (Marchesini et al., 2004; Nielsen et al., 1993) and nutritional therapy in hospitals is frequently inadequate (Campillo et al., 2003) due to either low awareness or insufficient nutritional knowledge of the staff.

14.2 CAUSES OF MALNUTRITION: REDUCED FOOD INTAKE

Reduced nutritional intake is a well-known phenomenon and is a major contributing factor in impaired nutritional status in liver cirrhosis. However, the etiology

TABLE 14.2

Potential Causes of Muscle Wasting and Malnutrition in Liver Disease

Causes	Consequences
Hypermetabolism[a]	Increased demand
Increased protein requirements	
Inflammation	
Loss of appetite	Decreased intake/altered resorption
Physical inactivity	
Portal hypertension/ascites	
Low hepatic glycogen stores	Disturbed metabolism/rapid onset of catabolic state
Disturbed GH/IGF axis	
Glucose intolerance/insulin resistance	

Note: Potential and evidenced causes for malnutrition and, in particular, muscle wasting in liver disease.

[a] Hypermetabolism is found in up to 34% of cirrhotic patients. The growth hormone (GH) insulin-like growth factor (IGF) is disturbed with high GH and low IGF-I, which indicates a state of severe GH resistance, which in turn might be a major contributing factor to protein catabolism and thus muscle wasting.

TABLE 14.3

Association of Malnutrition with Well-Being and Outcome in Liver Disease

Impact on body composition

    Decreased body cell mass

    Decreased muscle mass

    Decreased fat mass

Functionality and well-being

    Lower muscle strength

    Reduced quality of life

    Increased fatigue

Clinical features

    Higher incidence of encephalopathy

    Increased intestinal permeability

    Decreased immune function

Outcome

    Poor outcome after liver transplantation

    Decreased overall survival

Note: Malnutrition is associated with impaired well-being and decreased functionality as well as reduced
outcome in patients with liver disease.

of impaired nutritional intake is still not completely clear. The possible association between portal hypertension and disturbed gastric motility and accommodation might be one explanation. Studies on gastric relaxation, however, have yielded inconsistent results due to different methodologies or patient selection: Izbeki et al. (2002) found impaired accommodation of proximal stomach in patients with alcoholic liver disease and Aprile et al. (2002) demonstrated reduced gastric relaxation in patients with portal hypertension, whereas Kalatzaikis et al. (2007b) reported increased proximal stomach accommodation but an apparent disturbed relation between gastric accommodation and energy intake in cirrhotic patients. Aqel et al. (2005) investigated gastric accommodation in cirrhotic patients with ascites and found a reduced postprandial gastric volume and accommodation ratio, and also that large-volume paracentesis increased both fasting volumes and volumes ingested until maximal satiation as well as caloric intake.

Moreover, loss of appetite occurs frequently in patients with liver cirrhosis despite high ghrelin concentrations (Marchesini et al., 2004) and has been linked to increased brain tryptophan availability (Laviano et al., 1997).

14.3 ROLE OF INFLAMMATION

Most cachectic conditions are associated with underlying inflammatory processes, which are in part mediated by an increased production of proinflammatory cytokines such as interleukins 1 and 6 and tumor necrosis factor α. These cytokines are associated with anorexia and depression, and play a role in hypermetabolism, protein catabolism, and insulin resistance. However, events that trigger increased

production of cytokines in disease-related cachexia remain unclear. In liver cirrhosis, disturbed gut integrity allowing passage of bacterial endotoxins into the blood
has been reported (Pascual et al., 2003). The presence of endotoxins presents a potent
stimulus for cytokine production by mononuclear cells. The gut might, therefore,
play a significant role in the pathogenesis of the cachexia syndrome (Norman and
Pirlich, 2008). It has also been shown that malnourished patients with advanced liver
cirrhosis, in fact, exhibit increased small intestinal bowel permeability when compared to patients with liver cirrhosis with normal nutritional status (Norman et al.,
2007). Moreover, cytokine receptors have been shown to be higher in patients with
cachectic liver cirrhosis (Gerstner et al., 2000) and related with the resting energy
expenditure (REE) corrected for body cell mass.

14.4   METABOLIC ABNORMALITIES CONTRIBUTING
TO PROTEIN CATABOLISM

It has been demonstrated that patients with liver cirrhosis experience a catabolic state
of starvation more rapidly than healthy subjects. Owen et al. (1983) reported that cirrhotic patients are comparable to healthy people undergoing a 2- to 3-day period of
total starvation after just one overnight fast. Zillikens and colleagues (1993) observed
increased nocturnal protein turnover rates and increased early morning levels of free
fatty acids, lactate, insulin, glucagons, and growth hormone. Oral glucose administration at night improved nitrogen balance with a decrease in protein turnover rate
and decreased β-hydroxybutyrate, urea, and glucagon levels.

Similarly, Nakaya and colleagues (2002) also demonstrated significantly lower
respiratory quotient (RQ) after the overnight fast. The reduced quotient of produced
CO^2 and consumed O^2 indicates increased protein and fat oxidation. This suggests
that glycogen storage in liver cirrhosis is insufficient and cannot maintain blood glucose during the fasting period. The decreased nonprotein RQ is particularly harmful
to patients with liver cirrhosis who are already prone to malnutrition.

Hypermetabolism, which is associated with poorer outcome, is found in about
15–34% of patients with liver cirrhosis (Muller et al., 1999; Peng et al., 2007). Since
the REE is highly variable in these patients, it should be measured and not predicted
(Muller et al., 1999).

Furthermore, the growth hormone/insulin-like growth factor (GH/IGF) axis is
disturbed with high GH concentration and low IGF-I levels, indicating a state of
severe GH resistance, which might be a major contributing factor to the protein
catabolism and thus muscle wasting observed in liver cirrhosis (Plank et al., 2008).

14.4.1   GLUCOSE INTOLERANCE AND INSULIN RESISTANCE

Altered glucose metabolism is a common feature of chronic liver disease with 60–80%
of patients with cirrhosis showing impaired glucose tolerance and 10–35% developing overt diabetes (Bahr et al., 2008; Muller et al., 1994). In these patients, hyperglycemia results mainly from impaired nonoxidative glucose disposal in peripheral
tissues due to insulin resistance, whereas hepatic glucose output appears to play no

role. The current hypothesis on the pathogenesis of insulin resistance in patients with cirrhosis is based on persistent hyperinsulinemia observed frequently in these patients. Hyperinsulinemia results from both decreased hepatic first pass clearance of insulin due to capillarization of the hepatic sinusoids and extensive collateral blood flow as well as increased pancreatic insulin secretion (Bahr et al., 2008). Hyperinsulinemia, in turn, causes peripheral insulin receptor down-regulation or dysfunction, which might also contribute to muscle protein catabolism. Interestingly, these abnormalities persist even after liver transplantation (Tietge et al., 2004).

14.4.2 IMPAIRED GLYCOGEN STORES

Krahenbuhl et al. (2003) demonstrated decreased hepatic glycogen stores per volume of hepatocytes and per liver mass in both alcoholic and biliary liver cirrhosis. They concluded that both the loss of hepatocytes as well as impaired hepatocellular glycogen metabolism, such as decreased activity of glucokinase, are responsible for the inadequate glycogen stores, which in turn induces energy production from fatty acids as well as increased gluconeogenesis from amino acids.

14.4.3 INCREASED PROTEIN REQUIREMENTS

Postprandial albumin fractional synthesis rate as well as nonoxidative leucine disposal appears to be reduced in patients with stable liver cirrhosis (Tessari et al., 2002) as opposed to healthy subjects. Dichi et al. (2001) showed increased protein catabolism in fasting patients with advanced liver cirrhosis (Dichi et al., 2001) in contrast to patients with Child-Pugh class A cirrhosis (Dichi et al., 1996). When fed a high-protein diet, however, patients were able to significantly increase their nitrogen retention regardless of severity of disease, indicating enhanced protein requirements in liver cirrhosis. Swart et al. (1989a) concluded that 60 g of protein was sufficient to achieve a positive nitrogen balance in a small study with patients with liver cirrhosis, whereas 40 g was not. Other authors have also found evidence of increased protein requirements; Nielsen et al. (1995) reported efficient protein retention with increased protein intake that was dependent on energy balance.

A 50-g increase in daily protein intake, moreover, has been shown to increase the functional hepatic nitrogen clearance by approximately 40% in patients with alcoholic cirrhosis, which was comparable to that in healthy subjects (Hamberg et al., 1992).

Moreover, studies on high enteral protein administration have shown improvement of liver function parameters such as prothrombin time and albumin (Cabre et al. 1990; Kearns et al., 1992; Norman et al., 2008b) with no signs of hepatic encephalopathy.

Summarizing these data, there is strong evidence that a high protein intake might prevent and treat protein catabolism in liver cirrhosis. In the light of these findings, it is alarming that unnecessary low-protein diets are still regularly being prescribed as surveys in Great Britain, South Wales, and Australia by both Soulsby and Morgan (1999) and Heyman et al. (2006) show.

14.5   EFFECTS OF REGULAR DIET AND NUTRITIONAL COUNSELING

It is feasible to improve oral nutritional intake in patients with liver cirrhosis. Bories and Campillo (1994) reported increased energy and protein intake in patients with alcoholic cirrhosis ($n = 30$) after 1 month of regular oral diet in a hospital (providing 40 kcal/kg/day), which paralleled the improvement of liver function parameters such as albumin and prothrombin time. Moreover, in a small nonrandomized study, regular oral diet for 1 month, supervised by a dietitian in a rehabilitative unit, increased anthropometric parameters in severely malnourished cirrhotic patients ($n = 26$) (mean Child-Pugh score, 9.1 ± 0.5) (Campillo et al., 1995). In a further study, the authors were able to identify refractory ascites and hypometabolism as adverse factors for the improvement of nutritional status under oral nutritional therapy, whereas both nutritional status and liver function simultaneously improved after oral regular diet regardless of Child-Pugh class (Campillo et al., 1997).

The effects of 3-month ambulatory oral supplementation (approximately 370 kcal/day) and repeated nutritional counseling were observed in a small pilot study by Cunha et al. (2004) in patients with alcoholic cirrhosis ($n = 29$). It was shown that about two-thirds of patients accepted the nutritional therapy and anthropometric parameters, serum proteins as well as the Child-Pugh score, improved during the study period.

Manguso et al. (2005) studied the effect of an adequate oral diet (30–40 kcal/kg body weight; 16% protein) after individualized nutritional counseling in patients with hepatitis C virus–related liver cirrhosis ($n = 90$; Child A or B) in a randomized double-period crossover study design with a 3-month period of spontaneous nutritional intake followed by a controlled adequate oral diet or vice versa. They were able to report good compliance to the nutritional therapy and improved nutritional parameters as well as increased serum albumin in both groups after the periods with controlled diet.

These studies demonstrate that individualized dietary counseling is a useful means for achieving adequate energy intake and improvement of nutritional status in patients with liver cirrhosis in the ambulatory setting.

14.6   PREVENTION OF PROTEIN CATABOLISM: LATE EVENING SNACKS

To counter the rapid transition to the fasting state, Chang et al. (1997) studied the effects of a carbohydrate-rich late evening meal (50 g) on energy metabolism and substrate oxidation in a small randomized study in patients with liver cirrhosis. The group receiving the late evening snack experienced a significant increase in both RQ and carbon dioxide production, indicating shortened overnight fasting with more economic fuel utilization.

Swart and colleagues investigated the impact of a late evening meal on the nitrogen balance in patients with liver cirrhosis in a randomized crossover study comparing three meals a day with four and six meals a day, both including a late meal at 11 P.M. (20% of total daily protein and energy intake). The authors reported an improved nitrogen balance in the group receiving meal schedules including the late evening snack (Swart et al., 1989b). These results were recently confirmed by a 12-month randomized intervention study in 103 patients with liver cirrhosis, who received a supplement either at daytime (between 9:00 A.M. and 7:00 P.M.) or at night-time (between 9:00 P.M. and 7:00 A.M.). Nocturnal supplementation resulted in a significant accretion of total body protein, whereas daytime supplementation did not, although daily energy and protein intakes did not differ between groups. Quality of life also increased earlier in the nighttime group (at 6 vs. 12 months in the daytime group) (Plank et al., 2008).

14.7   LATE EVENING SNACK WITH BRANCHED-CHAIN AMINO ACIDS

Nakaya et al. (2002) compared the effects of late evening administration with oral glucose, a carbohydrate rich snack, or a mixture enriched with branched-chained amino acids (BCAA). Supplementation with carbohydrates and BCAA increased RQ and blood glucose to a similar degree, whereas oral administration of glucose resulted in a significantly greater rise of blood glucose. This might represent a problem, since many patients with liver cirrhosis suffer from glucose intolerance (Muller et al., 1994). In a recent study, however, simultaneous administration of the glucosidase inhibitor voglibose achieved blood sugar control in patients with impaired glucose tolerance (Korenaga et al., 2008).

Furthermore, administration of BCAA provides the possibility of nocturnal protein synthesis. Yamauchi et al. (2001) studied the effects of a late night snack with BCAA on protein metabolism in a randomized study. They demonstrated decreased excretion of 3-methylhistidine as well as decreased concentration of serum free fatty acid in the group receiving the late evening snack (10:30 P.M.) as compared to the group ingesting the BCAA supplement after dinner (7:00 P.M.), indicating improved protein metabolism and reduced lipolysis primarily after late night administration of BCAA supplements.

Okamoto et al. (2003) also reported reduced fat oxidation with increased RQ after a late evening snack containing BCAA. Although blood glucose levels did rise after the meal, fasting blood sugar did not change during the 7-day study. The same authors also compared the effects of a single late evening snack (10:00 P.M.) with BCAA to the provision of two snacks with BCAA (one between 10:00 A.M. and 3:00 P.M. and one at 10:00 P.M.). They observed comparable increased RQ and reduced fat oxidation in both groups as well as a correlation between the nonprotein RQ and the creatinine height index (Tsuchiya et al., 2005). Similarly, Fukushima et al. (2003) reported that nocturnal supplementation of BCAA improved serum albumin in patients over the course of 1 week, whereas the same dose did not alter serum albumin when given at daytime. This indicates that BCAA administered at night appear to be more beneficial by producing a higher nitrogen balance, presumably due to the lower consumption of BCAA for energy generation during the day.

Results from these small studies on short-term provision of late evening snacks with BCAA were confirmed in a larger, long-term randomized study in 48 patients with hepatitis C virus–related liver cirrhosis (Nakaya et al., 2007). During the 3-month period, fuel utilization as well as serum albumin and nitrogen balance was significantly improved in the group receiving the late evening snack containing BCAA compared to the control group, which received ordinary food as late evening snack. Their total energy intake was not different, although the protein intake was higher in the intervention patients. Neither diet, however, had a significant effect on quality of life.

Taken together, these studies indicate that late night provision of energy and protein is beneficial for reducing the catabolic state induced by the overnight fast in cirrhosis.

14.8 LONG-TERM EFFECTS OF BRANCHED-CHAIN AMINO ACIDS

Beside the above-mentioned findings, BCAA have long been the focus of research in liver disease. Patients with cirrhosis exhibit decreased BCAA levels in the plasma amino acid analysis, which is partly due to the enhanced BCAA uptake by the skeletal muscles for ammonia detoxification and energy generation (Moriwaki et al., 2004). However, BCAA appear to be beneficial not only for improving hepatic encephalopathy, but have also been demonstrated to improve nutritional parameters, event-free survival as well as quality of life of patients with liver cirrhosis in large multicenter trials on long-term BCAA supplementation (Marchesini et al., 2003; Muto et al., 2005).

14.9 SAFETY OF HIGH PROTEIN INTAKE REGARDING HEPATIC ENCEPHALOPATHY

Historically, nutrient protein was found to be associated with the occurrence of hepatic encephalopathy (Schwartz et al., 1954) leading to protein restriction as a common dietary practice even in nonencephalopathic subjects. However, current knowledge on hepatic encephalopathy enables a more differentiated view: in most patients, hepatic encephalopathy is triggered by other factors such as constipation, infection, bleeding, exsiccosis, or electrolyte imbalance, whereas high protein intake is very rarely a problem in patients with liver cirrhosis (Mas et al., 2006). As mentioned above, several tube-feeding studies with high-protein formulas demonstrated the safety in regard to the occurrence of hepatic encephalopathy.

Several studies have also compared the effects of equicaloric and equinitrogenous high-protein diets from animal versus vegetable origin (Bianchi et al., 1993; Uribe et al., 1982) in patients with various degrees of chronic encephalopathy. High-protein diets of vegetable origin were not only tolerated but consistently showed improvement of psychometric parameters.

A diet reduced in protein, on the contrary, may even be harmful to patients with liver damage due to their catabolic state. Moreover, it has even been suggested that malnutrition contributes to the onset of hepatic encephalopathy (Kalaitzakis et al., 2007a). In fact, a high protein intake is recommended and might actually prevent the occurrence of hepatic encephalopathy (Plauth et al., 2006).

TABLE 14.4
Practical Applications Modified from Evidence-Based ESPEN Guidelines on Enteral Nutrition in Liver Disease

Topic	Recommendation
Recommended energy intake	35–40 kcal/kg BW/day (147–168 kJ/kg BW/day)
Recommended protein intake	1.2–1.5 g/kg BW/day
Application	1. Oral food with adequate individualized nutritional advice (five to six small meals including a late evening snack with carbohydrates and protein)
	2. If patients cannot meet their caloric requirements through oral route, use supplemental enteral nutrition
Route	If patients are not able to maintain adequate oral intake from normal food, use
	1. Oral nutritional supplements
	2. Tube feeding (even in the presence of esophageal varices)
Type of formula	1. Whole protein formulae
	2. More concentrated high-energy formulae in patients with ascites
Hepatic encephalopathy	1. BCAA-enriched formulae
	2. Protein from vegetable origin

Note: Summary of evidence-based ESPEN guidelines on enteral nutrition in liver disease from 2006, and practical advice on nutritional therapy in patients with liver cirrhosis. ESPEN, European Society for Clinical Nutrition and Metabolism; BW, body weight; BCAA, branched-chain amino acids.

14.10 SUMMARY POINTS

- Malnutrition is frequent in liver cirrhosis and impairs outcome.
- Patients with liver cirrhosis need individualized dietary counseling.
- Nutritional therapy should include modification of the diet in regard to both a higher protein intake and a higher meal frequency including late evening snacks (Table 14.4).
- These snacks should be rich in carbohydrates and protein to reduce overnight catabolism.
- Furthermore, there is evidence that patients benefit from the long-term administration of branched-chain amino acids containing supplements.

REFERENCES

Aprile, L. R., U. G. Meneghelli, A. L. Martinelli, and C. R. Monteiro. 2002. Gastric motility in patients with presinusoidal portal hypertension. *Am J Gastroenterol* 97:3038–3044.

Aqel, B. A., J. S. Scolapio, R. C. Dickson, D. D. Burton, and E. P. Bouras. 2005. Contribution of ascites to impaired gastric function and nutritional intake in patients with cirrhosis and ascites. *Clin Gastroenterol Hepatol* 3:1095–1100.

Bahr, M. J., K. H. Boeker, M. P. Manns, and U. J. Tietge. 2008. Decreased hepatic RBP4 secretion is correlated with reduced hepatic glucose production but not associated with insulin resistance in patients with liver cirrhosis. *Clin Endocrinol (Oxf)*.

Bianchi, G. P., G. Marchesini, A. Fabbri, A. Rondelli, E. Bugianesi, M. Zoli, and E. Pisi. 1993. Vegetable versus animal protein diet in cirrhotic patients with chronic encephalopathy. A randomized cross-over comparison. *J Intern Med* 233:385–392.

Bories, P. N., and B. Campillo. 1994. One-month regular oral nutrition in alcoholic cirrhotic patients. Changes of nutritional status, hepatic function and serum lipid pattern. *Br J Nutr* 72:937–946.

Cabre, E., F. Gonzalez-Huix, A. Abad-Lacruz, M. Esteve, D. Acero, F. Fernandez-Banares, X. Xiol, and M. A. Gassull. 1990. Effect of total enteral nutrition on the short-term outcome of severely malnourished cirrhotics. A randomized controlled trial. *Gastroenterology* 98:715–720.

Campillo, B., P. N. Bories, M. Leluan, B. Pornin, M. Devanlay, and P. Fouet. 1995. Short-term changes in energy metabolism after 1 month of a regular oral diet in severely malnourished cirrhotic patients. *Metabolism* 44:765–770.

Campillo, B., P. N. Bories, B. Pornin, and M. Devanlay. 1997. Influence of liver failure, ascites, and energy expenditure on the response to oral nutrition in alcoholic liver cirrhosis. *Nutrition* 13:613–621.

Campillo, B., J. P. Richardet, E. Scherman, and P. N. Bories. 2003. Evaluation of nutritional practice in hospitalized cirrhotic patients: Results of a prospective study. *Nutrition* 19:515–521.

Chang, W. K., Y. C. Chao, H. S. Tang, H. F. Lang, and C. T. Hsu. 1997. Effects of extra-carbohydrate supplementation in the late evening on energy expenditure and substrate oxidation in patients with liver cirrhosis. *JPEN J Parenter Enteral Nutr* 21:96–99.

Cunha, L., N. M. Happi, A. L. Guibert, D. Nidegger, P. Beau, and M. Beauchant. 2004. Effects of prolonged oral nutritional support in malnourished cirrhotic patients: Results of a pilot study. *Gastroenterol Clin Biol* 28:36–39.

Dichi, I., J. B. Dichi, S. J. Papini-Berto, A. Y. Angeleli, M. H. Bicudo, T. A. Rezende, and R. C. Burini. 1996. Protein-energy status and 15N-glycine kinetic study of Child A cirrhotic patients fed low- to high-protein energy diets. *Nutrition* 12:519–523.

Dichi, J. B., I. Dichi, R. Maio, C. R. Correa, A. Y. Angeleli, M. H. Bicudo, T. A. Rezende, and R. C. Burini. 2001. Whole-body protein turnover in malnourished patients with Child class B and C cirrhosis on diets low to high in protein energy. *Nutrition* 17:239–242.

Fukushima, H., Y. Miwa, E. Ida, S. Kuriyama, K. Toda, Y. Shimomura, A. Sugiyama, J. Sugihara, E. Tomita, and H. Moriwaki. 2003. Nocturnal branched-chain amino acid administration improves protein metabolism in patients with liver cirrhosis: Comparison with daytime administration. *JPEN J Parenter Enteral Nutr* 27:315–322.

Gerstner, C., T. Schutz, A. Roské, and H. Lochs. 2000. Correlation between energy expenditure, nutrient intake, malnutrition and activation of the inflammatory system in patients with liver cirrhosis. *Clin Nutr* 19:7.

Hamberg, O., K. Nielsen, and H. Vilstrup. 1992. Effects of an increase in protein intake on hepatic efficacy for urea synthesis in healthy subjects and in patients with cirrhosis. *J Hepatol* 14:237–243.

Heyman, J. K., C. J. Whitfield, K. E. Brock, G. W. McCaughan, and A. J. Donaghy. 2006. Dietary protein intakes in patients with hepatic encephalopathy and cirrhosis: Current practice in NSW and ACT. *Med J Aust* 185:542–543.

Izbeki, F., I. Kiss, T. Wittmann, T. T. Varkonyi, P. Legrady, and J. Lonovics. 2002. Impaired accommodation of proximal stomach in patients with alcoholic liver cirrhosis. *Scand J Gastroenterol* 37:1403–1410.

Kalaitzakis, E., R. Olsson, P. Henfridsson, I. Hugosson, M. Bengtsson, R. Jalan, and E. Bjornsson. 2007a. Malnutrition and diabetes mellitus are related to hepatic encephalopathy in patients with liver cirrhosis. *Liver Int* 27:1194–1201.

Kalaitzakis, E., M. Simren, H. Abrahamsson, and E. Bjornsson. 2007b. Role of gastric sensorimotor dysfunction in gastrointestinal symptoms and energy intake in liver cirrhosis. *Scand J Gastroenterol* 42:237–246.

Kearns, P. J., H. Young, G. Garcia, T. Blaschke, G. O'Hanlon, M. Rinki, K. Sucher, and P. Gregory. 1992. Accelerated improvement of alcoholic liver disease with enteral nutrition. *Gastroenterology* 102:200–205.

Korenaga, K., M. Korenaga, K. Uchida, T. Yamasaki, and I. Sakaida. 2008. Effects of a late evening snack combined with alpha-glucosidase inhibitor on liver cirrhosis. *Hepatol Res* 38:1087–1097.

Krahenbuhl, L., C. Lang, S. Ludes, C. Seiler, M. Schafer, A. Zimmermann, and S. Krahenbuhl. 2003. Reduced hepatic glycogen stores in patients with liver cirrhosis. *Liver Int* 23:101–109.

Laviano, A., C. Cangiano, I. Preziosa, O. Riggio, L. Conversano, A. Cascino, S. Ariemma, and F. F. Rossi. 1997. Plasma tryptophan levels and anorexia in liver cirrhosis. *Int J Eat Disord* 21:181–186.

Manguso, F., G. D'Ambra, A. Menchise, R. Sollazzo, and L. D'Agostino. 2005. Effects of an appropriate oral diet on the nutritional status of patients with HCV-related liver cirrhosis: A prospective study. *Clin Nutr* 24:751–759.

Marchesini, G., G. Bianchi, P. Lucidi, N. Villanova, M. Zoli, and P. De Feo. 2004. Plasma ghrelin concentrations, food intake, and anorexia in liver failure. *J Clin Endocrinol Metab* 89:2136–2141.

Marchesini, G., G. Bianchi, M. Merli, P. Amodio, C. Panella, C. Loguercio, F. F. Rossi, and R. Abbiati. 2003. Nutritional supplementation with branched-chain amino acids in advanced cirrhosis: A double-blind, randomized trial. *Gastroenterology* 124:1792–1801.

Mas, A. 2006. Hepatic encephalopathy: From pathophysiology to treatment. *Digestion* 73:86–93.

Moriwaki, H., Y. Miwa, M. Tajika, M. Kato, H. Fukushima, and M. Shiraki. 2004. Branched-chain amino acids as a protein- and energy-source in liver cirrhosis. *Biochem Biophys Res Commun* 313:405–409.

Muller, M. J., J. Bottcher, O. Selberg, S. Weselmann, K. H. Boker, M. Schwarze, A. von zur Mühlen, and M. P. Manns. 1999. Hypermetabolism in clinically stable patients with liver cirrhosis. *Am J Clin Nutr* 69:1194–1201.

Muller, M. J., M. Pirlich, H. J. Balks, and O. Selberg. 1994. Glucose intolerance in liver cirrhosis: Role of hepatic and non-hepatic influences. *Eur J Clin Chem Clin Biochem* 32:749–758.

Muto, Y., S. Sato, A. Watanabe, H. Moriwaki, K. Suzuki, A. Kato, M. Kato, T. Nakamura, K. Higuchi, S. Nishiguchi, and H. Kumada. 2005. Effects of oral branched-chain amino acid granules on event-free survival in patients with liver cirrhosis. *Clin Gastroenterol Hepatol* 3:705–713.

Nakaya, Y., N. Harada, S. Kakui, K. Okada, A. Takahashi, J. Inoi, and S. Ito. 2002. Severe catabolic state after prolonged fasting in cirrhotic patients: Effect of oral branched-chain amino-acid–enriched nutrient mixture. *J Gastroenterol* 37:531–536.

Nakaya, Y., K. Okita, K. Suzuki, H. Moriwaki, A. Kato, Y. Miwa, K. Shiraishi, H. Okuda, M. Onji, H. Kanazawa, H. Tsubouchi, S. Kato, M. Kaito, A. Watanabe, D. Habu, S. Ito, T. Ishikawa, N. Kawamura, and Y. Arakawa. 2007. BCAA-enriched snack improves nutritional state of cirrhosis. *Nutrition* 23:113–120.

Nielsen, K., J. Kondrup, L. Martinsen, H. Dossing, B. Larsson, B. Stilling, and M. G. Jensen. 1995. Long-term oral refeeding of patients with cirrhosis of the liver. *Br J Nutr* 74:557–567.

Nielsen, K., J. Kondrup, L. Martinsen, B. Stilling, and B. Wikman. 1993. Nutritional assessment and adequacy of dietary intake in hospitalized patients with alcoholic liver cirrhosis. *Br J Nutr* 69:665–679.

Norman, K., S. Buhner, U. Friedrich, K. Schelwies, C. Moliner, H. Lochs, J. Ockenga, and M. Pirlich. 2007. Enhanced intestinal permeability in liver cachexia. *JPEN J Parenter Enteral Nutr* 31:35.

Norman, K., H. Kirchner, H. Lochs, and M. Pirlich. 2006. Malnutrition affects quality of life in gastroenterology patients. *World J Gastroenterol* 12:3380–3385.

Norman, K., C. Pichard, H. Lochs, and M. Pirlich. 2008a. Prognostic impact of disease-related malnutrition. *Clin Nutr* 27:5–15.

Norman, K., and M. Pirlich. 2008. Gastrointestinal tract in liver disease: Which organ is sick? *Curr Opin Clin Nutr Metab Care* 11:613–619.

Norman, K., C. Smoliner, N. Stobaeus, T. Schutz, H. Lochs, J. Ockenga, and M. Pirlich. 2008b. T1475 Early enteral nutrition improves functional parameters in liver cirrhosis. *Gastroenterology* 134:A-563.

Okamoto, M., I. Sakaida, M. Tsuchiya, C. Suzuki, and K. Okita. 2003. Effect of a late evening snack on the blood glucose level and energy metabolism in patients with liver cirrhosis. *Hepatol Res* 27:45–50.

Owen, O. E., V. E. Trapp, G. A. Reichard Jr., M. A. Mozzoli, J. Moctezuma, P. Paul, C. L. Skutches, and G. Boden. 1983. Nature and quantity of fuels consumed in patients with alcoholic cirrhosis. *J Clin Invest* 72:1821–1832.

Pascual, S., J. Such, A. Esteban, P. Zapater, J. A. Casellas, J. R. Aparicio, E. Girona, A. Gutierrez, F. Carnices, J. M. Palazon, J. Sola-Vera, and M. Perez-Mateo. 2003. Intestinal permeability is increased in patients with advanced cirrhosis. *Hepatogastroenterology* 50:1482–1486.

Peng, S., L. D. Plank, J. L. McCall, L. K. Gillanders, K. McIlroy, and E. J. Gane. 2007. Body composition, muscle function, and energy expenditure in patients with liver cirrhosis: A comprehensive study. *Am J Clin Nutr* 85:1257–1266.

Pirlich, M., T. Schutz, T. Spachos, S. Ertl, M. L. Weiss, H. Lochs, and M. Plauth. 2000. Bioelectrical impedance analysis is a useful bedside technique to assess malnutrition in cirrhotic patients with and without ascites. *Hepatology* 32:1208–1215.

Plank, L. D., E. J. Gane, S. Peng, C. Muthu, S. Mathur, L. Gillanders, K. McIlroy, A. J. Donaghy, and J. L. McCall. 2008. Nocturnal nutritional supplementation improves total body protein status of patients with liver cirrhosis: A randomized 12-month trial. *Hepatology* 48:557–566.

Plauth, M., E. Cabre, O. Riggio, M. Assis-Camilo, M. Pirlich, J. Kondrup, P. Ferenci, E. Holm, D. S. Vom, M. J. Muller, and W. Nolte. 2006. ESPEN guidelines on enteral nutrition: Liver disease. *Clin Nutr* 25:285–294.

Schwartz, R., G. B. Phillips, J. E. Seegmiller, G. J. Gabuzda Jr., and C. S. Davidson. 1954. Dietary protein in the genesis of hepatic coma. *N Engl J Med* 251:685–689.

Soulsby, C. T., and M. Y. Morgan. 1999. Dietary management of hepatic encephalopathy in cirrhotic patients: Survey of current practice in United Kingdom. *BMJ* 318:1391.

Swart, G. R., J. W. van den Berg, J. K. van Vuure, T. Rietveld, D. L. Wattimena, and M. Frenkel. 1989a. Minimum protein requirements in liver cirrhosis determined by nitrogen balance measurements at three levels of protein intake. *Clin Nutr* 8:329–336.

Swart, G. R., M. C. Zillikens, J. K. van Vuure, and J. W. van den Berg. 1989b. Effect of a late evening meal on nitrogen balance in patients with cirrhosis of the liver. *BMJ* 299:1202–1203.

Tessari, P., R. Barazzoni, E. Kiwanuka, G. Davanzo, G. De Pergola, R. Orlando, M. Vettore, and M. Zanetti. 2002. Impairment of albumin and whole body postprandial protein synthesis in compensated liver cirrhosis. *Am J Physiol Endocrinol Metab* 282:E304–E311.

Tietge, U. J., O. Selberg, A. Kreter, M. J. Bahr, M. Pirlich, W. Burchert, M. J. Muller, M. P. Manns, and K. H. Boker. 2004. Alterations in glucose metabolism associated with liver cirrhosis persist in the clinically stable long-term course after liver transplantation. *Liver Transpl* 10:1030–1040.

Tsuchiya, M., I. Sakaida, M. Okamoto, and K. Okita. 2005. The effect of a late evening snack in patients with liver cirrhosis. *Hepatol Res* 31:95–103.

Uribe, M., M. A. Marquez, R. G. Garcia, M. H. Ramos-Uribe, F. Vargas, A. Villalobos, and C. Ramos. 1982. Treatment of chronic portal-systemic encephalopathy with vegetable and animal protein diets. A controlled crossover study. *Dig Dis Sci* 27:1109–1116.

Yamauchi, M., K. Takeda, K. Sakamoto, M. Ohata, and G. Toda. 2001. Effect of oral branched chain amino acid supplementation in the late evening on the nutritional state of patients with liver cirrhosis. *Hepatol Res* 21:199–204.

Zillikens, M. C., J. W. van den Berg, J. L. Wattimena, T. Rietveld, and G. R. Swart. 1993. Nocturnal oral glucose supplementation. The effects on protein metabolism in cirrhotic patients and in healthy controls. *J Hepatol* 17:377–383.

15 General Dietary Management of Liver Cancer

Mazen Issa and Kia Saeian

CONTENTS

Primary liver cancer is the fifth most common malignancy in the world[1] and is known to result in alterations in host metabolism. These alterations are believed to result in malnutrition and cachexia[2,3] and to influence morbidity and mortality. The multifaceted relationship between general nutrition and liver cancer in particular is complex. More is known about the potential role of nutrition in the pathogenesis and prevention of liver cancer than nutritional intervention for treatment of liver cancer. In this chapter, we delineate the various components of the relationship between nutrition and liver cancer with a specific focus on the available knowledge on general dietary treatments for patients with liver cancer.

15.1   DIET AS RISK FACTOR FOR LIVER CANCER

Chronic infections with hepatitis B virus (HBV) and, to a lesser extent, hepatitis C virus (HCV)[4] are the major worldwide risk factors for development of hepatocellular carcinoma (HCC), the major type of liver cancer. However, the development of cirrhosis from whatever etiology remains a major risk factor for HCC. In fact, the risk of HCC in patients with chronic hepatitis C appears to be confined to those who have developed concomitant cirrhosis. It follows then that dietary factors resulting in the development of cirrhosis portend a substantial risk for development of HCC. Worldwide, diet is second only to tobacco as a preventable cause of all cancers and it is postulated that dietary factors may contribute to up to 30% of malignancies in Western countries.[5]

Excessive alcohol consumption remains the main diet-related risk factor for liver cancer in Western countries via the development of cirrhosis.[6] In developing countries, ingestion of foods contaminated with the mycotoxin aflatoxin[7,8] remains an important and best-studied risk.

Aflatoxin is a common and unavoidable contaminant of food staples in many developing countries. This toxin is produced by fungal action during production, harvest, storage, and food processing. The associated increased risk of HCC is caused by deletion mutations in the p53 tumor-suppressing gene and by activation of dominant oncogenes.[9] The risk of cancers due to exposure to the various forms of aflatoxin is well established[10] and is based on the cumulative lifetime dose. The International Cancer Research Institute identifies aflatoxin as a Class 1 carcinogen, resulting in the regulation of this toxin to very low concentrations in traded commodities (20 ppb in grains and 0.5 ppb in milk in the United States; 4 ppb in foods in some European countries[11]). A strong synergy has been reported between aflatoxin and chronic hepatitis B in the development of HCC. In hepatitis B surface antigen–positive subjects, aflatoxin is about 30 times more potent than in persons without the virus,[12] and the relative risk of cancer for HBV patients increases from approximately 5 with only HBV infection to about 60 when HBV infection and aflatoxin exposure are combined.[13] The magnitude of the impact of this synergy takes on epidemic proportions in developing countries in which HBV and HCV affect 8–20% of the population.

15.2   DIET AND PREVENTION OF LIVER CANCER

An important element in the relationship between diet and liver cancer is prevention. In this arena, there has been much interest in inquiry into foods having nonnutritive components that may provide protection against a variety of illnesses, including hepatic and gastrointestinal malignancies. Foremost among these agents have been antioxidants. Despite a number of preliminary experimental and epidemiological studies suggesting a preventive role for antioxidants,[14–18] randomized clinical trials have failed to confirm the beneficial effects of antioxidants.[19–21] Further large, randomized clinical trials are underway.

In a recent Cochrane review[22] of all the trials comparing antioxidant supplements with placebo or no intervention for the occurrence of gastrointestinal cancers, there was no evidence that the antioxidants studied (β-carotene, vitamin A, vitamin C, vitamin E, and selenium) prevent gastrointestinal cancers. Surprisingly, the antioxidants were actually associated with an increase in all-cause mortality.

A number of studies have reported the potential beneficial effects of coffee on abnormal liver enzymes, cirrhosis, and possibly HCC. The association between coffee consumption and improved liver function appears more robust than the association with decreased risk of HCC.[23] Nevertheless, an inverse association between coffee drinking and HCC risk has been suggested in three Japanese prospective studies.[24–26] Unfortunately, these studies did not control for HBV and HCV infection. Two recent meta-analyses based on these Japanese cohorts and five case-control studies have suggested that increased coffee consumption may reduce the risk of HCC.[27,28] A recent study[29] from Finland supports these findings. The mechanism of this beneficial effect is unclear, but one can certainly postulate that decreased rates of cirrhosis may result in decreased rates of HCC.

Epidemiological data suggest that for patients at higher risk for liver disease due to higher alcohol intake, diabetes, obesity, and elevated iron saturation, regular tea intake results in decreased risk of clinically significant chronic liver disease. Tea from the extract of the dry leaves of the plant *Camellia sinensis* is a popular beverage that has been shown, through its polyphenolic antioxidant property, to reduce cancer risk in a variety of animal tumor bioassay systems.[30,31] Despite abundant promising data from experimental and animal models of carcinogenesis, epidemiological data have been mixed as to the benefits of this extract.

Epidemiological studies suggest an association of high lycopene intake with lower risks of several types of malignancy.[32,33] *In vitro*, lycopene has been reported to inhibit the invasion of rat hepatoma AH109A cells in a dose-dependent manner up to 5 mmol/L.[34] Huang et al.[35] showed that lycopene inhibits the migration and invasion of human hepatoma SK-Hep-1 cells *in vitro* and that these effects are associated with the up-regulation of nm23-H1.[35] Cohort studies have demonstrated decreased risk of HCC in individuals with either high serum levels of lycopene or a regular and high intake of lycopene or tomatoes.

15.3 DIET AS THERAPY FOR LIVER CANCER

Diet as therapy can be separated in two aspects of care: (1) addressing malnutrition and cachexia and (2) using dietary modifications in an attempt to directly treat HCC. It is well established that cancer patients suffer from malnutrition, weight loss, and severe catabolic state, namely, cachexia. Cachexia is a major contributor to the morbidity and mortality of patients with advanced malignancy.[36,37] The syndrome of cachexia appears to result from a variety of metabolic alteration characterized by relative hypermetabolism, an acute-phase protein response, and a failure of anabolism compounded by inadequate food intake.[38] The mediators of this process are produced by both the tumor and the body in response to the tumor. Potential mediators include tumor necrosis factor, interleukin 1, interleukin 6, neuroendocrine hormones, and proteolysis-inducing factor.[39]

Addressing malnutrition and cachexia is a vital component of caring for patients with HCC. All patients with newly diagnosed HCC should undergo primary assessment of nutritional status and energy intake. Initial evaluation should provide data that will enable the clinician to stratify the patient's nutritional risk. The Subjective Global Assessment, one of the best-validated scores, assesses the nutritional status based on five features of history and three aspects of the physical examination.[40,41] Weight status is still the outcome parameter most relied upon in assessing the nutritional status of patients. Malnutrition is likely when a patient has lost more than 10% of his/her actual weight over the past 6 months or more than 5% over the past 3 months or when BMI is lower than 18.5 kg/m^2.[42,43]

O∖her important nutrition-related aspects that should be investigated early in the course are food intake patterns including dietary habits, use of supplements, food aversions, identifiable taste changes, actual food intake, pain, or discomfort encountered while eating as a result of mucositis, dysphagia, or early satiety. It would be imperative to address all these nutritional issues early in the course to minimize their negative impact on the disease course, quality of life, response to therapy, and prognosis.

Therapeutic goals of nutritional support in the individual patient change during the course of disease. Whereas at the start of treatment, maintenance of nutritional status and reduction of treatment associated morbidity are the central focus, improvement of subjective quality of life and palliative aspects of nutrition become more prominent as the disease progresses.

Despite the common usage of dietary supplements by patients during all phases of cancer treatment, evidence from human clinical studies that confirm supplement safety and benefit is limited. The American Institute for Cancer Research (AICR) resource advisory council published recommendations regarding the use of dietary supplements for cancer survivors who are under treatment.

15.3.1 SUPPLEMENTS WITH ANTIOXIDANT PROPERTIES

It has been proposed that oxidative stress is involved in the etiology and progression of cancers, including liver cancer.[44,45] Lipid oxidation products such as alondialdehyde may act as tumor promoters and cocarcinogenic agents via their high cytotoxicity action.[45] Several nonenzymatic antioxidants such as α-tocopherol, vitamin C, β-carotene, and other carotenoids possess antioxidative properties. However, clinical information about the benefits and risks of antioxidants in HCC is scarce, and it remains unclear whether antioxidants truly contribute to enhanced outcomes for HCC patients.

Two opposing views exist about the use of antioxidants in cancer therapy. The first one proposes a complementary approach in which multiple antioxidant together with low-fat, high-fiber diet and lifestyle modifications, including physical exercise, may markedly improve the efficacy of standard and experimental cancer therapies.[46] Proponents of supplementation with antioxidants argue that these agents provide a safe and effective means of enhancing the response to chemotherapy and improve quality of life by reducing or preventing side effects.[46–48] The contrarian view argues that supplemental antioxidants during chemotherapy may interfere with oxidative breakdown of cellular DNA and cell membranes necessary for the agents to work.[49,50] A further argument against the use of high-dose antioxidants is that apoptotic breakdown of tumor cells is selectively increased by the presence of reactive oxygen species within the tissue and that this process may be slowed down by an antioxidant-replete diet.[51]

The AICR discourages the use of individual or combined antioxidants in a dosing exceeding their Dietary Reference Intake (DRI).

Vitamin E is a lipid-soluble antioxidant, synthesized only by plants and predominantly found in edible polyunsaturated vegetable oils. It plays a role in preventing polyunsaturated fatty acid (PUFA) peroxidation. The recommended daily allowance (RDA) for vitamin E is 15 mg/day; the tolerable upper limit (UL) is 1000 IU.[52] Vitamin E has been touted as important for enhancing antineoplastic activity because of its role in preventing the peroxidation of lipids. This property is particularly attractive because it maintains the rapid proliferation of malignant cells, which is essential to the efficacy of chemotherapy, while preventing damage to normal cells and enhancing immune function. There is experimental evidence that in cancer cells vitamin E has a synergistic effect with chemotherapy and radiation.[48] In animal studies, combinations of high doses of vitamin E and chemotherapy have showed mixed results.[48] These findings have not been specific to HCC. However, using transgenic TGFα/c-myc mouse model of liver cancer, vitamin E was shown to protect liver tissue against oxidative stress and suppress tumorigenic potential of c-myc oncogene. Furthermore, vitamin E reduced liver dysplasia and increased viability of hepatocytes.[53]

There have been studies suggesting the beneficial effects of vitamin E at 1000 IU given in combination with vitamin C, leading to improvement of fibrosis in patients with nonalcoholic steatohepatitis[54]; however, other studies have failed to corroborate these benefits.

In considering the possible use of supplementary vitamin E, it is essential to remember that vitamin E may act as a prooxidant in cigarette smokers, particularly if they are following a diet with high amounts of (n-6) fatty acids.[55]

Despite the potential benefits of vitamin E outlined above, AICR has concluded that there is no sufficient evidence to warrant its routine use by patients undergoing chemotherapy or radiation therapy. Oversupplementation with vitamin E may be harmful and should be avoided.

15.3.1.1   Vitamin C

Vitamin C is a water-soluble nutrient that has antioxidant properties. It is common in a variety of fresh fruits and vegetables. The RDA for vitamin C is 90 mg/day for men and 75 mg/day for women; the UL is 2000 mg/day.[52] Some results show that recommendations for vitamin C intake should be several times higher to achieve tissue saturation in normal people.[56] Adverse effects of vitamin C (diarrhea, gastrointestinal disturbances, abdominal bloating) are rare and are associated with an intake of several grams daily.

Despite its wide use by cancer patients, its effect on conventional treatment is not known. Limited preclinical data suggest that vitamin C may either stimulate or inhibit tumor growth depending on the form, dose, and timing of supplementation, cancer site, and type of chemotherapy.

It has been reported that consuming excessive amounts of vitamin C could transform its protective antioxidant agent to a harmful pro-oxidant that may interfere with standard therapies.[57] Vitamin C can induce the decomposition of lipid hydroperoxides *in vitro*, which theoretically could give rise to DNA damage *in vivo*.[58] The investigators used concentrations of vitamin C comparable with what they thought would be found in the human body with an intake of 200 mg/day. Whether these same conditions actually prevail in the human body remains uncertain. There is no specific study to support or refute the use of vitamin C in HCC.

AICR recommends that cancer patients should follow a reasonable diet sufficient in fruits and vegetables that provide vitamin C at least at the RDA level, but that they should not take supplemental vitamin C more than the amount obtained in a reliable daily vitamin-mineral pill containing vitamin C at the level comparable with RDAs.

15.3.1.2   β-Carotene

β-Carotene is one of about 600 plant compounds classified as carotenoids. β-Carotene is the most abundant carotenoid and is found in orange vegetables and fruits and in dark green leafy vegetables. It is widely used as a supplement but its only defined role in nutrition is as a precursor for vitamin A.

Although β-carotene is an antioxidant, its importance to health in this role is not established. No DRI is proposed for β-carotene or other carotenoids,[52] but existing recommendations[59] for increased consumption of carotenoid-containing fruits and vegetables are supported.

Since β-carotene supplements have not been shown to confer any benefit for the prevention of cancer and may actually cause harm in certain subgroups, β-carotene supplements are not routinely advised for cancer patients. AICR recommends not taking β-carotene in quantities unattainable from a normal diet and that it is more beneficial to eat carotenoid-rich fruits and vegetables.

15.3.1.3   Selenium

The trace element selenium has an important role in the antioxidant defenses as a crucial component of selenoproteins, such as glutathione peroxidase. Phytochemicals with antioxidant properties also include some flavonoids, such as quercetin, and some polyphenols.

Selenium occurs naturally in cereal products, a wide variety of vegetables, and seafood. The richest source of selenium in a supplement is a selenium-enriched brewer's yeast. The RDA for selenium is 55 mg/day, and the UL is 400 mg/day.[52]

Animal studies have shown that selenium supplementation may enhance the effectiveness of various chemotherapeutic agents.[48,60] Thus, there is great interest in selenium as a preventive agent for cancer at a variety of sites. The suggested mechanism is that selenium (through glutathione peroxidase activity) acts as a scavenger for products of oxidation reactions induced by standard therapies. In addition, selenium supplementation may directly cause tumor cell apoptosis.

Based on animal and epidemiological studies suggesting an inverse association between selenium level and regional cancer incidence in a province in China, a placebo-controlled study was undertaken offering selenium supplementation of 200 μg daily with an 8-year follow-up looking at incidence of primary liver cancer. It showed reduced primary liver cancer incidence (by 35.1%) in selenium-supplemented versus the nonsupplemented population. Upon withdrawal of selenium from the treated group, the primary liver cancer incidence rate began to increase. However, the inhibitory response to HBV was sustained during the 3-year cessation of treatment.[61] Similar results were found in another study among chronic carriers of hepatitis B and/or C virus, where an inverse association was found between plasma selenium levels and HCC, especially among cigarette smokers and among subjects with low plasma levels of retinol or various carotenoids.[62]

In conclusion, there is no convincing evidence that antioxidants in the amounts obtained from fruits and vegetables in the diet have any deleterious effects on human health.[59] However, trials in which selected antioxidants are taken in amounts or combinations much higher than those normally found in foods have yielded conflicting data regarding cancer risk.[63–65] Specifically for HCC, only selenium supplementation has shown clear benefit. Cancer patients should try to eat sufficient fruits and vegetables daily to provide adequate levels of antioxidants, with the addition of a daily multivitamin-multimineral pill. The benefits of eating fruits and vegetables may be much greater than the effects of any of the individual antioxidants they contain because the various vitamins, minerals, and phytochemicals in these whole foods may act synergistically.[59,66] AICR and the World Cancer Research Fund advise that five or more servings of fruits and vegetables be consumed daily to reduce the risk of certain cancers.[59] The beneficial effects of fruits and vegetables for both healthy people and cancer survivors have sometimes been associated with the presence of various antioxidant micronutrients.

15.3.2 Dietary Supplements without Antioxidant Properties

The role of nonantioxidant supplements is controversial, but these agents, including (n-3) fatty acids, and vitamin D are commonly used.

15.3.2.1 Polyunsaturated Fatty Acids

Two families of PUFAs are essential: (n-6) and (n-3), which are grouped according to their chemical structures. Although plants can synthesize both the basic (n-6) and (n-3) structures, animals (including humans) cannot and must obtain them from dietary sources. Linoleic acid is the parent fatty acid of the (n-6) family and linolenic acid is the parent of the (n-3) family. Western diet is rich in (n-6) fatty acids and poor in (n-3) fatty acids because of the large amounts of vegetable oils and meats and relatively low amounts of fish in the diet. Both (n-6) and (n-3) PUFAs are important components of animal and plant cell membranes. α-Linolenic acid comes from green leafy vegetables, flaxseed, rapeseed, and walnuts.

According to animal studies, dietary n-3 PUFA can significantly retard the growth of tumors, whereas (n-6) fatty acids potentially can increase tumor development.[67,68] Furthermore, the efficacy of cancer chemotherapy drugs such as doxorubicin, epirubicin, CPT-11, 5-fluorouracil, and tamoxifen and of radiation therapy has been improved when the diet included omega-3 PUFAs.[69]

The effect of omega-3 and omega PUFAs on human HCC cells has been investigated. The researchers treated HCC with either the omega-3 fatty acids docosahexaenoic acid (DHA) and eicosapentaenoic acid (EPA) or the omega-6 fatty acid arachidonic acid (AA) for 12–48 hours. DHA and EPA treatment resulted in a dose-dependent inhibition of cell growth, whereas AA treatment exhibited no significant effect. According to the investigators, the effect of omega-3 fatty acids on cancer cells is likely due to the induction of apoptosis. Indeed, the investigators found that DHA treatment induced cleavage of poly (ADP-ribose) polymerase, which is involved in repairing DNA damage, mediating apoptosis, and regulating immune response. Furthermore, DHA and EPA treatment indirectly decreased the levels of another protein known as β-catenin, an overabundance of which has been linked to the development of various tumors.[70]

Despite the promising experimental data, a meta-analysis of more than 38 prospective high-quality cancer incidence studies found a large heterogeneity in reported outcome.[71] The authors of the meta-analysis concluded that little evidence exists to support the premise that n-3 PUFA intake reduces risk of cancer incidence.[71] Although it is difficult to demonstrate prophylactic effects in large populations, therapeutic effects have been reported by different groups.[58,60,72,73]

Several studies have documented the effect of dietary n-3 PUFA intake on the development of HCC in animal models. For example, Jelinska et al.[74] reported decreased liver tumor development in rats fed with fish and vegetable oils and treated with 7,12-dimethylbenz[a]anthracene, and decreased prostaglandin E2 concentrations in liver tumors and nontumorous liver tissue from these animals. Fish oil or corn oil also reduces the development of hepatocarcinoma induced by diethylnitrosamine in rats.[75,76] Similarly, administration of fish oil decreased the development of azoxymethane (AOM)-induced glutathione S-transferase placental form positive hepatocellular foci in male F344 rats.[77] Consistent with these observations, administration of highly purified EPA, one of the main components of the n-3 PUFA family, inhibits the growth of liver preneoplastic lesions.[78,79] These findings suggest that, in addition to inhibition of COX-2 signaling pathway, dietary intervention with n-3 fatty acids merit further clinical evaluation for the chemoprevention and treatment of HCC.[80]

AICR and other official organizations recommend that energy from dietary fat should be ≤ 30% of the total energy intake. Research indicates that the type of dietary fat is also important for normal growth and development and for treatment of cancer and other diseases. The ratio of (n-6) to (n-3) PUFA seems to be critical in some cases. It is recommended that cancer patients and healthy people should consume the recommended adequate intake for PUFAs.[81] Thus, consumption of omega-3 FA offers a nontoxic means to augment cancer therapy and support chemotherapy.[82]

15.3.2.2 Vitamin D

For more than a century, vitamin D has been recognized as essential for the normal development and mineralization of a healthy skeleton. However, the discovery of the vitamin D receptor in tissues that are not involved in calcium and phosphate metabolism has prompted an extensive reevaluation of the physiological and pharmacological actions of vitamin D.

Based on observational, case control, and cohort studies, a role of vitamin D in cancer prevention was suggested. Putative mechanisms for its protective role against cancer include $1\alpha,25$-$(OH)_2D_3$ inhibition of a variety of genes responsible for cellular proliferation, regulating cellular proliferation and enhancing apoptotic activities,[83] growth arrest at the G1 phase of the cell cycle, tumor cell differentiation, disruption of growth factor–mediated cell survival signals, and inhibition of angiogenesis and cell adhesion.

One of the drawbacks of $1\alpha,25$-$(OH)_2D_3$ supplementation use is the effect on calcium metabolism, which results in hypercalcemia and hypercalciuria. Newly developed vitamin D analogues with lower calcemic activity have been shown to retain many therapeutic properties of $1\alpha,25$-$(OH)_2D_3$. Several analogues are currently being tested in preclinical and clinical trials for the treatment of various types of cancer including phase I and phase II trials of hepatic arterial administration of $1\alpha,25$-$(OH)_2D_3$ and EB1089 daily oral supplement, respectively, for liver cancer.[84,85]

Definitive recommendations for vitamin D_3 and its analogues cannot be made for cancer patients at this time. Further scientific research is needed to provide a set of firm guidelines for use of additional vitamin D supplements by cancer patients during treatment.

15.3.2.3 Active Hexose-Correlated Compound

Active hexose-correlated compound (AHCC) is an extract of Basidiomycotina that is obtained through the hybridization of several types of mushroom. It was developed by the Amino Up Chemical Co. Ltd (Sapporo, Japan) in 1989 and labeled as "functional" food due to its additive health benefits to the expected nutritional value. It has been reported that AHCC enhances the natural killer (NK) cell activity of cancer patients and may be considered a potent biologic response modifier in the treatment of cancer patients.[86] It has been also suggested that NK cell activity may be associated with cancer incidence.[87] Furthermore, AHCC has been reported to reduce the metastasis rate of rat mammary adenocarcinomas,[88] to increase detoxification enzymes in the liver, and to protect the liver from CCl4-induced liver injury.[89] This prompted a prospective placebo-controlled trial studying the effect of AHCC supplementation in patients after liver resection secondary to a liver tumor. AHCC supplementation was associated with significantly longer recurrence-free period and increased overall survival rate when compared with the control group. It is premature to make definitive recommendations about AHCC use in HCC, but it is a promising agent.[90]

15.3.2.4 *S*-Adenosylmethionine

S-Adenosylmethionine (SAMe), a widely used supplement advocated for its beneficial effects on the liver, joints, and mental health, is being increasingly recognized for its role in hepatocyte growth, death, and malignant degeneration. There is increasing evidence that many of its actions are independent of its role as a methyl donor. SAMe inhibits the growth of both normal and cancerous hepatocytes, through two quite different mechanisms. Although SAMe is antiapoptotic in normal hepatocytes, it is proapoptotic in cancerous hepatocytes. The specific molecular mechanisms are still being elucidated, and there is increasing enthusiasm for the use of this agent in the chemoprevention and possibly treatment of HCC.[91]

15.3.2.5   *Silybum marianum*

Milk thistle (*S. marianum* [L.] Gaertn., plant family Asteraceae) seed is an herb commonly used by Western herbalists and naturopathic physicians in treating liver disorders in adults. The German Commission E currently recommends its use for dyspeptic complaints, toxin-induced liver damage, and hepatic cirrhosis and as a supportive therapy for chronic inflammatory liver conditions.[92] Furthermore, milk thistle has been increasingly used in research and clinical practice in adult and pediatric populations in the oncology setting. That would include detoxification after chemotherapy, as a hepatoprotectant during chemotherapy, as an adjunct to cancer treatment, and to ameliorate long-term effects of cancer treatment. Researchers are actively investigating its role as a chemopreventive agent and possible treatment of cancer.

In vitro and animal data suggest that milk thistle may increase the uptake and actions of chemotherapeutic agents. Silymarin increased daunomycin accumulation, potentiated doxorubicin toxicity, and inhibited efflux of these drugs from cancer cells.[93] It also potentiated the antitumor action of cisplatin *in vivo* and *in vitro* and reduced recovery time in mice administered with cisplatin.[94]

Another potential therapeutic indication of *S. marianum* has been explored by using MK-001, a standardized silymarin extract, in the management of hepatitis C. It displayed both prophylactic and therapeutic effects against HCV infection, and when combined with interferon α, it inhibited HCV replication more than interferon α alone. Commercial preparations of silymarin also displayed antiviral activity, although the effects were not as potent as MK-001. Antiviral effects of the extract are attributed in part to induction of Stat1 phosphorylation, whereas interferon-independent mechanisms were suggested when the extract was biochemically fractionated by high-performance liquid chromatography.[95]

These data indicate that silymarin exerts anti-inflammatory and antiviral effects and suggest that complementary and alternative medicine-based approaches may assist in the management of patients with chronic hepatitis C. Its use in liver cancer is still controversial, because several randomized trials have produced inconsistent results, most likely due to the unavailability of a standardized product. Moreover, the mechanisms of action of this botanical are not well characterized.

In summary, although diet has been implicated as a major risk factor for liver cancer, its role in prevention is still unclear. The current clinical evidence, pertaining to the potential benefits and risks associated with the use of dietary supplements and vitamins as therapy for liver cancer, remains scarce. Further data are needed to ultimately establish clear and comprehensive dietary guidelines.

REFERENCES

1. El-Serag, H. B. 2002. Hepatocellular carcinoma: An epidemiologic view. *J Clin Gastroenterol* 35:S72–S78.
2. Baracos, V. E. 2002. Hypercatabolism and hypermetabolism in wasting states. *Curr Opin Clin Nutr Metab Care* 5:237–239.
3. Vissers, Y. L., C. H. Dejong, Y. C. Luiking, K. C. Fearon, M. F. von Meyenfeldt, and N. E. Deutz. 2005. Plasma arginine concentrations are reduced in cancer patients: Evidence for arginine deficiency? *Am J Clin Nutr* 81:1142–1146.

4. IARC. 1994. Monographs on the evaluation of carcinogenic risks to humans, vol. 59. *Hepatitis Viruses.* Lyon, France: IARC.
5. Doll, R., and R. Peto. 1981. The causes of cancer: Quantitative estimates of avoidable risks of cancer in the United States today. *J Natl Cancer Inst* 66:1191–1308.
6. International Agency for Research on Cancer. 1990. *Cancer: Causes, Occurrence, and Control*, vol. 100. Lyon: IARC.
7. IARC. 1993. Monographs on the evaluation of carcinogenic risks to humans, vol. 56. *Some Naturally Occurring Substances: Food Items and Constituents, Heterocyclic Aromatic Amines and Mycotoxins.* Lyon: IARC.
8. Saracco, G. 1995. Primary liver cancer is of multifactorial origin: Importance of hepatitis B virus infection and dietary aflatoxin. *J Gastroenterol Hepatol* 10:604–608.
9. Dragan, Y. P., and H. C. Pitot. 1993. Aflatoxin carcinogenesis in the context of the multistage nature of cancer. In: *The Toxicology of Aflatoxins: Human Health, Veterinary, and Agricultural Significance*, 179. London: Academic Press.
10. Gorelick, N. J., R. D. Bruce, and M. S. Hoseyni. 1993. Human risk assessment based on animal data: Inconsistencies and alternatives. In: *The Toxicology of Aflatoxins: Human Health, Veterinary, and Agricultural Significance,* ed. D. L. Eaton and J. D. Groopman, 179. London: Academic Press.
11. Henry, S. H., F. X. Bosch, T. C. Troxell, and P. M. Bolger. 1999. Policy forum: Public health. Reducing liver cancer—global control of aflatoxin. *Science* 286:2453–2454.
12. Henry, S. H., F. X. Bosch, and J. C. Bowers. 2002. Aflatoxin, hepatitis and worldwide liver cancer risks. *Adv Exp Med Biol* 504:229–233.
13. Groopman, J. D. 1993. Molecular dosimetry methods for assessing human aflatoxin exposures. In: *The Toxicology of Aflatoxins: Human Health, Veterinary and Agricultural Significance,* ed. D. L. Eaton and J. D. Groopman, 259. London: Academic Press.
14. Lee, I. M. 1999. Antioxidant vitamins in the prevention of cancer. *Proc Assoc Am Physicians* 111:10–15.
15. Stanner, S. A., J. Hughes, C. N. Kelly, and J. Buttriss. 2004. A review of the epidemiological evidence for the 'antioxidant hypothesis'. *Public Health Nutr* 7:407–422.
16. Willcox, J. K., S. L. Ash, and G. L. Catignani. 2004. Antioxidants and prevention of chronic disease. *Crit Rev Food Sci Nutr* 44:275–295.
17. Gonzalez, C. A. 2006. Nutrition and cancer: The current epidemiological evidence. *Br J Nutr* 96:S42–S45.
18. Huang, H. Y., B. Caballero, S. Chang, et al. 2007. Multivitamin/Mineral supplements and prevention of chronic disease: Executive summary. *Am J Clin Nutr* 85: 265S–268S.
19. Shekelle, P. G., S. C. Morton, L. K. Jungvig, et al. 2004. Effect of supplemental vitamin E for the prevention and treatment of cardiovascular disease [see comment]. *J Gen Intern Med* 19:380–389.
20. Coulter, I. D., M. L. Hardy, S. C. Morton, et al. 2006. Antioxidants vitamin C and vitamin E for the prevention and treatment of cancer. *J Gen Intern Med* 21:735–744.
21. Greenwald, P., D. Anderson, S. A. Nelson, and P. R. Taylor. 2007. Clinical trials of vitamin and mineral supplements for cancer prevention. *Am J Clin Nutr* 85:314S–317S.
22. Bjelakovic, G., D. Nikolova, R. G. Simonetti, and C. Gluud. 2008. Systematic review: Primary and secondary prevention of gastrointestinal cancers with antioxidant supplements. *Aliment Pharmacol Ther* 28:689–703.
23. Ruhl, C. E., and J. E. Everhart. 2005. Coffee and caffeine consumption reduce the risk of elevated serum alanine aminotransferase activity in the United States. *Gastroenterology* 128:24–32.
24. Inoue, M., I. Yoshimi, T. Sobue, S. Tsugane, and the JPHC Study Group. 2005. Influence of coffee drinking on subsequent risk of hepatocellular carcinoma: A prospective study in Japan. *J Natl Cancer Inst* 97:293–300.

25. Shimazu, T., Y. Tsubono, S. Kuriyama, et al. 2005. Coffee consumption and the risk of primary liver cancer: Pooled analysis of two prospective studies in Japan. *Int J Cancer* 116:150–154.

26. Kurozawa, Y., I. Ogimoto, A. Shibata, et al. 2005. Coffee and risk of death from hepatocellular carcinoma in a large cohort study in Japan. *Br J Cancer* 93:607–610.

27. Larsson, S. C., and A. Wolk. 2007. Coffee consumption and risk of liver cancer: A meta-analysis. *Gastroenterology* 132:1740–1745.

28. Bravi, F., C. Bosetti, A. Tavani, et al. 2007. Coffee drinking and hepatocellular carcinoma risk: A meta-analysis. *Hepatology* 46:430–435.

29. Hu, G., J. Tuomilehto, E. Pukkala, et al. 2008. Joint effects of coffee consumption and serum gamma-glutamyltransferase on the risk of liver cancer. *Hepatology* 48:129–136.

30. Dreosti, I. E., M. J. Wargovich, and C. S. Yang. 1997. Inhibition of carcinogenesis by tea: The evidence from experimental studies. *Crit Rev Food Sci Nutr* 37:761–770.

31. Kohlmeier, L., K. G. Weterings, S. Steck, and F. J. Kok. 1997. Tea and cancer prevention: An evaluation of the epidemiologic literature. *Nutr Cancer* 27:1–13.

32. Clinton, S. K. 1998. Lycopene: Chemistry, biology, and implications for human health and disease. *Nutr Rev* 56:35–51.

33. Gerster, H. 1997. The potential role of lycopene for human health. *J Am Coll Nutr* 16:109–126.

34. Kozuki, Y., Y. Miura, and K. Yagasaki. 2000. Inhibitory effects of carotenoids on the invasion of rat ascites hepatoma cells in culture. *Cancer Lett* 151:111–115.

35. Huang, C. S., M. K. Shih, C. H. Chuang, and M. L. Hu. 2005. Lycopene inhibits cell migration and invasion and upregulates Nm23-H1 in a highly invasive hepatocarcinoma, SK-hep-1 cells. *J Nutr* 135:2119–2123.

36. Inagaki, J., V. Rodriguez, and G. P. Bodey. 1974. Proceedings: Causes of death in cancer patients. *Cancer* 33:568–573.

37. Dewys, W. D., C. Begg, P. T. Lavin, et al. 1980. Prognostic effect of weight loss prior to chemotherapy in cancer patients. Eastern Cooperative Oncology Group. *Am J Med* 69:491–497.

38. Fearon, K. C., M. D. Barber, and A. G. Moses. 2001. The cancer cachexia syndrome. *Surg Oncol Clin N Am* 10:109–126.

39. Tisdale, M. J. 2004. Tumor-host interactions. *J Cell Biochem* 93:871–877.

40. Detsky, A. S., J. P. Baker, K. O'Rourke, et al. 1987. Predicting nutrition-associated complications for patients undergoing gastrointestinal surgery. *JPEN J Parenter Enteral Nutr* 11:440–446.

41. Hirsch, S., N. de Obaldia, M. Petermann, et al. 1991. Subjective global assessment of nutritional status: Further validation. *Nutrition* 7:35–37.

42. Kotler, D. P. 2000. Cachexia. *Ann Intern Med* 133:622–634.

43. Kondrup, J., S. P. Allison, M. Elia, B. Vellas, and M. Plauth. 2003. Educational and Clinical Practice Committee, European Society of Parenteral and Enteral Nutrition (ESPEN). ESPEN Guidelines for Nutrition Screening 2002. *Clin Nutr* 22:415–421.

44. Ockner, R. K., R. M. Kaikaus, and N. M. Bass. 1993. Fatty-acid metabolism and the pathogenesis of hepatocellular carcinoma: Review and hypothesis. *Hepatology* 18:669–676.

45. Marnett, L. J. 1999. Lipid peroxidation-DNA damage by malondialdehyde. *Mutat Res* 424:83–95.

46. Prasad, K. N., A. Kumar, V. Kochupillai, and W. C. Cole. 1999. High doses of multiple antioxidant vitamins: Essential ingredients in improving the efficacy of standard cancer therapy. *J Am Coll Nutr* 18:13–25.

47. Lamson, D. W., and M. S. Brignall. 1999. Antioxidants in cancer therapy; their actions and interactions with oncologic therapies. *Altern Med Rev* 4:304–329.

48. Conklin, K. A. 2000. Dietary antioxidants during cancer therapy: Impact on chemo-therapeutic effectiveness and development of side effects. *Nutr Cancer* 37:1–18.
49. Labriola, D., and R. Livingston. 1999. Possible interactions between dietary antioxidants and chemotherapy. *Oncology (Williston)* 13:1003–1008.
50. Kong, Q., and K. O. Lillehei. 1998. Antioxidant inhibitors for cancer therapy. *Med Hypotheses* 51:405–409.
51. Salganik, R. I., C. D. Albright, J. Rodgers, et al. 2000. Dietary antioxidant depletion: Enhancement of tumor apoptosis and inhibition of brain tumor growth in transgenic mice. *Carcinogenesis* 21:909–914.
52. *Dietary Reference Intakes for Vitamin C, Vitamin E, Selenium, and Carotenoids.* 2000. Washington, DC: National Academy Press.
53. Calvisi, D. F., S. Ladu, K. Hironaka, V. M. Factor, and S. S. Thorgeirsson. 2004. Vitamin E down-modulates iNOS and NADPH oxidase in c-Myc/TGF-alpha transgenic mouse model of liver cancer. *J Hepatol* 41:815–822.
54. Harrison, S. A., S. Torgerson, P. Hayashi, J. Ward, and S. Schenker. 2003. Vitamin E and vitamin C treatment improves fibrosis in patients with nonalcoholic steatohepatitis. *Am J Gastroenterol* 98:2485–2490.
55. Weinberg, R. B., B. S. VanderWerken, R. A. Anderson, J. E. Stegner, and M. J. Thomas. 2001. Pro-oxidant effect of vitamin E in cigarette smokers consuming a high polyunsaturated fat diet. *Arterioscler Thromb Vasc Biol* 21:1029–1033.
56. Levine, M., S. C. Rumsey, R. Daruwala, J. B. Park, and Y. Wang. 1999. Criteria and recommendations for vitamin C intake. *JAMA* 281:1415–1423.
57. Vitamin C publication. 2001. Nutrition. *Harv Health Lett* 26:4–5.
58. Lee, S. H., T. Oe, and I. A. Blair. 2001. Vitamin C–induced decomposition of lipid hydroperoxides to endogenous genotoxins. *Science* 292:2083–2086.
59. AICR/WCRF. 1997. *Food, Nutrition and the Prevention of Cancer: A Global Perspective.* Washington, DC: AICR.
60. Vadgama, J. V., Y. Wu, D. Shen, S. Hsia, and J. Block. 2000. Effect of selenium in combination with adriamycin or taxol on several different cancer cells. *Anticancer Res* 20:1391–1414.
61. Yu, S. Y., Y. J. Zhu, and W. G. Li. 1997. Protective role of selenium against hepatitis B virus and primary liver cancer in Qidong. *Biol Trace Elem Res* 56:117–124.
62. Yu, M. W., I. S. Horng, K. H. Hsu, Y. C. Chiang, Y. F. Liaw, and C. J. Chen. 1999. Plasma selenium levels and risk of hepatocellular carcinoma among men with chronic hepatitis virus infection. *Am J Epidemiol* 150:367–374.
63. Lee, I. M. 1999. Antioxidant vitamins in the prevention of cancer. *Proc Assoc Am Physicians* 111:10–15.
64. Maxwell, S. R. 1999. Antioxidant vitamin supplements: Update of their potential benefits and possible risks. *Drug Saf* 21:253–266.
65. Ruffin, M. T., and C. L Rock. 2001. Do antioxidants still have a role in the prevention of human cancer? *Curr Oncol Rep* 3:306–313.
66. Brown, J., T. Byers, K. Thompson, et al. 2001. Nutrition during and after cancer treatment: A guide for informed choices by cancer survivors. *CA Cancer J Clin* 51:153–187.
67. Simopoulos, A. P. 2001. The Mediterranean diets: What is so special about the diet of Greece? The scientific evidence. *J Nutr* 131:3065S–3073S.
68. Fay, M. P., L. S. Freedman, C. K. Clifford, and D. N. Midthune. 1997. Effect of different types and amounts of fat on the development of mammary tumors in rodents: A review. *Cancer Res* 57:3979–3988.
69. Hardman, W. E. 2004. (n-3) Fatty acids and cancer therapy. *J Nutr* 134:3427S–3430S.
70. Lim, K., C. Han, L. Xu, and T. Wu. 2006. Omega-3 polyunsaturated fatty acids inhibit hepatocellular carcinoma cell growth through downregulation of β-catenin/wnt signaling pathway. *Cancer Res* 68:553–560.

71. Heuser, G., and A. Vojdani. 1997. Enhancement of natural killer cell activity and T and B cell function by buffered vitamin C in patients exposed to toxic chemicals: The role of protein kinase-C. *Immunopharmacol Immunotoxicol* 19:291–312.

72. van der Vliet, A. 2000. Cigarettes, cancer, and carotenoids: A continuing, unresolved antioxidant paradox. *Am J Clin Nutr* 72:1421–1423.

73. Caffrey, P. B., and G. D. Frenkel. 2000. Selenium compounds prevent the induction of drug resistance by cisplatin in human ovarian tumor xenografts in vivo. *Cancer Chemother Pharmacol* 46:74–78.

74. Jelinska, M., A. Tokarz, R. Oledzka, and A. Czorniuk-Sliwa. 2003. Effects of dietary linseed, evening primrose or fish oils on fatty acid and prostaglandin E_2 contents in the rat livers and 7,12-dimethylbenz[*a*]anthracene-induced tumours. *Biochim Biophys Acta* 1637:193–199.

75. Kim, Y., S. K. Ji, and H. Choi. 2000. Modulation of liver microsomal monooxygenase system by dietary n-6/n-3 ratios in rat hepatocarcinogenesis. *Nutr Cancer* 37:65–72.

76. Rahman, K. M., S. Sugie, K. Okamoto, T. Watanabe, T. Tanaka, and H. Mori. 1999. Modulating effects of diets high in omega-3 and omega-6 fatty acids in initiation and postinitiation stages of diethylnitrosamine-induced hepatocarcinogenesis in rats. *Jpn J Cancer Res* 90:31–39.

77. Sugie, S., K. Okamoto, T. Tanaka, H. Mori, B. S. Reddy, and K. Satoh. 1995. Effect of fish oil on the development of AOM-induced glutathione *S*-transferase placental form positive hepatocellular foci in male F344 rats. *Nutr Cancer* 24:187–195.

78. Calviello, G., P. Palozza, P. Franceschelli, et al. 1999. Eicosapentaenoic acid inhibits the growth of liver preneoplastic lesions and alters membrane phospholipid composition and peroxisomal β-oxidation. *Nutr Cancer* 34:206–212.

79. Calviello, G., P. Palozza, E. Piccioni, et al. 1998. Dietary supplementation with eicosa-pentaenoic and docosahexaenoic acid inhibits growth of Morris hepatocarcinoma 3924A in rats: Effects on proliferation and apoptosis. *Int J Cancer* 75:699–705.

80. Wu, T. 2006. Cyclooxygenase-2 in hepatocellular carcinoma. *Cancer Treat Rev* 32:28–44.

81. Simopoulos, A. P., A. Leaf, and N. Salem Jr. 1999. Workshop on the essentiality of and recommended dietary intakes for omega-6 and omega-3 fatty acids. *J Am Coll Nutr* 18:487–489.

82. Stehr, S. N., and A. R. Heller. 2006. Omega-3 fatty acid effects on biochemical indices following cancer surgery. *Clin Chim Acta* 373:1–8.

83. Hager, G., J. Kornfehl, B. Knerer, G. Weigel, and M. Formanek. 2004. Molecular analy-sis of p21 promoter activity isolated from squamous carcinoma cell lines of the head and neck under the influence of 1,25(OH)$_2$ vitamin D3 and its analogs. *Acta Otolaryngol (Stockh)* 124:90–96.

84. Finlay, I. G., G. J. Stewart, J. Ahkter, and D. L. Morris. 2001. A phase one study of the hepatic arterial administration of 1,25-dihydroxyvitamin D3 for liver cancers. *J Gastroenterol Hepatol* 16:333–337.

85. Dalhoff, K., J. Dancey, L. Astrup, et al. 2003. A phase II study of the vitamin D ana-logue seocalcitol in patients with inoperable hepatocellular carcinoma. *Br J Cancer* 89:252–257.

86. Ghoneum, M., Y. Ninomiya, M. Torabi, G. Gill, and A. Wojdani. 1992. Active hemicel-lulose compound (AHCC) enhances NK cell activity of aged mice in vivo. *FASEB J* 6.

87. Imai, K., S. Matsuyama, S. Miyake, K. Suga, and K. Nakachi. 2000. Natural cytotoxic activity of peripheral-blood lymphocytes and cancer incidence: An 11-year follow-up study of a general population. *Lancet* 356:1795–1799.

88. Matsushita, K., Y. Kuramitsu, Y. Ohiro, et al. 1998. Combination therapy of active hexose correlated compound plus UFT significantly reduces the metastasis of rat mam-mary adenocarcinoma. *Anticancer Drugs* 9:343–350.

89. Sun, B., K. Wakame, T. Mukoda, A. Toyoshima, T. Kanazawa, and K. Kosuna. 1997. Protective effects of AHCC on carbon tetrachloride induced liver injury in mice. *Nat Med* 51:310–315.

90. Matsui, Y., J. Uhara, S. Satoi, et al. 2002. Improved prognosis of postoperative hepatocellular carcinoma patients when treated with functional foods: A prospective cohort study. *J Hepatol* 37:78–86.

91. Lu, S. C., and J. M. Mato. 2008. *S*-Adenosylmethionine in cell growth, apoptosis and liver cancer. *J Gastroenterol Hepatol* 23:S73–S77.

92. *The Complete German Commission E Monographs: Therapeutic Guide to Herbal Medicines.* Baltimore, MD: Lippincott Williams & Wilkins; 1998.

93. Zhang, S., and M. E. Morris. 2003. Effects of the flavonoids biochanin A, morin, phloretin, and silymarin on P-glycoprotein–mediated transport. *J Pharmacol Exp Ther* 304:1258–1267.

94. Giacomelli, S., D. Gallo, P. Apollonio, et al. 2002. Silybin and its bioavailable phospholipid complex (IdB 1016) potentiate in vitro and in vivo the activity of cisplatin. *Life Sci* 70:1447–1459.

95. Polyak, S. J., C. Morishima, M. C. Shuhart, C. C. Wang, Y. Liu, and D. Y. Lee. 2007. Inhibition of T-cell inflammatory cytokines, hepatocyte NF-kappaB signaling, and HCV infection by standardized silymarin. *Gastroenterology* 132:1925–1936.

16 Vitamins in Hepatocellular Carcinoma

Akihiro Tamori and Susumu Shiomi

CONTENTS

16.1 INTRODUCTION

Hepatocellular carcinoma (HCC) is a major health care problem worldwide because it is the fifth leading cause of cancer mortality and the third most common cause of cancer-related death. HCC has two major clinical characteristics: (1) HCC develops from chronic hepatitis or liver cirrhosis at a high constant incidence (about 5–7%) per year; (2) even when HCC is initially detected at an early stage and can be treated radically, disease recurrence or secondary hepatic cancers develop at a high incidence (10–25%) per year [1,2]. Because of these features, HCC remains one of the cancers with the poorest outcomes, despite recent advances in diagnosis and treatment. Epidemiological studies predict that the number of deaths from HCC will increase by 2010–2015 [3].

The incidence of cancer developing from the unresected part of the liver after surgical treatment of the first cancer is much higher than the incidence of cancer developing from liver cirrhosis. Therefore, the unresected liver is the most important factor to consider when devising "measures to prevent recurrence of HCC." The high incidence of HCC onset and recurrence seems to be associated with the fact that the buds (clones) of cancer arise in a multicentric manner throughout the entire liver (a "field" exposed to stimuli for carcinogenesis). If these clones can be effectively eliminated, recurrence of HCC may be suppressed, considerably improving the outcomes of patients with HCC. However, it is practically impossible to locate all microscopic clones (potentially cancerous cells or precancerous cells possibly present in large numbers throughout the liver) macroscopically and visually and to remove them by invasive techniques (surgical resection, etc.).

In recent years, the concept of "cancer chemoprevention" has begun to attract considerable attention in the research and clinical management of various cancers, including HCC. This concept was first proposed by Michael B. Sporn and implies the "prevention of progression of precancerous cells into cancer by arresting the cells in the precancerous stage or reversing the direction of their progression toward cancer into the direction toward normal cells" [4]. Chemoprevention with active interventions is expected to be indicated for hepatic cancer in high-risk patients (i.e., those with chronic hepatitis, liver cirrhosis, or unresected liver expected to contain clones for HCC after treatment of a first cancer). In practice, interferon (IFN) [5,6], Sho-saiko-to [7], glycyrrhizin [8], vitamin K [9], and acyclic retinoid [10] have been reported to be effective for preventing primary cancer in patients with hepatic cirrhosis and recurrent cancer, or the onset of a secondary cancer in patients with a complete response to treatment of a first HCC. Advances in prophylactic therapy are expected to play an important role in improving the outcomes of HCC and in eventually eradicating HCC [11]. In this chapter, we review the effects of vitamins A and K in the chemoprevention of HCC.

16.2   VITAMIN A

Vitamin A is essential for growth, retinoic function, and development of blood cells, including immune response cells. Loss of vitamin A is known to induce night blindness or corneal dryness. Recently, vitamin A was found to play important roles in cell development and maintenance of normal cell function. Clinical studies have revealed a relation between vitamin A metabolism and carcinogenesis and provided evidence that vitamin A derivatives contribute to the prevention of cancer.

"Retinoid" is a collective term for vitamin A and its derivatives and analogues. In the body, retinoid is converted into retinoic acid and binds as a ligand to retinoic acid receptor (RAR) and retinoid X receptor (RXR), which comprise the intranuclear receptor family. Retinoid bound to these receptors regulates transcription. Three subunits (α, β, and γ) are known for each of RAR and RXR. RXR forms a homodimer with RXR or a heterodimer with RAR and binds to retinoid X response element and retinoic acid response element, both of which are response regions on DNA. Expression of various target genes is regulated in this manner. Typical phenotypes regulated by retinoid are tissue morphogenesis, cell differentiation, and apoptosis. These functions are closely related to the proliferation and death of cells. Therefore, abnormalities in the functions and expression of retinoid, RXR, and RAR can lead to a departure from normal cell differentiation, proliferation, and death, that is, to the appearance of atypical, malignant, or immortal cells. Retinoid, RXR, and RAR may thus be important targets for the prevention and treatment of various malignant tumors [12].

Studies conducted to date have yielded the following findings: (1) Retinoid metabolism is abnormal, and retinoid concentrations are markedly lower in HCC cells than in normal liver cells [13]. (2) RXR-α, one of the retinoid nuclear receptors, usually undergoes phosphorylation by Ras/Erk/MAPK at a particular amino acid residue, resulting in loss of its transcription-related function [14]. (3) Phosphorylated RXR-α accumulates abnormally in cells without undergoing degradation by the ubiquitin/proteosome system, thus inhibiting the function of normal RXR in a dominant-negative manner [15]. Because RXR can form heterodimers not only with RAR, but also with thyroid hormone receptor, vitamin D receptor, peroxisome growth factor activation receptor, and other molecules, and can bind to various response sequences, RXR acts as the most important "master regulator" in various nuclear receptor families [16]. It is speculated that dysfunction of RXR-α protein due to abnormal modification (phosphorylation) and lack of response to retinoid are involved in the onset of hepatic cancer. In other words, loss of RXR-mediated control of normal cell proliferation or death is apparently an important mechanism leading to the development of hepatic cancer. Attempts have thus been made to synthesize new retinoids capable of simulating normal signals of retinoid receptors (particularly RXR), with the goal of preventing the onset of hepatic cancer. One such compound is acyclic retinoid, which lacks a cyclic structure (Figure 16.1). Acyclic retinoid serves as a ligand that acts on and binds to RXR and RAR (particularly RXR), similar to other retinoic acids [17]. Acyclic retinoid also inhibits Ras activity, thereby suppressing RXR-α phosphorylation in HCC cells under the activity of the Ras-Erk system and stimulating resumption of RXR function [18]. Moreover, *in vivo* and *in vitro* studies have shown that acyclic retinoid suppresses activation of the Ras-Erk system mediated by EGFR, a receptor type tyrosine kinase. That is, acyclic retinoid is considered to regulate normal proliferation and apoptosis of cells, and suppress the proliferation of tumor cells through the following actions: (1) inhibition of RXR phosphorylation by acting on receptor type tyrosine kinase and the Ras-Erk system, (2) stimulation of resumption of the function of RXR as a nuclear receptor, and (3) by serving as a ligand that acts on and binds to RXR, acyclic retinoid stimulates recovery of the

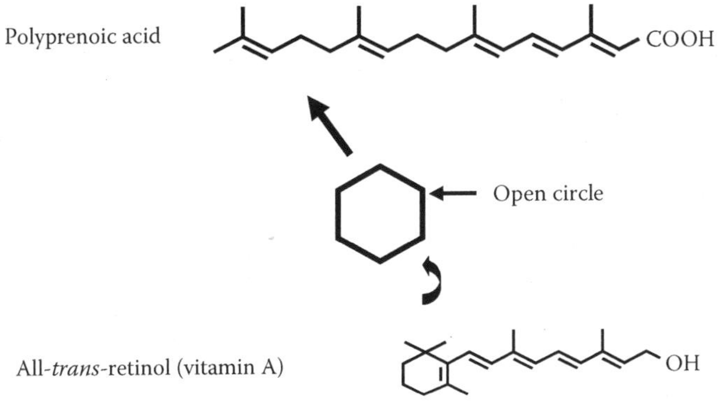

FIGURE 16.1 Chemical structure of acyclic retinoid.

dimer-forming capability of RXR and induces the expression of RXR-α target genes such as STAT-1 [19] and p21 [20].

16.3   EFFICACY OF ACYCLIC RETINOID IN CLINICAL STUDIES

As stated above, one feature of hepatic cancer is "multicentric onset," attributed to the presence of independent, multiple clones of HCC throughout the entire liver affected by chronic hepatitis or cirrhosis after viral infection; these clones advance within the liver. It is practically impossible to remove all these clones surgically. Consequently, "clonal deletion with a chemical agent has been proposed, and acyclic retinoid" has become a basic concept in prevention of the development and recurrence of hepatic cancer. To test this concept, Muto et al. [10] carried out an interventional clinical study using acyclic retinoid, with the goal of preventing recurrence of HCC. Patients who had undergone radical treatment (surgical resection, etc.) of a first HCC received acyclic retinoid for 1 year. These patients had a significantly decreased incidence of secondary hepatic cancer and a markedly improved survival rate [10] (Figure 16.2). In addition, the study showed that the serum level of AFP-L3 (possibly produced by microscopic clones) decreased to the negative range after treatment with acyclic retinoid, and that treatment with acyclic retinoid suppressed the reappearance of AFP-L3 in patients in whom AFP-L3 had disappeared. Interestingly, secondary hepatic cancer subsequently developed in patients in whom serum AFP-L3 became positive or higher [21]. Long-term follow-up showed that the development of hepatic cancer remained suppressed for about 4 years after the end of acyclic retinoid treatment [22]. These results suggest that once microscopic cancer cell clones (abundantly present across the intensely cancer-affected liver) are eradicated by acyclic retinoid, many years

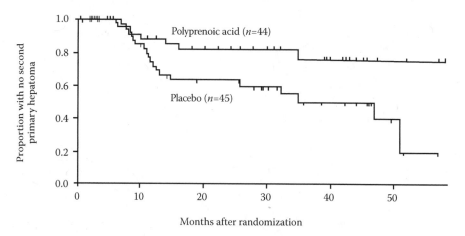

FIGURE 16.2   Kaplan–Meier estimates of the proportion of patients without second primary HCCs. The treatment period lasted for 12 months, beginning with month 0. $p = .04$ for the comparison between groups by the log-rank test. Tick marks indicate patients who withdrew or were excluded from the study. (From Muto, Y., Moriwaki, H., Ninomiya, M., et al., *N Engl J Med*, 334, 1561–1567, 1996. With permission.)

are required for the development (or recurrence) of clinically detectable secondary hepatic cancer. This notion clinically supports the concept of "clonal deletion."

16.4   FUTURE STRATEGIES FOR SECONDARY CHEMOPREVENTION BY ACYCLIC RETINOID

In addition to acyclic retinoid, IFN [6] and vitamin K [9] have been shown to contribute to prevention of the onset and recurrence of hepatic cancer in liver containing abundant HCC clones, that is, liver affected by cirrhosis or the unresected part of the liver after surgical treatment of a first HCC. One possibility for the future clinical application of these drugs is combined administration, with the hope of "synergistically" preventing hepatic cancer. In experiments, acyclic retinoid has been demonstrated to increase the sensitivity of HCC cells to IFN by stimulating the expression of IFN receptor (located downstream of RXR-α) and STAT-1 (a molecule involved in signal transduction for IFN receptor). Acyclic retinoid combined with IFN thereby synergistically induces apoptosis of HCC cells and suppresses tumor cell proliferation [19]. Treatment with a combination of acyclic retinoid and vitamin K also synergistically suppresses HCC cell proliferation. Kanamori et al. [23] are currently investigating the mechanisms underlying such effects. One comprehensive program for preventing hepatic cancer that merits attention is "combined-drug cancer prevention," which combines acyclic retinoid not only with IFN or vitamin K, but also with liver-protective agents (glycyrrhizin, ursodeoxycholic acid, etc.) or other synthetic or natural compounds (e.g., Sho-saiko-to). Given possible mechanisms of action, maximum synergistic benefits are expected when acyclic retinoid is used in combination with drugs that target the Ras-Erk system (involved in abnormal modification, i.e., phosphorylation, of RXR-α), growth factors and receptors located upstream (receptor type tyrosine kinase), and factors associated with transcription. Further development of more effective retinoids that can be used in combination with other classes of anticancer drugs, including immunopreventive agents, may lead to better strategies for cancer prevention.

16.5   VITAMIN K

Vitamin K is an essential cofactor for the converting enzyme γ-glutamyl-carboxylase, which converts glutamate residues into γ-carboxy-glutamate. Vitamin K–dependent proteins include coagulation factors II (prothrombin), VII, IX, and X, proteins C and S, osteocalcin, surfactant-associated proteins, and bone matrix protein. Vitamin K plays an important role in hemostasis by activating blood coagulation and anticoagulation factors in the liver. Some vitamin K–dependent proteins are present in extrahepatic tissues, such as bone and vascular tissue. Matrix Gla protein (MGP) was identified in human atherosclerotic plaque, where it may prevent calcium precipitation, as it similarly does in bone. This effect is clearly demonstrated in MGP knockout mice, which die of massive aortic and coronary calcification shortly after birth. The vitamin K family of molecules comprises the natural forms vitamin K_1 (phylloquinone) and vitamin K_2 (menaquinones), as well as the synthetic form vitamin K_3 (menadione). These naphthoquinone-containing molecules inhibit tumor cell growth in culture, with vitamin K_3 being more potent than either vitamin K_1 or K_2. Vitamin K_2 inhibits growth of human cancer cell lines and suppresses induction of differentiation in various human myeloid leukemia cell lines [24,25]. Clinically, myelodysplastic syndrome has been successfully treated with vitamin K_2 [26]. However, the mechanisms of this clinical effect have yet to be fully explored. Recently, vitamin K_2 has attracted attention as a new chemopreventive agent against HCC.

16.6 ROLE OF VITAMIN K IN CELL GROWTH

A number of findings suggest that vitamin K participates in controlling cell growth. Underlying mechanisms may involve redox cycling (as known for vitamin K_3), proteins with growth inhibitory properties induced by vitamin K (e.g., prothrombin [27]), previously unidentified pathways involving arylation [28], or growth arrest genes such as gas 6 [29]. Geranylgeraniol (GGO), a side chain of vitamin K_2, strongly induces apoptosis of tumor cells, suggesting that GGO might inhibit cell growth [30] (Figure 16.3).

Recently, microarray analysis has shown that several genes are induced by treatment with vitamin K_2 [31]. Protein kinase A (PKA) is a common activator of related signaling pathways, identified by microarray analysis. Vitamin K_2 is thought to activate PKA, which inhibits RhoA activation. Alterations caused by high-dose treatment with vitamin K_2 result in cell cycle arrest at the G1 and G2/M phases, accompanied by inhibition of tumor invasion. The effects of vitamin K_2 in doses used to treat osteoporosis are poorly understood, especially in the liver. However, the results of *in vitro* studies suggest that vitamin K_2 is one of the most promising agents for the chemoprevention of HCC.

16.7 CHEMOPREVENTION WITH VITAMIN K_2

We previously reported a 2-year study showing that vitamin K_2 helps to prevent bone loss in women with viral cirrhosis of the liver [32]. Most of the subjects agreed to

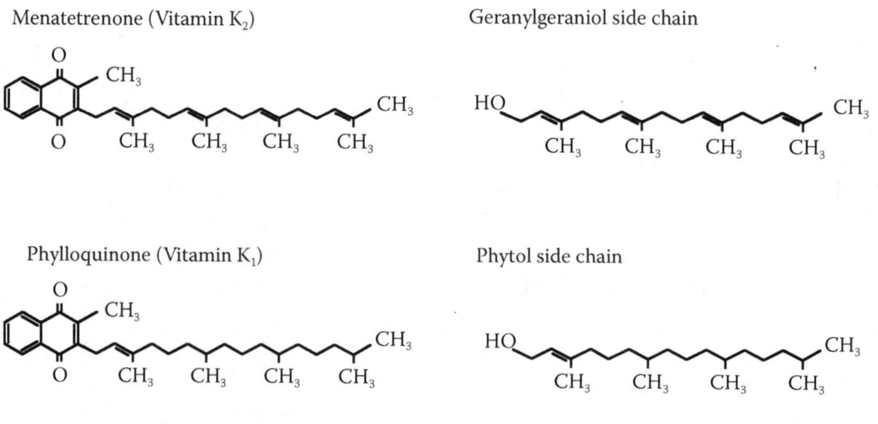

FIGURE 16.3 Chemical structure of vitamin K.

participate in an extended study designed to clarify the long-term effects of vitamin K_2 on bone loss associated with cirrhosis. The incidence of HCC was found to differ between women who received vitamin K_2 and those who did not [33]. In detail, the subjects of the initial 2-year study were 50 women with viral liver cirrhosis who were admitted to our department between 1996 and 1998. If the results of abdominal dynamic computed tomography and abdominal ultrasonography suggested the presence of HCC, abdominal angiography or needle biopsy was performed to confirm the diagnosis. Three patients in the treated group and four in the control group were confirmed to have HCC, and were subsequently excluded from further study. The remaining 43 patients were randomly assigned by means of sealed envelopes to receive 45 mg/day of vitamin K_2 (Glakay; Eisai Co., Tokyo, Japan) orally (treated group) or no vitamin K_2 (control group). At the end of the first study (after 2 years of treatment), 21 patients in the treated group and 19 in the control group consented to participate in a longer trial. In this trial, all but one patient in each group had hepatitis C virus (HCV) infection; two other patients had hepatitis B infection. Seven patients, four in the control group and three in the treated group, had previously received IFN-α for their HCV infections, but HCV was not eradicated. No patient was given IFN therapy after study entry. Surveillance for HCC was done according to detailed guidelines for the follow-up of patients with liver cirrhosis in Japan [5]. Compliance with vitamin K_2 in the treated group was good; no patient had adverse reactions or dropped out of the study. The two groups were similar with respect to age, virus type, platelets, alanine aminotransferase (ALT), α-fetoprotein (AFP), and other clinical findings (Table 16.1). After the first study commenced, HCC was detected in 2 of the 21 patients given vitamin K_2 as compared with 9 of the 19 controls; the cumulative proportion of patients with HCC was smaller in the treated group (log-rank test, $p = .024$; Figure 16.4). On univariate analysis, the risk ratio for the development of HCC in the treated group versus the control group was 0.195

TABLE 16.1
Baseline Characteristics

	Treatment ($n = 21$)	Control ($n = 19$)	p Value
Average age (years)	59.8 ± 8.7	61.4 ± 7.1	.54
HBV/HCV	1/20	1/18	.94
Albumin (g/dL)	3.9 ± 0.3	3.9 ± 0.3	.87
Platelets (10^4/mm³)	14.7 ± 5.4	12.1 ± 5.2	.13
Total bilirubin (mg/dL)	0.8 ± 0.2	0.9 ± 0.4	.47
ALT (IU/mL)	81.7 ± 42.7	70.4 ± 33.4	.36
AFP (ng/mL)	13.4 ± 17.7	13.3 ± 8.7	.99
IFN (+/−)	4/17	3/16	.79

Source: Data from Habu, D., Shiomi, S., Tamori, A., et al., JAMA, 292, 358–361, 2004.

Note: Mann-Whitney U test for age, serum albumin, platelets, total bilirubin, ALT, and AFP; χ² test for HBV/HCV. ALT, alanine aminotransferase; AFP, α-fetoprotein. IFN (+/−), patients who received interferon (IFN) before enrollment; +, yes; −, no.

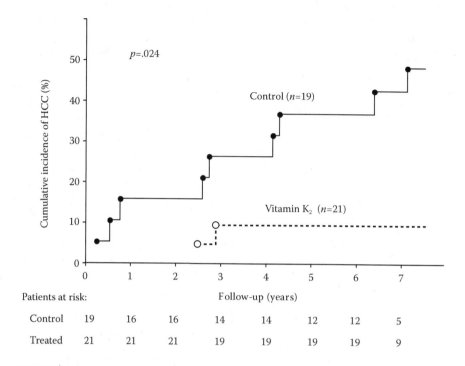

FIGURE 16.4 Cumulative incidence of HCC diagnosed in patients treated with vitamin K_2 and in a control group (cited from Habu et al. [33]). All patients were followed up for at least 6 years. Vertical marks on curves show the latest follow-up to date for the 15 patients monitored for less than 7 years. (From Habu, D., Shiomi, S., Tamori, A., et al., *JAMA* 292, 358–361, 2004. With permission.)

(0.042–0.913; $p = .038$). On multivariate analysis with adjustment for age, ALT activity, serum albumin, total bilirubin, platelet count, AFP, and history of treatment with IFN-α, the risk ratio for the development of HCC in patients given vitamin K_2 was 0.126 (0.016–0.992; $p = .049$) (Table 16.2).

The original goal of our trial was to assess the long-term effects of vitamin K_2 on bone loss in women with viral liver cirrhosis. Our trial thus had several important limitations when the data are used to assess the value of vitamin K_2 for the primary prevention of HCC in patients with liver cirrhosis. Factors limiting the value of our findings included the small study group, the inclusion of women only, and the participation of only one center. However, similar to previously reported, randomized controlled studies of cirrhosis in which the primary endpoint was the development of HCC, patients with evidence of HCC on highly sensitive imaging studies were excluded, and the two study groups were similar with respect to risk factors for HCC, including age, severity of cirrhosis, history of IFN therapy, and type of hepatitis virus infection. Our results indicate that vitamin K_2 decreases the risk of HCC to about 20% as compared with control, suggesting that vitamin K_2 may delay the onset of hepatocarcinogenesis.

TABLE 16.2
Adjusted Odds Ratios for the Development of HCC

	Odds Ratio	95% CI	p Value
VK$_2$/Control	0.126	0.016–0.992	.0491
Total bilirubin (mg/dL) (1.0 +/< 1.0)	0.294	0.042–2.044	.2161
Albumin (g/dL) (< 3.5/3.5+)	33.434	2.362–473.352	.0094
Platelets (10^4/mm^3) (< 100/100+)	2.235	0.458–10.900	.3200
ALT (IU/mL) (< 80/80+)	0.393	0.071–2.164	.2831
AFP (ng/mL) (20+/< 20)	1.689	0.306–9.335	.5477
IFN (+/−)	1.260	0.201–7.903	.8053

Source: Data from Habu, D., Shiomi, S., Tamori, A., et al., *JAMA*, 292, 358–361, 2004.

Note: Adjusted for age and all other variables in this table. ALT, alanine aminotransferase; AFP, α-fetoprotein; IFN (+/−), patients who received interferon (IFN) before enrolment; +, yes; −, no.

Before our study of primary chemoprevention, vitamin K$_2$ had been used to prevent the development of second primary malignancies after curative therapy for HCC. Koike et al. [34] showed that treatment with vitamin K$_2$ decreases the risk of portal vein invasion by tumor in patients with HCC who have high levels of des-γ-carboxy prothrombin. Preliminary results of a study being conducted by Mizuta et al. [35] suggest that vitamin K$_2$ inhibits the recurrence of HCC, especially in patients with HCV. However, these clinical studies of vitamin K$_2$ have focused on patients with specific characteristics or risk factors for HCC, including only women or patients with high levels of des-γ-carboxy prothrombin. Recent multicenter randomized controlled studies in Japan have suggested that monotherapy with vitamin K$_2$ could not prevent the occurrence of HCC (unpublished results).

16.8   COMBINATION THERAPY WITH VITAMIN K IN CHEMOPREVENTION

Previous studies have evaluated the effectiveness of single agents for preventing HCC in patients with chronic liver diseases. To our knowledge, studies assessing the value of combination therapy for chemoprevention have not been reported. One of the reasons for the lack of studies evaluating combined treatment is concern about adverse effects associated with different agents. For example, adverse effects of IFN therapy include fever, leukopenia, and thrombocytopenia. In contrast, vitamin K$_2$ has not been associated with serious side effects in patients with osteoporosis. One of the effects of vitamin K$_2$ that requires caution is a decrease in serum levels of des-γ-carboxy prothrombin, a useful marker of HCC, in patients with or without

HCC. In patients given vitamin K_2, des-γ-carboxy prothrombin would thus be an unreliable screening marker for HCC. Moreover, the administration of vitamin K_2 to patients treated with warfarin is contraindicated.

Yoshiji et al. [36] reported that a combination of vitamin K_2 and perindopril, an angiotensin-converting enzyme inhibitor (ACE), was more effective for chemoprevention than either agent alone in a rat model of diethylnitrosamine-induced hepatocarcinogenesis. The number and size of enzyme-altered preneoplastic lesions were both significantly reduced, and the expression of CD31, a marker of neovascularization, was decreased in rats given combination treatment. Their findings suggested that a low dose of vitamin K_2 (1 μM) inhibits the proliferation of endothelial cells. Clinical trials examining whether vitamin K_2 plus an ACE inhibitor prevents HCC in patients with chronic liver diseases thus appear to be warranted. Vitamin K_2 may therefore be used concomitantly with other chemopreventive agents, without increasing the risk of adverse reactions. The safety, relatively low cost, and ease of use of vitamin K_2 have led to good compliance with treatment. These properties make vitamin K_2 a suitable candidate for clinical trials assessing the value of combination treatment for chemoprevention or chemotherapy in patients at risk for, or with a confirmed diagnosis of, HCC.

The results of preliminary trials are intriguing and suggest a potential role for vitamin K_2 in the prevention of primary and second hepatocarcinogenesis in patients with hepatic cirrhosis.

16.9   CONCLUSION

HCC has a high incidence rate in Asia and Africa, and its incidence has been rising sharply over the past decade in Europe and the United States. Eradication of HCC is an urgent health issue. As of May 2007, an interventional clinical (phase II/III) study of acyclic retinoid is under way in Japan to evaluate whether acyclic retinoid suppresses the onset of HCC or its recurrence after radical treatment of a first HCC. We hope that the results of this interventional clinical study will provide further hope for the prevention of hepatic cancer recurrence. The results of basic and clinical studies conducted to date, designed to test the validity of the concept of "clonal deletion," suggest that acyclic retinoid can serve as an "agent for cancer treatment" that can actively eradicate precancerous lesions (clones), rather than simply serving as a "cancer preventive drug." Acyclic retinoid and vitamin K_2 are expected to play important roles in establishing more widely applicable and effective means of preventing the recurrence of hepatic cancer.

REFERENCES

1. Tsukuma, H., T. Hiyama, S. Tanaka, et al. 1993. Risk factors for hepatocelluar carcinoma among patients with chronic liver disease. *N Engl J Med* 328:1797–1801.
2. Kumada, T., S. Nakano, I. Takeda, et al. 1997. Patterns of recurrence after initial treatment in patients with small hepatocellular carcinoma. *Hepatology* 25:87–92.
3. Shibuya, K., and E. Yano. 2005. Regression analysis of trends in mortality from hepatocellular carcinoma in Japan, 1972–2001. *Int J Epidemiol* 34:397–402.

4. Sporn, M. B., and D. L. Newton. 1979. Chemoprevention of cancer with retinoids. *Fed Proc* 38:2528–2534.

5. Nishiguchi, S., T. Kuroki, S. Nakatani, et al. 1995. Randomised trial of effects of interferon-α on incidence of hepatocellular carcinoma in chronic active hepatitis C with cirrhosis. *Lancet* 346:1051–1055.

6. Kubo, S., S. Nishiguchi, K. Hirohashi, et al. 2001. Effects of long-term postoperative interferon-alpha therapy on intrahepatic recurrence after resection of hepatitis C virus–related hepatocellular carcinoma. A randomized, controlled trial. *Ann Intern Med.* 134:963–967.

7. Oka, H., S. Yamamoto, T. Kuroki, et al. 1995. Prospective study of chemoprevention of hepatocellular carcinoma with Sho-saiko-to (TJ-9). *Cancer* 76:743–749.

8. Kumada, H. 2002. Long-term treatment of chronic hepatitis C with glycyrrhizin [stronger neo-minophagen C (SNMC)] for preventing liver cirrhosis and hepatocellular carcinoma. *Oncology* 62 Suppl 1:94–100.

9. Mizuta, T., I. Ozaki, Y. Eguchi, et al. 2006. The effect of mentrenone, a vitamin K_2 analog, on disease recurrence and survival in patients with hepatocellular carcinoma after curative treatment: A pilot study. *Cancer* 106:867–872.

10. Muto, Y., H. Moriwaki, M. Ninomiya, et al. 1996. Prevention of second primary tumors by an acyclic retinoid, polyprenoic acid, in patients with hepatocellular carcinoma. Hepatoma Prevention Study Group. *N Engl J Med* 334:1561–1567.

11. Moriwaki, H. 2002. Prevention of liver cancer: Basic and clinical aspects. *Exp Mol Med* 34:319–325.

12. Altucci, L., and H. Gronemeyer. 2001. The promise of retinoids to fight against cancer. *Nat Rev Cancer* 1:181–193.

13. Muto, Y., and H. Moriwaki. 1984. Antitumor activity of vitamin A and its derivatives. *J Natl Cancer Inst* 73:1389–1393.

14. Matsushima-Nishiwaki, R., M. Okuno, S. Adachi, et al. 2001. Phosphorylation of retinoid X receptor alpha at serine 260 impairs its metabolism and function in human hepatocellular carcinoma. *Cancer Res* 61:7675–7682.

15. Adachi, S., M. Okuno, R. Matsushima-Nishiwaki, et al. 2002. Phosphorylation of retinoid X receptor suppresses its ubiquitionation in human hepatocellular carcinoma. *Hepatology* 35:332–340.

16. Chambon, P. 1996. A decade of molecular biology of retinoic acid receptors. *FASEB J* 10:940–954.

17. Araki, H., Y. Shidoji, Y. Yamada, et al. 1995. Retinoid agonist activities of synthetic geranyl geranoic acid derivatives. *Biochem Biophys Res Commun* 209:66–72.

18. Matsushima-Nishiwaki, R., M. Okuno, Y. Takano, et al. 2003. Molecular mechanism for growth suppression of human hepatocellular carcinoma cells by acyclic retinoid. *Carcinogenesis* 24:1353–1359.

19. Obora, A., Y. Shiratori, M. Okuno, et al. 2002. Synergistic induction of apoptosis by acyclic retinoid and interferon-beta in human hepatocellular carcinoma cells. *Hepatology* 36:1115–1124.

20. Suzuki, M., M. Masuda, J. Y. Lim, et al. 2002. Growth inhibition of human hepatoma cells by acyclic retinoid is associated with induction of p21 (CIP1) and inhibition of expression of cyclin D1. *Cancer* 62:3997–4006.

21. Moriwaki, H., I. Yasuda, Y. Shiratori, et al. 1997. Deletion of serum lectin-reactive alpha-fetoprotein by acyclic retinoid: A potent biomarker in the chemoprevention of second primary hepatoma. *Clin Cancer Res* 3:727–731.

22. Takai, K., M. Okuno, I. Yasuda, et al. 2005. Prevention of second primary tumors by an acyclic retinoid in patients with hepatocellular carcinoma. Updated analysis of the long-term follow-up data. *Intervirology* 48:39–45.

23. Kanamori, T., M. Shimizu, M. Okuno, et al. 2007. Synergistic growth inhibition by acyclic retinoid and vitamin K$_2$ in human hepatocellular carcinoma cells. *Cancer Sci* 98:431–437.
24. Sasaki, I., S. Hashimoto, M. Yoda, et al. 1994. Novel role of vitamin K$_2$: A potent inducer of differentiation of various human myeloid leukemia cell lines. *Biochem Biophys Res Commun* 205:1305–1310.
25. Nishimaki, J., K. Miyazawa, M. Yamaguchi, et al. 1999. Vitamin K$_2$ induces apoptosis of a novel cell line established from patients with myelodysplastic syndrome in blastic formation. *Leukemia* 13:1399–1405.
26. Takami, A., S. Nakao, Y. Ontachi, et al. 1999. Successful therapy of myelodysplastic syndrome with menatetrenone, a vitamin K$_2$ analog. *Int J Hematol* 69:24–26.
27. Carr, B. I., Z. Wang, S. Kar, and M. Wang. 1995. Prothrombin inhibits hepatocyte DNA synthesis and expression of the α5 integrin gene. *Proc AACR* 36:266.
28. Kar, S., and B. I. Carr. 2000. Growth inhibition and protein tyrosine phosphorylation in MCF breast cancer cells by a novel K vitamin. *J Cell Physiol* 185:386–393.
29. Varnum, B. C., C. Young, G. Elliott, A. Garcia, T. D. Bartley, Y.-W. Fridell, et al. 1995. Axl receptor tyrosine kinase stimulated by the vitamin K–dependent protein encoded by growth-arrest–specific gene 6. *Nature* 373:623–626.
30. Ohizumi, H., Y. Masuda, S. Nakajo, I. Sakai, S. Ohsawa, and K. Nakaya. 1995. Geranylgeraniol is a potent inducer of apoptosis in tumor cells. *J Biochem* 117:11–13.
31. Otsuka, M., N. Kato, R. X. Shao, et al. 2004. Vitamin K2 inhibits the growth and invasiveness of hepatocellular carcinoma cells via protein kinase A activation. *Hepatology* 40:243–251.
32. Shiomi, S., S. Nishiguchi, S. Kubo, et al. 2002. Vitamin K$_2$ (menatetrenone) for bone loss in patients with cirrhosis of the liver. *Am J Gastroenterol* 97:978–981.
33. Habu, D., S. Shiomi, A. Tamori, et al. 2004. Role of vitamin K$_2$ in the development of hepatocellular carcinoma in women with viral cirrhosis of the liver. *JAMA* 292:358–361.
34. Koike, Y., Y. Shiratori, S. Shiina et al. 2002. Randomized prospective study of prevention from tumor invasion into portal vein in 120 patients with hepatocellular carcinoma by vitamin K–II administration [Abstract]. *Gastroenterology* 122:643a.
35. Mizuta, T., I. Ozaki, Y. Eguchi, et al. 2006. The effect of menatetrenone, a vitamin K$_2$ analog, on disease recurrence and survival in patients with hepatocellular carcinoma after curative treatment: A pilot study. *Cancer* 106:867–872.
36. Yoshiji, H., S. Kuriyama, R. Noguchi, et al. 2005. Combination of vitamin K$_2$ and the angiotensin-converting enzyme inhibitor, perindopril, attenuates the liver enzyme-altered preneoplastic lesions in rats via angiogenesis suppression. *J Hepatol* 42:687–693.

17 Supplementation with High Doses of Vitamins E and C in Chronic Hepatitis C

Yasunori Kawaguchi and Toshihiko Mizuta

CONTENTS

17.1 INTRODUCTION

It has been reported that more than 170 million people worldwide are infected with chronic hepatitis C (CHC) [1], which is the leading cause of cirrhosis and hepatocellular carcinoma (HCC) [2]. Thus, the first goal of treatment for patients with CHC is the eradication of the hepatitis C virus (HCV) by interferon (IFN) therapy.

The addition of ribavirin (RBV) to interferon α (IFN-α) leads to marked improvements in the sustained virological response (SVR) rates [3–5]. However, reversible hemolytic anemia is one of the main side effects, reinforcing the need for dose reduction and/or suspension of combination therapy [4–7]. It was reported that half of the patients who received combination therapy with IFN-α plus RBV experienced a hemoglobin decrease of more than 3 g/dL [8], and dose reduction and treatment discontinuation as a result of anemia were 27.6% and 7.3%, respectively [7].

It has been speculated that oxidative stress to red blood cell membranes is related to RBV-induced hemolysis [9]. Because vitamins E and C have important roles on antioxidant defense systems in the cell membranes [10–13], it is worth investigating whether these micronutrients can protect against oxidative stress to the red cell membrane due to RBV.

17.2   HCV INFECTION AND OXIDATIVE STRESS

The HCV genome comprises genes for 10 viral proteins. The amino-terminal one-third of the genome encodes four structural proteins (core, E1, E2, and p7), and the remainder of the genome encodes six nonstructural proteins (NS2, NS3, NS4A, NS4B, NS5A, and NS5B) [14]. It has been reported that some HCV proteins cause oxidative stress [15–17]. An HCV core transgenic mouse model revealed that the core protein caused oxidative stress by altering the oxidant/antioxidant state in the liver without inflammation, which seems to be a result of mitochondrial damage [15]. The NS3 protein was reported to induce the production of reactive oxygen species (ROS) in human monocytes via the activation of nicotinamide adenine dinucleotide phosphate (NADPH) oxidase [16]. An experimental study using a cell culture system showed that NS5A induced calcium release from the endoplasmic reticulum, which led to ROS production in mitochondria [17].

Furthermore, experiments using transgenic mice expressing the HCV polyprotein showed that HCV-induced ROS led to hepatic iron accumulation via the downregulation of hepcidin transcription [18]. Since excess divalent iron levels can produce highly reactive hydroxyl radicals through the Fenton reaction [19], HCV infection is in a vicious circle of oxidative stress. Indeed, it has been clinically reported that oxidative stress is a key feature of HCV infection in asymptomatic carriers as well as patients with cirrhosis [20,21].

17.3   LIVER SUPPORTIVE THERAPIES INCLUDING
ANTIOXIDANTS FOR CHC

The first goal of treating patients with CHC is the eradication of HCV by IFN therapy. However, if this is not possible, the second goal is the normalization of liver function tests, which may delay disease progression.

Stronger Neo-Minophagen C (SNMC), which consists of 0.2% glycyrrhizin, 0.1% cysteine, and 2.0% glycine in physiological solution, is intravenously administered at doses ranging from 40 mL three times a week to 100 mL daily as liver supportive therapy for patients with CHC. Experiments using transgenic mice expressing the HCV polyprotein revealed that SNMC could protect hepatocytes against carbon tetrachloride–induced oxidative stress and mitochondrial injury by restoring depleted cellular glutathione [22]. A randomized, double-blind controlled trial showed that SNMC suppressed serum transaminase in patients with CHC [23]. Furthermore, it was reported that long-term administration of SNMC for HCV-infected patients could attenuate the incidence of HCC [24].

Ursodeoxycholic acid (UDCA), as well as SNMC, was reported to decrease serum thioredoxin levels, a marker of oxidative stress, in HCV-infected patients [25]. A large-scale, multicenter, double-blind trial demonstrated that 600 mg of UDCA daily was optimal to decrease serum aminotransferase levels in CHC patients, whereas a daily dose of 900 mg decreased serum γ-glutamyl transpeptidase levels further [26].

A pilot study showed that long-term iron removal by phlebotomy, to remove oxidative stress, could maintain lower serum aminotransferase levels and suppress the progression of liver fibrosis in CHC patients without any major side effects [27].

The effect of the antioxidant vitamins E and C in CHC is controversial. Short-term administration of vitamin E (745 IU/day for 3 months [28]; 800 IU/day for 3 months [29]) was reported to improve serum aminotransferase in patients with CHC and protect against liver damage caused by oxidative stress. In contrast, a randomized, controlled trial among HCV-infected patients showed that supplementation with vitamin C (500 mg), vitamin E (945 IU), and selenium (200 μg) daily for 6 months had no effects on alanine aminotransferase, viral load, or oxidative stress [30]. Furthermore, a recent meta-analysis showed that long-term administration of high-dose vitamin E ($\geq$ 400 IU/day, 1.4–8.2 years) might increase all-cause mortality [31]. Based on the reports mentioned above, the long-term administration of high doses of vitamins E and C is not recommended in patients with CHC.

17.4 RBV AND OXIDATIVE STRESS

1-β-D-Ribofuranosyl-1,2,4-triazole-3-carboxamide (RBV) is a water-soluble synthetic guanosine analogue that possesses antiviral activity against several RNA and DNA viruses [32]. Although RBV monotherapy cannot eradicate HCV, the addition of RBV to IFN-α leads to marked improvements in SVR rates [3–5]. How RBV augments the response rate to IFN has not been fully elucidated, but some mechanisms have been reported [6]. RBV is phosphorylated intracellularly to form monophosphate (RMP), diphosphate (RDP), and triphosphate (RTP). The misincorporation of RTP by RNA polymerases leads to early chain termination and the inhibition of replication. RMP is a competitive inhibitor of inosine monophosphate dehydrogenase, which leads to depletion of the guanosine triphosphate necessary for viral RNA synthesis. Furthermore, RBV has been reported to exhibit its antiviral activity by increasing the mutation frequency of HCV and by altering the Th1/Th2 balance, favoring a Th1 response.

The major side effect of RBV treatment is reversible hemolytic anemia, although the mechanisms of RBV-induced hemolytic anemia have not been clearly demonstrated. The accumulation of RBV-phosphorylated metabolites in erythrocytes produces a relative adenosine triphosphate (ATP) deficiency [33]. The lowered ATP level might indirectly cause oxidative damage to red blood cell membranes and induce erythrophagocytic removal via the reticuloendothelial system, resulting in hemolytic anemia [9].

17.5 INTERACTIONS BETWEEN ANTIOXIDANT DEFENSE SYSTEMS IN THE BIOLOGIC MEMBRANE

Vitamin E is a fat-soluble vitamin that is mainly located in the biologic membrane and stabilizes the membrane via its antioxidant property [10] (Figure 17.1). It converts peroxyl free radicals of polyunsaturated fatty acid (PUFA-OO•) into hydroperoxy PUFA (PUFA-OOH) before PUFA-OO• can establish a chain reaction. Vitamin E is more effective than other antioxidants in scavenging radicals in membranes and lipoproteins. The vitamin E radical is relatively unreactive and ultimately forms nonradical compounds with other antioxidants. In particular, vitamin C reduces the vitamin E radical efficiently to regenerate vitamin E and to inhibit oxidation induced

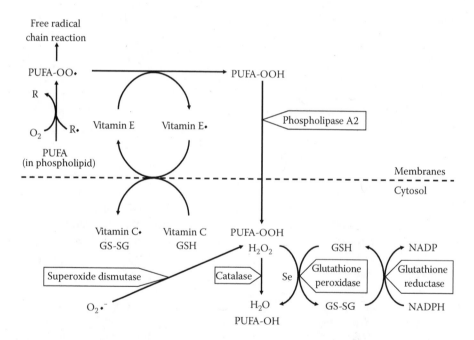

FIGURE 17.1 Interaction and synergism between antioxidant defense systems in biologic membranes (lipid phase) and in the cytosol (aqueous phase). R•, free radical; PUFA, polyunsaturated fatty acid; PUFA-OO•, peroxyl free radical of polyunsaturated fatty acid in membrane phospholipid; PUFA-OOH, hydroperoxy polyunsaturated fatty acid in membrane phospholipid; PUFA-OH, hydroxy polyunsaturated fatty acid; vitamin E•, vitamin E radical; vitamin C•, vitamin C radical; Se, selenium; GSH, reduced glutathione; GS-SG, oxidized glutathione. (Modified from Bender, D. A., and Mayes, P. A., in *Harper's Illustrated Biochemistry*, 26th ed., eds. R. K. Murray, D. K. Granner, P. A. Mayes, and V. W. Rodwell,. New York: McGraw-Hill, pp. 481–497, 2003.)

by vitamin E radicals. The resultant monodehydroascorbate free radical is subjected to enzymic or nonenzymic reaction to produce ascorbate and dehydroascorbate, neither of which is a free radical [12,13]. As a result, vitamin C accelerates the antioxidant action of vitamin E [11]. PUFA-OOH in the membrane is released into the cytosol by the action of phospholipase A_2. In the cytosol, PUFA-OOH and hydrogen peroxide (H_2O_2) generated from superoxide ($O_2\cdot^-$) are converted into hydroxy PUFA (PUFA-OH), water, and oxygen by catalase or selenium-dependent glutathione peroxidase. Oxidized glutathione returns to the reduced state after reacting with NADPH, a process that is catalyzed by glutathione reductase [12,13].

17.6 ANTIOXIDANTS FOR RBV-INDUCED HEMOLYTIC ANEMIA

It was reported that supplementation with vitamin E (800 IU/day) did not diminish RBV-associated hemolysis [34]. On the other hand, supplementation of vitamins E (500 mg/day) and C (750 mg/day) was reported to attenuate the RBV-induced decrease of eicosapentaenoic acid in erythrocyte membrane in CHC patients but failed to inhibit RBV-induced anemia [35]. Furthermore, one report in an abstract form suggested that supplementation with vitamins E (800 IU/day) and C (1000 mg/day) attenuated the severity of RBV-induced hemolytic anemia [36]. Therefore, we thought that enrichment of antioxidants in the red blood cell membrane might prevent RBV-induced hemolytic anemia [37].

17.7 EFFECTS OF SUPPLEMENTATION WITH HIGH DOSES OF VITAMINS E AND C ON RBV-INDUCED HEMOLYTIC ANEMIA

17.7.1 PATIENTS

To examine the effect of supplementation with high doses of vitamins E and C on RBV-induced hemolytic anemia, 21 consecutive patients with CHC were enrolled in the current study (vitamins E/C group).

Twenty-one sex- and age-matched patients who received a standard regimen of IFN-α-2b plus RBV combination therapy for CHC were included as a control group. No differences were found in the baseline characteristics between the two groups.

17.7.2 DOSE SETTINGS OF VITAMINS E AND C

A review article involving a large number of subjects showed that high oral doses of up to 3,200 IU/day led to no consistent adverse effects, but oral intakes of high levels of vitamin E could exacerbate the blood coagulation defect of vitamin K deficiency caused by malabsorption or anticoagulation therapy [38]. Although there is no clear safe standard dose range of vitamin E for chronic hepatitis, vitamin E at 300–1000 IU/day (3 months–1 year) was reported to be safe for chronic hepatitis [35,36,39,40]. Because it is thought that the prevention of RBV-induced hemolytic anemia requires a higher dose of vitamin E than in previous reports, we set the dose of vitamin E at 2,000 mg (2000 IU)/day, considering its efficacy and safety. Vitamin C was set to 2,000 mg, the upper limit for a standard dose.

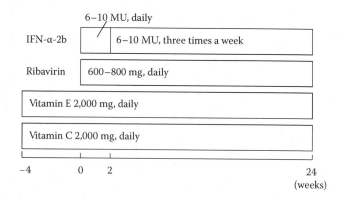

FIGURE 17.2 Treatment schedule in the vitamin E/C group. (From Kawaguchi, Y., Mizuta, T., Takahashi, H., et al., *Hepatol Res*, 37:317–324, 2007. Erratum in *Hepatol Res*, 38:114, 2008. With permission.)

17.7.3 TREATMENT REGIMENS

Patients in the vitamin E/C group received daily oral doses of vitamin E (Juvela N; Eisai Co., Ltd., Tokyo, Japan) at 2,000 mg and vitamin C (Hicee, Takeda Pharmaceutical Co., Tokyo, Japan) at 2,000 mg, starting at 4 weeks before the initiation of antiviral treatment. The patients then started antiviral therapy, namely, daily intramuscular administrations of 6 or 10 million units (MU) of IFN-α-2b for 2 weeks, and then three times a week for 22 weeks, in combination with daily oral doses of RBV of 600 or 800 mg depending on body weight (≤ 60 or > 60 kg, respectively). The patients continued to take vitamins E and C at the same doses daily during the antiviral combination therapy (Figure 17.2).

Patients in the control group received the above-mentioned antiviral combination therapy without supplementation with vitamins E and C.

17.7.4 TOLERABILITY OF TREATMENT

Sixteen (76.2%) patients in the vitamin E/C group and 15 (71.4%) patients in the control group completed the protocol. The dropout rates in the two groups were not different. Anemia was the most frequent reason for reducing the dose of antiviral drugs or dropping out in the control group; no patient in the vitamin E/C group experienced dose reduction or dropout owing to anemia.

No patient showed complications with HCC during the treatment period. Patients in the vitamin E/C group did not report any adverse events such as gastrointestinal symptoms or blood coagulation disorders as a result of vitamins E and C.

We administered vitamins E and C from 4 weeks before IFN plus RBV treatment to evaluate their effects on liver function or potential adverse effects. We found that there were no effects on liver function or blood cell counts, and there were no adverse effects during the period when only vitamins E and C were administered.

17.7.5 TRANSITIONS OF DATA

Transitions between values from the commencement of antiviral therapy and each time point were analyzed with regard to serum ALT levels, leukocyte counts, hemoglobin levels, and platelet counts by analysis of variance with repeated measures (Figure 17.3). Monthly monitoring showed that decreases in hemoglobin levels and platelet counts were significantly recovered in the vitamin E/C group compared with the control group ($p = .029$ and $p = .049$, respectively). Unexpectedly, this study revealed that vitamins E and C could prevent a decrease in serum platelet counts, but the detailed mechanism is unknown. Their actions as antioxidants may be involved in this process.

17.8 EFFECTS OF SUPPLEMENTATION WITH HIGH DOSES OF VITAMINS E AND C ON THE ANTIVIRAL RESPONSE

Of the nine patients with SVR, 5 (23.8%) were in the vitamin E/C group and 5 (19%) were in the control group, using an intention-to-treat analysis. With on-treatment

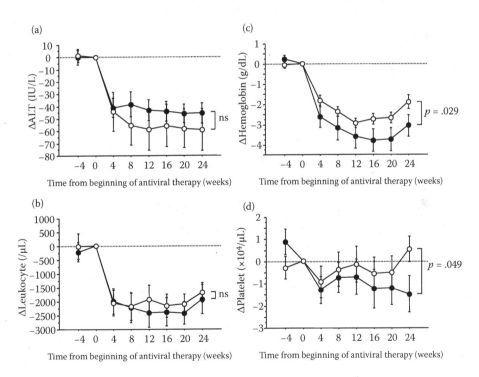

FIGURE 17.3 Time courses of (a) serum ALT levels, (b) leukocyte counts, (c) hemoglobin levels, and (d) platelet counts in the vitamin E/C group (open circles) and the control group (closed circles). Δs represent differences between values from commencement of antiviral therapy and each time point. ns, not significant. (From Kawaguchi, Y., Mizuta, T., Takahashi, H., et al., *Hepatol Res* 37:317–324, 2007. Erratum in *Hepatol Res*, 38:114, 2008. With permission.)

analysis, 4 (25%) patients with SVR were in the vitamin E/C group and 3 (20%) were in the control group. There were no significant differences between the two groups.

17.9 CONCLUSIONS

In this work, we found that supplementation with high doses of vitamins E and C can safely improve RBV-induced hemolytic anemia during IFN-α-2b and RBV therapy in CHC, indicating that short-term administration of strong antioxidants might be a good option to prevent drug-induced adverse effects.

Combination therapy with pegylated IFN and RBV is currently recommended as standard therapy for patients with CHC. In HCV genotype 1 patients, pegylated IFN and RBV combination therapy for 48 weeks has achieved SVR rates of 42–52% [41,42]. Moreover, several recent studies demonstrated that extending the treatment duration from 48 to 72 weeks could improve the SVR rates in HCV genotype 1 patients, with a slow virologic response defined as HCV-RNA positive at week 12 but negative at week 24 [43,44]. With the extension of the treatment period, the safety and efficacy of long-term supplementation with high doses of vitamins E and C must be carefully examined in future studies.

17.10 SUMMARY POINTS

- Oxidative stress is a key feature of HCV infection in asymptomatic carriers as well as cirrhotic patients.
- The first goal of treating patients with CHC is the eradication of HCV by IFN therapy. The second goal is normalization of the liver function tests, which may delay disease progression.
- Although liver supportive therapies such as SNMC, UDCA, and phlebotomy for CHC patients are effective through attenuation of oxidative stress, the safety and efficacy of high-dose vitamins E and C are controversial.
- RBV augments the response rate to IFN but often causes hemolytic anemia as a side effect. The accumulation of RBV-phosphorylated metabolites in erythrocytes might be induced by the relative depletion of ATP, which causes oxidative damage to red blood cell membranes, resulting in hemolytic anemia.
- Vitamin E, a fat-soluble vitamin mainly located in the biologic membrane, stabilizes the membrane through its antioxidant property. Vitamin C accelerates the antioxidant action of vitamin E.
- Supplementation with high-dose vitamins E (2000 mg) and C (2000 mg) can safely improve RBV-induced hemolytic anemia during IFN-α-2b and RBV combination therapy for 24 weeks in CHC.
- Combination therapy with pegylated IFN and RBV for 48 weeks has been recommended as a standard therapy in refractory CHC. Recently, extending the treatment duration to 72 weeks has been reported to improve the SVR rates in slow virologic responders.
- The safety and efficacy of long-term supplementation with high doses of vitamins E and C for CHC patients remain to be elucidated.

REFERENCES

1. Lauer, G., and B. D. Walker. 2001. Hepatitis C virus infection. *N Engl J Med* 345: 41–52.
2. Poynard, T., M. F. Yuen, V. Ratziu, and C. L. Lai. 2003. Viral hepatitis C. *Lancet* 362:2095–2100.
3. Feld, J. J., and J. H. Hoofnagle. 2005. Mechanism of action of interferon and ribavirin in treatment of hepatitis C. *Nature* 436:967–972.
4. McHutchison, J. G., S. C. Gordon, E. R. Schiff, M. L. Shiffman, W. M. Lee, V. K. Rustgi, et al. 1998. Interferon alpha-2b alone or in combination with ribavirin as initial treatment for chronic hepatitis C. The Hepatitis International Therapy Group. *N Engl J Med* 339:1485–1492.
5. Davis, G. L., R. Esteban-Mur, V. Rustgi, J. Hoefs, S. C. Gordon, C. Trepo, et al. 1998. Interferon alpha-2b alone or in combination with ribavirin for the treatment of relapse of chronic hepatitis C. The Hepatitis International Therapy Group. *N Engl J Med* 339:1493–1499.
6. Poynard, T., P. Marcellin, S. S. Lee, C. Niederau, G. S. Minuk, G. Ideo, et al. 1998. Randomized trial of interferon alpha–2b plus ribavirin for 48 weeks or for 24 weeks versus interferon alpha–2b plus placebo for 48 weeks for treatment of chronic infection with hepatitis C virus. The International Hepatitis Interventional Therapy Group. *Lancet* 352:1426–1432.
7. Takaki, S., A. Tsubota, T. Hosaka, N. Akuta, T. Someya, M. Kobayashi, et al. 2004. Factors contributing to ribavirin dose reduction due to anemia during interferon alpha2b and ribavirin combination therapy for chronic hepatitis C. *J Gastroenterol* 39:668–673.
8. Sulkowski, M. S., R. Wasserman, L. Brooks, L. Ball, and R. Gish. 2004. Changes in haemoglobin during interferon alpha–2b plus ribavirin combination therapy for chronic hepatitis C virus infection. *J Viral Hepatol* 11:243–250.
9. Franceschi, L. D., G. Fattovich, F. Turrini, K. Ayi, C. Brugnara, F. Manzato, et al. 2000. Hemolytic anemia induced by ribavirin therapy in patients with chronic hepatitis C virus infection: Role of membrane oxidative damage. *Hepatology* 31:997–1004.
10. Meydani, M. 1995. Vitamin E. *Lancet* 345:170–175.
11. Rifici, V. A., and A. K. Khachadurian. 1993. Dietary supplementation with vitamins C and E inhibits in vitro oxidation of lipoproteins. *J Am Coll Nutr* 12:631–637.
12. Bwnder, D. A., and P. A. Mayes. 2003. Vitamins and minerals. In *Harper's Illustrated Biochemistry*, 26th ed., ed. R. K. Murray, D. K. Granner, P. A. Mayes, and V. W. Rodwell, 481–497. New York: McGraw-Hill.
13. Machlin, L. J., and A. Bendich. 1987. Free radical tissue damage: Protective role of antioxidant nutrients. *FASEB J* 1:441–445.
14. Lindenbach, B. D., and C. M. Rice. 2005. Unravelling hepatitis C virus replication from genome to function. *Nature* 436:933–938.
15. Moriya, K., K. Nakagawa, T. Santa, Y. Shintani, H. Fujie, H. Miyoshi, et al. 2001. Oxidative stress in the absence of inflammation in a mouse model for hepatitis C virus–associated hepatocarcinogenesis. *Cancer Res* 61:4365–4370.
16. Bureau, C., J. Bernad, N. Chaouche, C. Orfila, M. Béraud, C. Gonindard, et al. 2001. Nonstructural 3 protein of hepatitis C virus triggers an oxidative burst in human monocytes via activation of NADPH oxidase. *J Biol Chem* 276:23077–23083.
17. Gong, G., G. Waris, R. Tanveer, and A. Siddiqui. 2001. Human hepatitis C virus NS5A protein alters intracellular calcium levels, induces oxidative stress, and activates STAT-3 and NF-κB. *Proc Natl Acad Sci U S A* 96:9599–9604.
18. Nishina, S., K. Hino, M. Korenaga, C. Vecchi, A. Pietrangelo, Y. Mizukami, et al. 2008. Hepatitis C virus–induced reactive oxygen species raise hepatic iron level in mice by reducing hepcidin transcription. *Gastroenterology* 134:226–238.

19. Fenton, H. J. H. 1894. Oxidation of tartaric acid in presence of iron. *J Chem Soc* 65:899–910.

20. Vendemiale, G., I. Grattagliano, P. Portincasa, G. Serviddio, G. Palasciamo, and E. Altomare. 2001. Oxidative stress in symptom-free HCV carriers: Relation with ALT flare-up. *Eur J Clin Invest* 31:54–63.

21. Jain, S. K., P. W. Pemberton, A. Smith, R. F. T. McMahon, P. C. Burrows, A. Aboutwerat, et al. 2002. Oxidative stress in chronic hepatitis C: Not just a feature of late stage disease. *J Hepatol* 36:805–811.

22. Hidaka, I., K. Hino, M. Korenaga, T. Gondo, S. Nishina, M. Ando, et al. 2007. Stronger Neo-Minophagen C™, a glycyrrhizin-containing preparation, protects liver against carbon tetrachloride-induced oxidative stress in transgenic mice expressing the hepatitis C virus polyprotein. *Liver Int* 27:845–853.

23. Suzuki, H., T. Ohta, T. Takino, K. Fujisawa, and C. Hirayama. 1983. Effects of glycyrrhizin on biochemical tests in patients with chronic hepatitis. Double-blind trial. *Asian Med J* 26:423–438.

24. Arase, Y., K. Ikeda, N. Murashima, K. Chayama, A. Tsubota, I. Koida, et al. 1997. The long term efficacy of glycyrrhizin in chronic hepatitis C patients. *Cancer* 79: 1494–1500.

25. Nakashima, T., Y. Sumida, T. Yoh, Y. Kakisaka, Y. Nakajima, H. Ishikawa, et al. 2000. Thioredoxin levels in the sera of untreated viral hepatitis patients and those treated with glycyrrhizin or ursodeoxycholic acid. *Antioxid Redox Signal* 2:687–694.

26. Omata, M., H. Yoshida, J. Toyota, E. Tomita, S. Nishiguchi, N. Hayashi, et al. 2007. A large-scale, multicentre, double-blind trial of ursodeoxycholic acid in patients with chronic hepatitis C. Japanese C-Viral Hepatitis Network. *Gut* 56:1747–1753.

27. Yano, M., H. Hayashi, S. Wakusawa, F. Sanae, T. Takikawa, Y. Shiono, et al. 2002. Long term effects of phlebotomy on biochemical and histological parameters of chronic hepatitis C. *Am J Gastroenterol* 97:133–137.

28. Mahmood, S., G. Yamada, G. Niiyama, M. Kawanaka, K. Togawa, M. Sho, et al. 2003. Effect of vitamin E on serum aminotransferase and thioredoxin levels in patients with viral hepatitis C. *Free Radic Res* 37:781–785.

29. Herbay, A. V., W. Stahl, C. Niederau, and H. Sies. 1997. Vitamin E improves the aminotransferase status of patients suffering from viral hepatitis C: A randomized, double-blind, placebo-controlled study. *Free Radic Res* 27:599–605.

30. Groenbaek, K., H. Friis, M. Hansen, H. Ring-Larsen, and H. B. Krarup. 2006. The effect of antioxidant supplementation on hepatitis C viral load, transaminases and oxidative status: A randomized trial among chronic hepatitis C virus–infected patients. *Eur J Gastroenterol Hepatol* 18:985–989.

31. Miller, E. R. 3rd, R. Pastor-Barriuso, D. Dalal, R. A. Riemersma, L. J. Appel, and E. Guallar. 2005. Meta-analysis: High-dosage vitamin E supplementation may increase all-cause mortality. *Ann Intern Med* 142:37–46.

32. Patterson, J. L., and R. Fernandez-Larsson. 1990. Molecular mechanisms of action of ribavirin. *Rev Infect Dis* 12:1139–1146.

33. Page, T., and J. D. Connor. 1990. The mechanism of ribavirin in erythrocytes and nucleated cells. *Int J Biochem* 22:379–383.

34. Saeian, K., J. S. Bajaj, J. Franco, J. F. Knox, J. Daniel, C. Peine, et al. 2004. High-dose vitamin E supplementation does not diminish ribavirin-associated haemolysis in hepatitis C treatment with combination standard alpha-interferon and ribavirin. Midwest Hepatitis Group. *Aliment Pharmacol Ther* 20:1189–1193.

35. Hino, K., Y. Murakami, A. Nagai, A. Kitase, Y. Hara, T. Furutani, et al. 2006. Alpha-tocopherol [corrected] and ascorbic acid attenuates the ribavirin [corrected] induced decrease of eicosapentaenoic acid in erythrocyte membrane in chronic hepatitis C patients. *J Gastroenterol Hepatol* 21:1269–1275. Erratum in *J Gastroenterol Hepatol* 21:1640.

36. Brass, C. A., and E. Piken. 1999. Do antioxidants ameliorate ribavirin related anemia in HCV patients? *Gastroenterology* 116:L0056.
37. Kawaguchi, Y., T. Mizuta, H. Takahashi [corrected], S. Iwane, K. Ario, H. Kawasoe, et al. 2007. High-dose vitamins E and C supplementation prevents ribavirin-induced hemolytic anemia in patients with chronic hepatitis C. *Hepatol Res* 37:317–324. Erratum in *Hepatol Res* 2008;38:114.
38. Kappus, H., and A. T. Diplock. 1992. Tolerance and safety of vitamin E: A toxicological position report. *Free Radic Biol Med* 13:55–74.
39. Hasegawa, T., M. Yoneda, K. Nakamura, I. Makino, and A. Terano. 2001. Plasma transforming growth factor–beta1 level and efficacy of alpha-tocopherol in patients with nonalcoholic steatohepatitis: A pilot study. *Aliment Pharmacol Ther* 15:1667–1672.
40. Mezey, E., J. J. Potter, L. Rennie-Tankersley, J. Caballeria, and A. Pares. 2004. A randomized placebo controlled trial of vitamin E for alcoholic hepatitis. *J Hepatol* 40:40–46.
41. Manns, M. P., J. G. McHutchison, S. C. Gordon, V. K. Rustgi, M. Shiffman, R. Reindollar, et al. 2001. Peginterferon alpha-2b plus ribavirin compared with interferon alpha-2b plus ribavirin for initial treatment of chronic hepatitis C: A randomised trial. The International Hepatitis Interventional Therapy Group. *Lancet* 358:958–965.
42. Hadziyannis, S. J., H. Sette Jr., T. R. Morgan, V. Balan, M. Diago, P. Marcellin, et al. 2004. Peginterferon-α2a and ribavirin combination therapy in chronic hepatitis C: A randomized study of treatment duration and ribavirin dose. The PEGASYS International Study Group. *Ann Intern Med* 140:346–355.
43. Pearlman, B. L., C. Ehleben, and S. Saifee. 2007. Treatment extension to 72 weeks of peginterferon and ribavirin in hepatitis C genotype 1–infected slow responders. *Hepatology* 46:1688–1694.
44. Berg, T., M. von Wagner, S. Nasser, C. Sarrazin, T. Heintges, T. Gerlach, et al. 2006. Extended treatment duration for hepatitis C virus type 1: Comparing 48 versus 72 weeks of peginterferon-alpha-2a plus ribavirin. *Gastroenterology* 130:1086–1097.

18 Diet Therapy in Virus-Related Liver Disease

Francesco Manguso and Luciano D'Agostino

CONTENTS

18.1 INTRODUCTION

There has been an increasing interest in the role of diet in virus-related liver disease. In patients chronically affected by hepatitis B virus (HBV) and hepatitis C virus (HCV) infection, some nutritional aspects are considered factors that can increase the risk of progression of liver disease, promoting or accelerating the course to the end stages. Overweight and obesity seem to influence this clinical course negatively, and protein-energy malnutrition, a frequent finding in patients with liver cirrhosis, represents a risk factor influencing survival [1]. The correction of these factors has practical consequences because it can improve the quality of life of these patients and of their families and reduce the social costs of chronic viral liver disease.

The aim of this chapter is to briefly examine the relationships between the nutritional aspects and HBV- and HCV-related diseases. In particular, we will look at (1) the influence of nutritional comorbidities on viral liver disease progression, (2) the impact of the nutritional status on viral liver disease outcome, and (3) the therapeutic role of nutrition on chronic liver disease.

The key functions of the liver, the features of virus-related liver disease, and the basic concepts of protein-energy malnutrition in cirrhosis are summarized in Table 18.1.

TABLE 18.1
Key Concepts in Virus-Related Liver Disease

1. The liver plays a pivotal role in metabolic homeostasis, regulating energy metabolism by taking up and processing ingested nutrients. These functions assure a controlled distribution of vital molecules to the cells of the entire organism. Moreover, the liver synthesizes enzymes, essential proteins, and cofactors necessary for digestion. Finally, the liver detoxifies and eliminates many endogenous and exogenous compounds.

2. There are five major hepatotropic viruses that cause hepatitis. Hepatitis A and E viruses cause acute hepatitis only, and their prevalence varies widely from country to country, as well as in different areas of the same country. HBV (with or without hepatitis D virus coinfection or superinfection) and HCV also cause acute hepatitis, which turns into chronic infections in a high percentage of cases.

3. Patients with acute viral liver disease do not require specific nutritional management, with the exception of acute viral fulminant liver disease in which nutrition assumes a main relevance among the resuscitative and conservative procedures that should be undertaken.

4. Besides viral- and host-related factors, other factors such as alcohol consumption and metabolic and environmental factors affect the progression of chronic viral liver disease. Among the metabolic factors, NAFLD, diabetes, and obesity may increase the risk of progression of chronic liver disease. The spectrum NAFLD—a liver disease that occurs in individuals who are not alcohol abusers—encompasses simple fatty liver, NASH (fatty liver plus parenchymal inflammation with or without accompanying focal necrosis), and varying degrees of fibrosis, including cirrhosis (NAFLD-associated cirrhosis).

5. The evolution of chronic liver disease is characterized by the appearance of fibrosis. With its progression, groups of hepatocytes become completely surrounded by fibrous substance, so developing a new cell organization, the nodule, which replaces the normal lobular structure. The final stage of this liver disease is cirrhosis.

6. HBV and HCV infection may eventually result in liver cirrhosis, with decompensation and hepatocellular carcinoma. In chronically affected patients, an antiviral treatment should be attempted with the aim of stopping the progression of the disease. Hepatic steatosis appears to be an independent predictor of poor response to antiviral therapy in patients with chronic active HCV infection. Hence, the correction of hepatic steatosis should be pursued to optimize the effect of antiviral therapy.

7. Protein-energy malnutrition is a frequent finding in HBV/HCV cirrhotic patients, affecting the 15–20% of compensated and higher percentages of decompensated diseases.

8. Several extrametabolic factors contribute to the establishment of protein-energy malnutrition during cirrhosis: decreased food intake due to anorexia, nausea, impaired taste ability, gastric fullness, and dyspepsia. These symptoms are frequently observed when a conspicuous peritoneal fluid is present.

9. The nutritional status should be assessed in all cirrhotic patients. An appropriate diet, aimed at changing the patients' eating habits and not simply at compensating single deficiencies, can improve the indexes of malnutrition and positively influence the clinical outcome of the disease.

Note: Key functions of the liver, features of virus-related liver disease, and basic concepts of protein-energy malnutrition in cirrhosis. HBV, hepatitis B virus; HCV, hepatitis C virus; NAFLD, nonalcoholic fatty liver disease; NASH, nonalcoholic steatohepatitis.

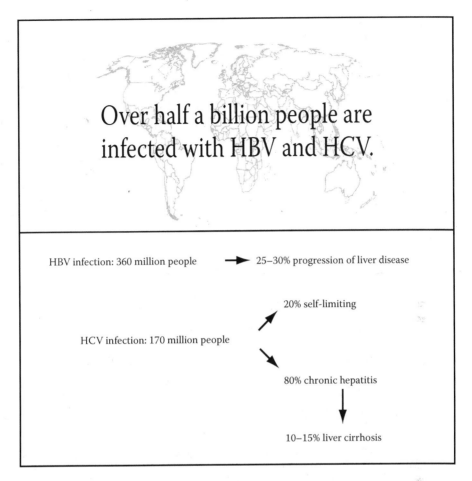

Over half a billion people are infected with HBV and HCV.

HBV infection: 360 million people ⟶ 25–30% progression of liver disease

HCV infection: 170 million people

20% self-limiting

80% chronic hepatitis

10–15% liver cirrhosis

FIGURE 18.1 Worldwide distribution of HBV and HCV infection. There are over half a billion HBV and HCV carriers in the world, and about 20% of them will die from the chronic sequelae of these infections: cirrhosis and primary liver cancer. In particular, according to the WHO, approximately 360 million and 170 million individuals worldwide are chronically infected with HBV and HCV, respectively. HBV infection is declining because of a wider use of prophylactic strategies, including vaccination. On the other hand, HCV infection rate remains unchanged. Patients in whom there is a persistence of hepatitis HBsAg in serum for more than 6 months are referred to as "chronic HBsAg carriers." The frequency of progression from acute to chronic HBV infection is primarily determined by age at the time of infection, but other risk factors have been described. Between one-third and one-quarter of individuals chronically infected with HBV are expected to develop progressive liver disease. HCV infection is self-limiting in only about 20% of individuals, but in the remaining 80%, chronic hepatitis develops. Liver cirrhosis occurs in about 10–15% of chronically infected patients. Host factors contribute to the disease progression. HBsAg, hepatitis B surface antigen; HBV, hepatitis B virus; HCV, hepatitis C virus; WHO, World Health Organization.

18.2 THE EPIDEMIOLOGICAL SCENARIO

There are five major hepatotropic viruses that cause hepatitis [2,3]. Hepatitis A and E viruses cause acute illness only, and their prevalence varies widely from country to country, as well as in different areas of the same country [3,4]. HBV (with or without hepatitis D virus coinfection or superinfection) and HCV viruses also cause acute hepatitis but may lead to chronic infection [2].

The worldwide distribution of HBV and HCV infection is shown in Figure 18.1. Roughly, one-quarter of individuals chronically infected with HBV are expected to develop progressive liver disease [5]. The frequency of the progression from acute to chronic HBV infection is primarily determined by the patient's age at infection, but other risk factors have been described [6,7]. HCV infection is self-limiting in only about 20% of patients, and approximately 80% of infected patients do not clear the virus within 6 months, thus developing chronic hepatitis [8]. Liver cirrhosis is the endpoint of the 10–15% of patients infected by HCV [8]. HCV and HBV infections are the most common disorders leading to liver transplantation and their late-stage complications. These infections, in combination with alcohol intake, obesity, diabetes, insulin resistance, and alteration of lipid metabolism, have high prevalence in southern Europe, giving us the chance to observe the global impact of these major risk factors.

18.3 NUTRITION AND ACUTE VIRAL LIVER DISEASE

Patients with acute viral liver disease do not require specific nutritional management. Factors such as anorexia, vomiting, and diarrhea may lead to acute weight loss, but malnutrition is unusual. During the acute phase of the infection, patients should maintain a high-caloric diet because the body is in a high catabolic state. No data are available regarding a possible relation between nutrition and the progression of HCV and HBV into chronic stage.

Acute viral fulminant liver disease is an uncommon but potentially lethal illness [9]. Nutrition assumes a main relevance among the resuscitative and conservative procedures that should be undertaken. There is a surprising lack of consensus about the appropriate feeding regimes, and in liver units nutritional support is offered to critical cases with a wide variability in terms of method of feeding (parenteral or enteral), solution composition, dosage, metabolic monitoring, and insulin usage [10]. However, the discussion of these items overwhelms the scopes of this chapter.

18.4 NUTRITIONAL FACTORS INVOLVED IN THE PROGRESSION OF CHRONIC LIVER DISEASE

The sequence of chronic hepatitis, cirrhosis, and hepatocellular carcinoma (HCC) has been extensively studied. Besides viral- and host-related factors, other factors such as alcohol consumption, metabolic, and environmental factors seem related to the progression of chronic viral liver disease (Figure 18.2). Alcohol consumption appears to be one of the most influential factors driving fibrosis progression in patients with chronic viral hepatitis, and it is acknowledged that its excessive consumption

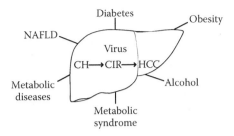

FIGURE 18.2   Factors influencing the progression of chronic viral liver disease. Progression of the viral liver disease, from chronic hepatitis to cirrhosis and hepatocellular carcinoma, is influenced by several factors. CH, chronic hepatitis; CIR, cirrhosis; HCC, hepatocellular carcinoma; NAFLD, nonalcoholic fatty liver disease.

contributes to the development of progressive liver disease [11,12]. Furthermore, a higher risk for HCC has been reported for patients with chronic HBV infection and concomitant alcohol intake > 50 g/day [13,14].

Metabolic factors, such as nonalcoholic fatty liver disease (NAFLD), diabetes, and obesity can increase the risk of progression of chronic viral liver disease [7,15,16], sometimes synergistically [17]. NAFLD and hepatotropic viruses seem to cooperate in modifying the cytokine production pathway, thereby producing a synergistic effect that results in increased liver damage [18,19] (Figure 18.3). Some studies reported that advanced NAFLD, responsible for cirrhosis in 5% of cases, is rare before the age of 45–50 years [18], indicating that an adequate duration is necessary for the progression to the NAFLD-associated cirrhosis. Interestingly, both NAFLD and its progressive subtype, nonalcoholic steatohepatitis (NASH), are considered hepatic manifestations of the metabolic syndrome [20], since an association between insulin resistance and NAFLD has been demonstrated [21].

HCV, and not HBV, has been linked with the derangement of glucose homeostasis and induction of insulin resistance [21–23]. A study demonstrated that HCV-associated insulin resistance depends on the virus itself, since adipocytokines were elevated in the sera of HCV-infected subjects when compared to healthy controls matched for age, body mass index, and waist/hip ratio [24]. In contrast, in patients with chronic HBV, superimposed NAFLD seems more related to the components of the metabolic syndrome (obesity, dyslipidemia, hypertension, and insulin resistance) [25–27], and clinical data do not support a "steatogenic" role for HBV, even though the prevalence of steatosis ranges from 20% to 70% in liver biopsies [25,26,28].

Hepatic steatosis is a common finding in chronic HCV infection; for patients infected with genotype 3, steatosis is directly ascribed to the virus, whereas other mechanisms are supposed for genotypes 1 and 4 [29].

There is no conclusive evidence about the causal association between hepatic steatosis and fibrosis progression in chronic hepatitis B: two cross-sectional studies found that hepatic steatosis was not correlated with severity of fibrosis [24,28], whereas an Italian longitudinal study reported that steatosis was associated with a

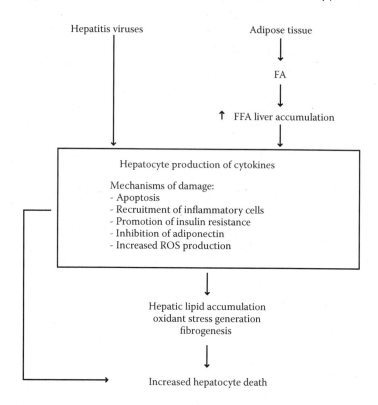

FIGURE 18.3 Liver damage: possible interaction between NAFLD and virus infection. The mechanisms by which fat-derived factors regulate hepatic inflammatory responses have been in part elucidated. FA, adiponectin, and TNF-α promote NAFLD by modulating the hepatic inflammatory response. Increases in hepatic FFA activate signals that increase hepatocyte production of TNF-α. TNF-α, in turn, inhibits adiponectin. This promotes hepatic lipid accumulation and insulin resistance. Efforts to remove these excess lipids increase hepatocyte lipid metabolism, and this process increases the generation of ROS. TNF-α itself also increases hepatocyte ROS production. Increased hepatocyte exposure to ROS generates a state of oxidant stress. This cytokine-dependent pathway is also triggered by hepatotropic viruses. FA, fatty acids; FFA, free fatty acids; NAFLD, nonalcoholic fatty liver disease; TNF, tumor necrosis factor; ROS, reactive oxygen species.

twofold increased risk of progression to overt cirrhosis [30]. On the other hand, a clearer link is recognizable for HCV; several studies are in favor of a contributory role of steatosis in the progression of liver fibrosis [31].

Taking these evidences together, in patients with chronic HCV disease, hepatic steatosis is a reflection of the viral infection and only in part of the host metabolic profile, whereas in chronic HBV disease, the host metabolic profile seems to prevail.

Finally, besides the observation that alcohol intake may influence the progression toward virus-related HCC [13,14], some researchers affirm that diabetes is strictly associated with an increased risk for HCC in viral hepatitis patients [32].

18.5   MALNUTRITION IN VIRUS-RELATED LIVER CIRRHOSIS: MAGNITUDE OF THE PROBLEM

Protein-energy malnutrition is a frequent finding in HBV/HCV cirrhotic patients, and it is correlated to the degree of liver disease, reaching 15–20% in compensated cirrhosis and higher percentages in decompensated cirrhosis, regardless of the origin of the disease [33–35]. Malnutrition is an independent risk factor influencing survival in patients with this disease and can modify their prognosis [36,37]. Moreover, abnormalities in nutritional status are associated with a higher risk of clinical complications and a higher mortality rate, together with complicated transplantation and other abdominal surgery outcomes, by increasing perioperative mortality and morbidity [38,39].

The mechanisms of protein-energy malnutrition during cirrhosis involve many factors that are summarized in Figure 18.4. Cirrhotic patients frequently experience decreased food intake due to anorexia, nausea, a decrease in the ability to taste, gastric fullness, and dyspepsia especially in the presence of conspicuous peritoneal fluid. Anorexia, even if more unusual than in alcoholic patients, can play a role, since the liver is an organ primarily involved in the metabolic control of eating, because of the activation of hepatic metabolic signals to the brain stem [40]. Cirrhosis complications, such as ascites and hepatic encephalopathy, make malnutrition worse. In fact, the therapy for these complications, such as diuretics, water restriction, or reduced nitrogen intake for encephalopathy, could potentially represent another cause of malnutrition. The prescription of a no-added-salt diet may contribute to the anorexia, reducing the protein intake and worsening the malnutrition. Moreover, exudative enteropathy together with cholestasis may contribute to malabsorption in the course of liver cirrhosis. Metabolic abnormalities are also observed in the course of liver disease and are represented by an increased energy expenditure during rest, insulin resistance, alterations of substrate oxidation (reduced glucose oxidation and increased lipid oxidation), accelerated protein breakdown, and inefficient protein synthesis [41,42].

The degree of the increased rate of metabolic activity in patients with liver cirrhosis is directly correlated to the Child score class. Several studies indicate that cirrhotic patients belonging to class B or C of Child classification, corresponding to those with moderate or severe liver disease, are hypercatabolic, having a deficient whole-body protein turnover [43]. Finally, patients with liver cirrhosis often have low plasma levels of vitamins and trace minerals [44]. Water- and lipid-soluble vitamin deficiency is observed during the course of liver cirrhosis. As regards essential trace minerals, zinc and selenium deficiency are also frequently observed.

In patients with chronic liver disease, the assessment of the nutritional status is very inaccurate especially in the presence of tissue edema and ascites, and most of the traditional biological and clinical parameters, together with morphological tools, used to estimate the nutritional state have considerable limitations [45].

The European Society for Clinical Nutrition and Metabolism (ESPEN) recently issued specific guidelines for the assessment of malnutrition in liver disease [46]. The guidelines recommend the use of simple bedside methods such as the Subjective Global Assessment [47] or anthropometry to identify patients at risk for undernutrition. To quantify undernutrition, the phase angle or body cell mass measured by

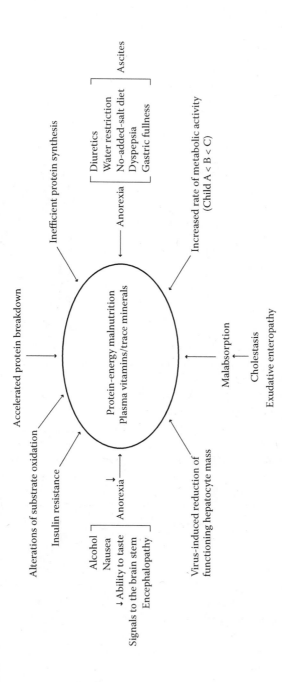

FIGURE 18.4   The mechanisms of protein-energy malnutrition and plasma vitamin and trace mineral reduction during viral liver cirrhosis. Metabolic factors, anorexia, clinical manifestations of decompensated disease (ascites, encephalopathy, and malabsorption), and virus-induced reduction of functioning hepatocyte mass, contribute to a decreased food intake and to the development of protein-energy malnutrition and reduction of plasma vitamins and trace minerals.

bioelectrical impedance analysis is considered adequate, despite some limitations described in patients with ascites [46].

18.6 THERAPEUTIC ROLE OF NUTRITION ON CHRONIC VIRAL LIVER DISEASE

18.6.1 CHRONIC HEPATITIS

Although a great amount of information concerning the mechanisms of the progression of chronic viral liver disease has accumulated in the past decade, there is still a long way to go in understanding who are the patients at risk for progressive disease that have to be treated and how to treat them. Since it is well established that the coexistence of viral chronic hepatitis together with metabolic factors (NAFLD, diabetes, and obesity) may increase the risk of progression of chronic liver disease, it is reasonable to promote strategies limiting their impact in the attempt to prevent or to slow down the progression toward more severe stages of the disease. Our opinion is that, in the presence of adjunctive damaging factors, it is mandatory to counsel lifestyle modification. Furthermore, despite the absence of long-term data concerning a histological improvement in patients treated for NAFLD, we believe that it is prudent to advise the chronically infected patients with a coexistent NAFDL about the risk of not abandoning a diet favoring the accumulation of lipids in the liver. This belief is based on clinical trials showing a significant alanine aminotransferase activity reduction in NAFLD patients put on restrictive diet with or without exercise [48,49].

Insulin resistance is associated with NASH or NASH-related fibrosis [20]. For this reason, treatment strategies are focusing on reversing or improving the insulin resistance. In overweight/obese patients, weight reduction results in the loss of adipose tissue with a decreasing of insulin resistance. It is noteworthy that hepatic steatosis, mild, moderate, or severe, appears to be an independent predictor of poor response to antiviral therapy in patients with chronic active HCV infection [50,51]. Hence, in these patients, the correction of hepatic steatosis could be of benefit in obtaining an optimal effect of antiviral therapy when it is planned. As regards specific medications, much evidence suggested that the decreased insulin resistance and reduced hyperinsulinemia may facilitate the efficacy of antiviral drugs on HCV replication. In Italy, an ongoing study is investigating the efficacy and safety of pegylated interferon and ribavirin plus metformin versus pegylated interferon and ribavirin alone in the treatment of naive patients with genotype 1 chronic HCV infection and insulin resistance, and data will be available early in 2009. At the moment, the use of insulin sensitizers such as metformin and the glitazones should be reserved for patients at risk for progression [52]. Of note, metformin seems safer because it is lacking in liver toxicity, being excreted unchanged in the urine without any hepatic metabolism [53], whereas thiazolidinediones have shown liver toxicity [54].

In conclusion, at present there is no established diet treatment for patients with concomitant chronic viral hepatitis and metabolic risk factors. However, prudent measures for these patients could be, apart from the generally accepted recommendation of the alcohol abstinence, the prescription of an appropriate equilibrate diet intended to reduce the liver fat accumulation, together with advice for a change in lifestyle. Explicitly, nutritional counseling and physical exercise planning should be considered crucial therapeutic and preventive measures.

18.6.2   LIVER CIRRHOSIS

There is no specific consensus that can drive the reader as to when to give nutrition support to patients with liver cirrhosis [55]. An interesting meta-analysis showed that the rates of complications, infections, and mortality in inpatients with different diseases, including liver disease, were significantly reduced when an appropriate oral or tube feeding was started [56]. Because patients with cirrhosis are part of the malnourished population in hospitals, it may be argued that nutrition support also improves the clinical outcomes of these patients. Moreover, nutrition plays a key role especially in those patients awaiting liver transplantation [57].

The restriction of dietary protein intake in patients with viral liver cirrhosis with or without hepatic encephalopathy became common practice in the 1970s and 1980s but was clearly not evidence-based. Conversely, in the past decade, the ESPEN guidelines have recommended higher protein intakes. In fact, the primary goal in patients with liver cirrhosis is to achieve an energy intake of 35–40 kcal/kg body weight (BW)/day (147–168 kJ/kg BW/day) and a protein intake of 1.2–1.5 g/kg BW/day [46]. Unfortunately, until now, these indications are still difficult to

TABLE 18.2
Characteristics of the Diet Prescribed to Cirrhotic Patients

Components

kcal/kg of desirable body weight/day (kcal)	30–40
kcal of total protein (%)	16
Vegetable protein (%)	10
Animal protein (%)	6
kcal of total carbohydrate (%)	55
Soluble carbohydrate (%)	15
Complex carbohydrate (%)	40
kcal of total lipid (%)	28–30
Calcium (mg/day)[a]	500–600
Iron (mg/day)	18
Sodium (mg/day)	1000
Potassium (mg/day)	2000–3000
Phosphorus (mg/day)	1200–1400

Source: From Manguso, F., D'Ambra, G., Menchise, A., Sollazzo, R., and D'Agostino, L., *Clin Nutr*, 24, 751–759. With permission.

Note: Composition of the prescribed diet in patients with liver cirrhosis of viral origin. Data are percentages of total caloric intake (%) except when otherwise indicated.

[a] Oral calcium (500 mg/day) supplement was prescribed to all patients.

TABLE 18.3

Example of Diet Recommended for Cirrhotic Patients without Ascites

Breakfast

- Coffee or barley without sugar
- Partially skimmed milk (150 g) or light yogurt (125 g)
- Seven whole wheat crackers (ship's biscuit)

Snack

- Unsalted crackers (25 g) or four whole wheat crackers, or fresh fruit (150 g)

Lunch

- Pulses (chickpeas, lentils, broad beans, etc.; 100 g) with wholemeal bread (30 g) at least two times a week or pasta or rice (50 g) with pulses (60 g) or vegetable soup (200 g) with pulses (40 g) and pasta or rice (40 g) or pasta or rice (60 g) with cooked vegetables (250 g) or no more than once a week pasta or rice (80 g) with tomato sauce or potatoes (350 g) or potatoes (150 g) with cooked vegetables (250 g) or potatoes (200 g) with raw vegetables (150 g)
- Meat, whichever type, sliced meat (120 g) or at least two times a week fish (150 g) or no more than two times a week 2 eggs or mozzarella cheese (80 g), ricotta (cottage cheese; 150 g), fresh or seasoned cheese (45 g)
- Vegetable salad (100 g) or cooked vegetables (200 g)
- Wholemeal bread (50 g)
- Fresh fruit (150 g)

Dinner

- Pasta or rice or semolina or "polenta" or maize (60 g) or potato gnocchi (140 g) or potatoes (260 g) or pizza with tomatoes (100 g) or wholemeal bread (70 g)
- Vegetable salad (150 g) or cooked vegetables (250 g)
- Wholemeal bread (50 g)
- Fresh fruit (150 g)

For each day: 3 tablespoons of extra virgin olive oil

Daily example

Breakfast: 1 coffee, milk partially skimmed (150 g), 7 whole wheat crackers

Snack: unsalted crackers (25 g)

Lunch: Pasta (50 g) with lentils (60 g), codfish with tomato sauce (150 g), vegetable salad (100 g), wholemeal bread (50 g), apple (150 g)

Dinner: wholemeal bread (120 g), boiled courgettes (250 g), pear (150 g)

Condiment: 3 tablespoons of extra virgin olive oil (used for cooking and/or salad dressing)

Note: Characteristics of diet proposed for patients with liver cirrhosis without ascites. This diet takes into account the dietary habits of our country. The authors are indebted to Giovanna D'Ambra for the preparation of the diet.

achieve. More recent studies have shown that long-term oral supplementation with a branched-chain amino acid (BCAA) mixture is better than ordinary food in a late evening snack at improving the serum albumin level and the energy metabolism in patients with cirrhosis [58]. A recent Cochrane review on the use of intravenous and oral BCAA for hepatic encephalopathy has shown that patients receiving BCAA are more likely to recover from hepatic encephalopathy than patients treated with other regimens but without convincing evidence on survival [59].

Even though a considerable amount of data demonstrated malnutrition and specific deficiencies in patients with liver cirrhosis, only a few studies investigated nutritional improvement after dietary intervention [1]. In our experience, in patients with liver cirrhosis of viral origin, an appropriate diet may improve the nutritional status and protein malnutrition [1]. Since we found that, in the majority of patients with cirrhosis, malnutrition was associated with the assumption of an inadequate diet, we believe that the prescribed diet should be aimed at changing the patients' eating habits and not simply at compensating single deficiency. This approach is, in our experience, successful, as indicated by the very good compliance observed among patients during the monitored phases of our study [1]. In prescribing the diet, we pay attention to the fact that diet has to be varied, well balanced, palatable, and able to assure an adequate caloric and protein intake, with prevalence of vegetable proteins. In Tables 18.2 and 18.3, it is possible to see the characteristics of the diet and a standard daily regimen we propose for cirrhotic patients. The diet is supplied on an average 30–40 kcal/kg of desirable body weight, of which 16% derived from proteins, 28–30% from lipids, and 55% carbohydrates (simple carbohydrate, not more than 10%). The diet is modified according to the presence of diabetes mellitus. Patients with diabetes receive calories spread over six meals. Oral calcium (500 mg/day) is prescribed for all patients in order to compensate for its reduced content in the diet.

Our experience emphasizes the importance of evaluating the nutritional status in patients with cirrhosis of viral origin because they often present a poor caloric and protein intake, demonstrating that a rational and simple nutritional approach can improve the indexes of malnutrition, and positively influence the clinical outcome. Consequently, we are convinced that nutritional care represents a complementary, but not secondary, therapy that can improve the quality of life of patients with chronic viral liver disease.

18.7 SUMMARY POINTS

- Nutritional management of patients with acute viral liver disease does not require specific management.
- In acute viral fulminant liver disease, nutrition assumes a main relevance among the resuscitative and conservative procedures.
- Alcohol consumption as well as metabolic and environmental factors seems related to the progression of chronic viral hepatitis.
- In patients with chronic viral hepatitis, adjunctive factors potentially injuring the liver tissue should be avoided in the attempt to prevent or to slow down the progression toward more severe stages of the disease.
- In the presence of adjunctive damaging factors, the initial management of viral chronic liver disease must include lifestyle modification.
- Malnutrition is a complication of viral liver cirrhosis with important prognostic implications.
- Nutrition problems are related to the clinical course even in patients with cirrhosis with mild disease.

- Etiology of malnutrition in liver cirrhosis includes poor oral intake, malabsorption, increased energy expenditure, and an altered pattern of fuel consumption.
- In all cirrhotic patients, the nutritional status should be assessed.
- An appropriate diet can improve the indexes of malnutrition and positively influence the clinical outcome of viral cirrhosis.

REFERENCES

1. Manguso, F., G. D'Ambra, A. Menchise, R. Sollazzo, and L. D'Agostino. 2005. Effects of an appropriate oral diet on the nutritional status of patients with HCV-related liver cirrhosis: A prospective study. *Clin Nutr* 24:751–759.
2. Blackard, J. T., M. T. Shata, N. J. Shire, and K. E. Sherman. 2008. Acute hepatitis C virus infection: A chronic problem. *Hepatology* 47:321–331.
3. Wasley, A., S. Grytdal, K. Gallagher, and Centers for Disease Control and Prevention (CDC). 2008. Surveillance for acute viral hepatitis—United States, 2006. *MMWR Surveill Summ* 57:1–24.
4. Nguyen, G. C., and P. J. Thuluvath. 2008. Racial disparity in liver disease: Biological, cultural, or socioeconomic factors. *Hepatology* 47:1058–1066.
5. Pungpapong, S., W. R. Kim, and J. J. Poterucha. 2007. Natural history of hepatitis B virus infection: An update for clinicians. *Mayo Clin Proc* 82:967–975.
6. de Franchis, R., A. Hadengue, G. Lau, et al., EASL Jury. 2003. EASL International Consensus Conference on Hepatitis B. 13–14 September, 2002 Geneva, Switzerland. Consensus statement (long version). *J Hepatol* 39 (Suppl 1):S3–S25.
7. Fattovich, G., F. Bortolotti, and F. Donato. 2008. Natural history of chronic hepatitis B: Special emphasis on disease progression and prognostic factors. *J Hepatol* 48:335–352.
8. National Institutes of Health Consensus Development Conference Statement: Management of Hepatitis C: 2002 (June 10–12, 2002). *Gastroenterology* 123:2082–2099.
9. Taylor, R. M., T. Davern, S. Munoz, et al., US Acute Liver Failure Study Group. 2006. Fulminant hepatitis A virus infection in the United States: Incidence, prognosis, and outcomes. *Hepatology* 44:1589–1597.
10. Schütz, T., W. O. Bechstein, P. Neuhaus, H. Lochs, and M. Plauth. 2004. Clinical practice of nutrition in acute liver failure—A European survey. *Clin Nutr* 23:975–982.
11. Bellentani, S., G. Pozzato, G. Saccoccio, et al. 1999. Clinical course and risk factors of hepatitis C virus related liver disease in the general population: Report from the Dionysos study. *Gut* 44:874–880.
12. Corrao, G., P. A. Ferrari, and G. Galatola. 1995. Exploring the role of diet in modifying the effect of known disease determinants: Application to risk factors of liver cirrhosis. *Am J Epidemiol* 142:1136–1146.
13. Donato, F., U. Gelatti, R. M. Limina, and G. Fattovich. 2006. Southern Europe as an example of interaction between various environmental factors: A systematic review of the epidemiologic evidence. *Oncogene* 25:3756–3770.
14. Jee, S. H., H. Ohrr, J. W. Sull, and J. M. Samet. 2004. Cigarette smoking, alcohol drinking, hepatitis B, and risk for hepatocellular carcinoma in Korea. *J Natl Cancer Inst* 96:1851–1856.
15. Huo, T. I., J. C. Wu, S. J. Hwang, et al. 2000. Factors predictive of liver cirrhosis in patients with chronic hepatitis B: A multivariate analysis in a longitudinal study. *Eur J Gastroenterol Hepatol* 12:687–693.
16. Moscatiello, S., R. Manini, and G. Marchesini. 2007. Diabetes and liver disease: An ominous association. *Nutr Metab Cardiovasc Dis* 17:63–70.

17. Cimino, L., G. Oriani, A. D'Arienzo, et al. 2001. Interactions between metabolic disorders (diabetes, gallstones, and dyslipidaemia) and the progression of chronic hepatitis C virus infection to cirrhosis and hepatocellular carcinoma. A cross-sectional multicentre survey. *Dig Liver Dis* 33:240–246.

18. Ratziu, V., P. Giral, F. Charlotte, et al. 2000. Liver fibrosis in overweight patients. *Gastroenterology* 118:1117–1123.

19. Tacke, F., T. Luedde, and C. Trautwein. 2008. Inflammatory pathways in liver homeostasis and liver injury. *Clin Rev Allergy Immunol* doi:10.1007/s12016-008-8091-0.

20. Younossi, Z. M. 2008. Review Article: Current management of nonalcoholic fatty liver disease and non-alcoholic steatohepatitis (NAFLD and NASH). *Aliment Pharmacol Ther* 28:2–12.

21. Angelico, F., M. Del Ben, R. Conti, et al. 2005. Insulin resistance, the metabolic syndrome, and nonalcoholic fatty liver disease. *J Clin Endocrinol Metab* 90:1578–1582.

22. Fan, J. G., and S. Chitturi. 2008. Hepatitis B and fatty liver: Causal or coincidental? *J Gastroenterol Hepatol* 23:679–681.

23. Wang, C. C., C. S. Hsu, C. J. Liu, J. H. Kao, and D. S. Chen. 2008. Association of chronic hepatitis B virus infection with insulin resistance and hepatic steatosis. *J Gastroenterol Hepatol* 23:779–782.

24. Cua, I. H., J. M. Hui, P. Bandara, et al. 2007. Insulin resistance and liver injury in hepatitis C is not associated with virus-specific changes in adipocytokines. *Hepatology* 46:66–73.

25. Thomopoulos, K. C., V. Arvaniti, A. C. Tsamantas, et al. 2006. Prevalence of liver steatosis in patients with chronic hepatitis B: A study of associated factors and of relationship with fibrosis. *Eur J Gastroenterol Hepatol* 18:233–237.

26. Bondini, S., J. Kallman, A. Wheeler, et al. 2007. Impact of non-alcoholic fatty liver disease on chronic hepatitis B. *Liver Int* 27:607–611.

27. Tsochatzis, E., G. V. Papatheodoridis, E. K. Manesis, N. Chrysanthos, G. Kafiri, and A. J. Archimandritis. 2007. Hepatic steatosis in chronic hepatitis B develops due to host metabolic factors: A comparative approach with genotype 1 chronic hepatitis C. *Dig Liver Dis* 39:936–942.

28. Gordon, A., C. A. McLean, J. S. Pedersen, M. J. Bailey, and S. K. Roberts. 2005. Hepatic steatosis in chronic hepatitis B and C: Predictors, distribution and effect on fibrosis. *J Hepatol* 43:38–44.

29. Adinolfi, L. E., E. Durante-Mangoni, R. Zampino, and G. Ruggiero. 2005. Review article: Hepatitis C virus–associated steatosis—Pathogenic mechanisms and clinical implications. *Aliment Pharmacol Ther* 22 (Suppl 2):52–55.

30. Brunetto, M. R., F. Oliveri, B. Coco, et al. 2002. Outcome of anti-HBe positive chronic hepatitis B in alpha-interferon treated and untreated patients: A long term cohort study. *J Hepatol* 36:263–270.

31. Ortiz, V., M. Berenguer, J. M. Rayón, D. Carrasco, and J. Berenguer. 2002. Contribution of obesity to hepatitis C–related fibrosis progression. *Am J Gastroenterol* 97:2408–2414.

32. Davila, J. A., R. O. Morgan, Y. Shaib, K. A. McGlynn, and H. B. El-Serag. 2005. Diabetes increases the risk of hepatocellular carcinoma in the United States: A population based case control study. *Gut* 54:533–539.

33. Guglielmi, F. W., C. Panella, A. Buda, et al. 2005. Nutritional state and energy balance in cirrhotic patients with or without hypermetabolism. Multicentre prospective study by the 'Nutritional Problems in Gastroenterology' Section of the Italian Society of Gastroenterology (SIGE). *Dig Liver Dis* 37:681–688.

34. Lautz, H. U., O. Selberg, J. Körber, M. Bürger, and M. J. Müller. 1992. Protein-calorie malnutrition in liver cirrhosis. *Clin Investig* 70:478–486.

35. Carvalho, L., and E. R. Parise. 2006. Evaluation of nutritional status of nonhospitalized patients with liver cirrhosis. *Arq Gastroenterol* 43:269–274.

36. Caregaro, L., F. Alberino, P. Amodio, et al. 1996. Malnutrition in alcoholic and virus-related cirrhosis. *Am J Clin Nutr* 63:602–609.
37. Alberino, F., A. Gatta, P. Amodio, et al. 2001. Nutrition and survival in patients with liver cirrhosis. *Nutrition* 17:445–450.
38. Porayko, M. K., S. DiCecco, and S. J. O'Keefe. 1991. Impact of malnutrition and its therapy on liver transplantation. *Semin Liver Dis* 11:305–314.
39. Child, T. C., and J. G. Turcotte. 1964. *Surgery in Portal Hypertension*. Philadelphia: WB Saunders.
40. Friedman, M. I., and P. E. Sawchenko. 1984. Evidence for hepatic involvement in control of *ad libitum* food intake in rats. *Am J Physiol* 247(1 Pt 2):R106–R113.
41. Marsano, L., and C. J. McClain. 1991. Nutrition and alcoholic liver disease. *J Parenter Enteral Nutr* 15:337–344.
42. Riggio, O., S. Angeloni, L. Ciuffa, et al. 2003. Malnutrition is not related to alterations in energy balance in patients with stable liver cirrhosis. *Clin Nutr* 22:553–559.
43. Dichi, J. B., I. Dichi, R. Maio, et al. 2001. Whole-body protein turnover in malnourished patients with Child class B and C cirrhosis on diets low to high in protein energy. *Nutrition* 17:239–242.
44. Loguercio, C., V. De Girolamo, A. Federico, et al. 1997. Trace elements and chronic liver diseases. *J Trace Elem Med Biol* 11:158–161.
45. Merli, M., A. Romiti, O. Riggio, and L. Capocaccia. 1987. Optimal nutritional indexes in chronic liver disease. *J Parenter Enteral Nutr* 11(Suppl 5):130S–134S.
46. Plauth, M., E. Cabré, O. Riggio, et al. 2006. ESPEN Guidelines on Enteral Nutrition: Liver disease. *Clin Nutr* 25:285–294.
47. Hasse, J., S. Strong, M. A. Gorman, and G. Liepa. 1993. Subjective global assessment: Alternative nutrition-assessment technique for liver-transplant candidates. *Nutrition* 9:339–343.
48. Kadayifci, A., R. Merriman, and N. Bass. 2007. Medical treatment of non-alcoholic steatohepatitis. *Clin Liver Dis* 11:119–140.
49. Ueno, T., H. Sugawara, K. Sujaka, et al. 1997. Therapeutic effects of restricted diet and exercise in obese patients with fatty liver. *J Hepatol* 27:103–107.
50. Poustchi, H., F. Negro, J. Hui, et al. 2008. Insulin resistance and response to therapy in patients infected with chronic hepatitis C virus genotypes 2 and 3. *J Hepatol* 48:28–34.
51. Soresi, M., S. Tripi, V. Franco, et al. 2006. Impact of liver steatosis on the antiviral response in the hepatitis C virus–associated chronic hepatitis. *Liver Int* 26:1119–1125.
52. Cortez-Pinto, H. 2005. Concluding remarks: Metabolic syndrome, liver and HCV. *Aliment Pharmacol Ther* 22 (Suppl 2):83–85.
53. Sirtori, C. R., G. Franceschini, M. Galli-Kienle, et al. 1978. Disposition of metformin (*N,N*-dimethylbiguanide) in man. *Clin Pharmacol Ther* 24:683–693.
54. Scheen, A. J. 2001. Thiazolidinediones and liver toxicity. *Diabetes Metab (Paris)* 27:305–313.
55. Kondrup, J. 2006. Nutrition in end stage liver disease. *Best Pract Res Clin Gastroenterol* 20:547–560.
56. Stratton, R. J., C. J. Green, and M. Elia. 2003. Combined analysis of the effects of oral nutritional supplements and enteral tube feeding. In *Disease-Related Malnutrition: An Evidence-Based Approach to Treatment*. Wallingford: CABI Publishing, pp. 276–287.
57. Stickel, F., D. Inderbitzin, and D. Candinas. 2008. Role of nutrition in liver transplantation for end-stage chronic liver disease. *Nutr Rev* 66:47–54.
58. Tsiaousi, E. T., A. I. Hatzitolios, S. K. Trygonis, and C. G. Savopoulos. 2008. Malnutrition in end stage liver disease: Recommendations and nutritional support. *J Gastroenterol Hepatol* 23:527–533.
59. Als-Nielsen, B., R. L. Koretz, L. L. Kjaergard, and C. Gluud. 2003. Branched-chain amino acids for hepatic encephalopathy. *Cochrane Database Syst Rev* CD001939.

Section IV

The Young and Aging Liver,
End-Stage, and Transplantation

19 Nutritional Care for Infants with Cholestatic Liver Diseases

Alastair Baker

CONTENTS

19.1 INTRODUCTION

Pediatric liver disease is uncommon. A summary of the most common conditions presenting to specialist services in infancy with liver disease severe enough to justify nutritional support is shown in Table 19.1. Of these, the most common single condition causing cholestasis is biliary atresia occurring in 1 in 9,000–16,000 births in every population. All cases will require nutritional management and perhaps half will require intensive input including nasogastric tube (NGT) feeding. Other hepatological patients requiring nutritional care include those with parenteral nutrition

TABLE 19.1

Causes of Neonatal Cholestatic Liver Disease Encountered in Pediatric Hepatological Practice

Cholangiopathies

    Biliary atresia—particularly after failed Kasai portoenterostomy

    Variants of progressive familial intrahepatic cholestasis (bile salt export pump deficiency, PFIC1
        disease)

    Alagille syndrome

    Neonatal sclerosing cholangitis

    Neonatal Caroli disease

Metabolic conditions

    α-1-Antitrypsin deficiency

    Inborn errors of bile acid synthesis

    Storage disorders, e.g., Niemann-Pick C disease

Causes of inspissated bile syndrome

    Sepsis, especially gram negative and fungal

    Shock—septic shock, asphyxia, and cardiac failure

    Parenteral nutrition

    Prematurity

    Intrauterine growth restriction

Source: Baker A., Stevenson, R., Dhawan, A., Goncalves, I., Socha, P., and Sokal, E., *Pediatr Transplant*,
        11, 825–834, 2007. With permission.

associated cholestasis (PNAC) and metabolic conditions. In total, perhaps 1 infant with liver disease requiring intensive feeding could be anticipated for every 5,000–10,000 births. In the UK, this may represent 50–100 infants per year.

Liver transplantation is a curative option in a significant proportion of infants with established liver disease. Outcome of transplantation is related to nutritional status; therefore, all patients with cholestatic liver disease approaching liver transplantation will require nutritional supervision and most will require intervention. After transplantation, good nutritional recovery is anticipated but with the help of medical rehabilitation.

Cholestatic patients are typically jaundiced and may itch as soon as they reach 5 months if cholestasis is profound. The physical characteristics of severe liver disease, including body habitus with thin limbs and a prominent abdomen, will be evident in anthropometric measurements. Mid upper-arm circumference tends to become depleted earliest in the course of progressive disease, followed by triceps skin-fold thickness. Abdominal girth becomes equal to or exceeds thoracic girth measured at the nipples. Height growth failure tends to occur last unless severe rickets is present. Weight is affected by fluid balance abnormalities and visceromegaly is thus an insensitive indicator of nutritional state [2–4]. Clinical nutritional assessment includes the above anthropometry with assessment of dietary intake by history.

Nutritional impairment correlates broadly with liver function tests, suggesting that the former might have prognostic value [2]. Children with better nutritional status have fewer complications, including infections and rejection, and lower mortality at orthotopic liver transplantation (OLT), where a height standard deviation (SD or Z) score of less than −1 is associated with increased mortality at OLT [5,6], and those with height SD score of < 1.5 have double the hospital stay at transplantation of those with > 1.5 SD [7]. Although with the exception of liver transplantation (OLT), no treatment has been clearly shown to improve the prognosis of chronic liver disease (CLD), complications related to fat-soluble vitamin deficiency can be readily prevented by regular monitoring of plasma levels and diligent enteral, or if necessary, parenteral replacement. Nutrition is optimized in the expectation of reducing complications of the disease and improving outcome at OLT. The sense of well-being in malnourished children with liver disease, as perceived by the parents, improves with intensive enteral feeding, thereby justifying aggressive management [8]. Refractory failure to thrive is an important indication for early OLT [9]. Fifty-seven percent of a small series of patients who underwent transplantation before they were 3 years old had adverse developmental consequences apparently related to their previous nutritional impairments [10]. Therefore, nutritional care should also seek to optimize long-term neurodevelopmental outcomes.

Regular, planned multidisciplinary clinical nutritional review should be undertaken with a frequency appropriate to the patient's clinical course. A multidisciplinary nutritional care team consisting of a consultant pediatric gastroenterologist/nutritionist, a dietitian, a nutritional care nurse, a speech therapist, and, for parenteral nutrition (PN), a pharmacist, will assess and plan optimal care. Units managing cholestatic liver disease should have a comprehensive nutritional protocol for the assessment, management, and follow-up of cholestatic liver disease that can be subjected to audit. That protocol should require that all children with cholestatic liver disease have a clinical nutritional review with an intervention and follow-up plan including the frequency of review documented in their care records. The nutritional care team should liaise with local services to ensure adherence to the patient's plan in primary care.

19.2   MECHANISMS OF GROWTH IMPAIRMENT

Normal growth is controlled by a complex interaction of nutritional, hormonal, and genetic factors. Cholestasis implies severe depletion of intraluminal bile acid concentration with secondary fat malabsorption. Although malabsorption of lipid is the likely primary nutritional problem, malabsorption associated with portal hypertension and effects related to metabolic and endocrine consequences of hepatocellular dysfunction may contribute. Anorexia is attributed to organomegaly or pressure effects of ascites, but may be equally due to a congested gastric mucosa or reduced gastrointestinal (GI) motility of portal hypertension giving a feeling of satiety, or central effects of unidentified toxins. In adults, severity of GI symptoms is associated with recent weight loss and impaired health-related quality of life with the severity of GI symptoms related to the severity of cirrhosis [11]. When present, severe pruritus may appear to distract the child from eating.

Increased energy expenditure has been suggested as a cause of failure to thrive and is elevated by 40% or more for body weight in malnutrition [12], but is normal when expressed in terms independent of body composition including for Alagille syndrome [7,13,14]. Children with liver disease do not exhibit the hypometabolism of children with starvation from reduced intake alone. Thus, malnourished children with liver disease have high energy expenditure for their size, but not for their age [15]. Patients with cirrhosis show evidence of catabolism as soon as 8 hours after fasting comparable with that seen after 48 hours in normal adults [16].

The interaction of growth hormone (GH) with insulin and the downstream effects of insulin-like growth factor 1 (IGF-1) and its binding proteins (IGF-BPs) constitute an important mechanism linking nutrition and growth. The liver is the major source of plasma IGFs and IGF-BPs in response to circulating GH. Normal IGF-1 and IGF-BP responses to exogenous GH are lost with increasing severity of liver disease and associated malnutrition. Reduced responses are also seen in portal hypertension with good liver function. Although Alagille syndrome and progressive familial intrahepatic cholestasis 1 are associated with short stature after successful liver transplantation, nonconstitutional abnormalities correct rapidly after liver transplantation, but are often resistant to hyperalimentation before transplantation [17,18].

19.3   LIPIDS

Lipids play an important role in nutrition as an energy dense nutrient with low osmolarity and as the source of essential constituents of cell membranes: polyunsaturated fatty acids (PUFA). Increasing total fat intake may increase the overall quantity of fat absorbed and improve growth despite steatorrhea [19]. Medium-chain triglycerides (MCTs) are carried into the portal venous system without need for formation of mixed micelles and can be readily used as an energy source [20]. The addition of 30–50% of total lipids as MCT can be useful in cases with intraluminal bile salt deficiency [21,22] when large proportion of ingested MCTs can be absorbed, thereby reducing steatorrhea. The ideal dietary fat content and ratio of MCT to long-chain triglycerides (LCT) is unclear. Limited data point to better fat solubilization and growth of cholestatic infants fed with 30% or 70% MCT against a 50:50 mixture of MCT/LCT [23]. Caution is required when administering feeds with MCT in high proportions. Very high proportion of MCT to total lipid (> 80%) risks essential fatty acid deficiency [24,25]. MCT given as a supplement contributes to total energy ingested, but nutrient intake is controlled by appetite related to total energy intake, so that MCT-rich feeds may not increase intake while risking PUFA deficiency. In practice, the major feeds for infants with CLD contain MCT as 50%+ of fat, supplemented with essential fatty acids (e.g., Caprilon 75% MCT). Lipid intake and MCT ratio should be titrated between best possible weight gain and growth and against intolerance of nutrients, particularly, in diarrhea. In older children, MCT oil can be added to meals but must be balanced by other fat of high PUFA content. They may also make the feeds unpalatable, thereby reducing intake.

In summary, lipid should be used to increase dietary calorie density, and the proportion of lipid energy to total dietary energy of at least that for healthy age-matched children (from 30% to 50%) seems to be reasonable. If the taste of MCT/

LCT formula (leading to decreased energy intake) is not tolerated by the child, regular formula is preferable with MCT oil supplementation if necessary. High MCT/LCT formula should be used in children with significant malnutrition and signs of lipid malabsorption, with probable need for nasogastric feeding because of the palatability and volume required.

19.4 POLYUNSATURATED FATTY ACIDS

Long-chain PUFAs (LCPs, i.e., PUFA with carbon chain length > 18) such as arachidonic acid (AA) and docosahexaenoic acid (DHA) are important for early human growth and particularly in the development of the brain and the retina [26]. Omega 12-6 and omega 12-3 PUFAs are also precursors of eicosanoids with important biological roles such as mediators of immune and vascular functions and platelet aggregation, making PUFA deficiency a concern in CLD, especially from the ω-6 series [27–30]. Several factors contributing to PUFA and LCP deficiency include low PUFA intake (from dietary constituents and anorexia), malabsorption, and disturbed hepatic metabolism of PUFA to long-chain derivatives. Extra PUFA intake should be given (e.g., soybean or rapeseed oil) in higher proportion than normal, exceeding 10% of total energy [30], but even this may not be sufficient to correct LCP status [24]. LCP supplementation can be given in dietary products such as egg yolk (rich in AA) or fish oil (rich in DHA). Infants may be given conventional LCP-supplemented formulas available for healthy term and preterm infants [29]. Increased lipid peroxidation due to low vitamin E levels in cholestasis can also impair fatty acid status, but there is no direct relationship between PUFA and lipid peroxides [26,27]. Early dietary intervention seems to be important as the LCP status is not normalized up to a year after OLT [30]. Requirements for ideal intake remain unknown. It is reasonable in clinical practice to use PUFA-rich vegetable oils and/or egg yolk as dietary supplements to increase energy density and PUFA intake. In infants with cholestasis who receive regular infant formulas and do not require MCT-enriched feeds, LCP-supplemented infant formulas may be used.

19.5 ENERGY/CARBOHYDRATES

Carbohydrate (CHO) is the major source of dietary energy, contributing about two-thirds of the nonprotein energy. CHO can be used in feeds in three forms: monomer, short-chain polymer, or starch. Glucose is generally preferred in all three forms to avoid intolerance of galactose or other sugars. Short-chain polymers effect a compromise between osmotic load with diarrhea potentially seen in high monomer content feeds and malabsorbed starch reaching the colon and being fermented with bloating and diarrhea.

Side effects and complications of feeding with CHO, principally bloating and diarrhea, derive from its osmotic content. It is often difficult to attribute side effects to any specific element of the feed. Despite insulin resistance, hyperglycemia is uncommon except in patients who already have endocrine pancreatic insufficiency such as those with cystic fibrosis. Forms of CHO do not have the aversive flavors found in some protein and lipid preparations.

Given the calorimetric findings described above, in assessing energy requirements to prescribe a feed, assume it to be either normal for weight for age if there is evidence of an early growth pattern to establish the child's ideal growth before failing to thrive, or estimate it to be up to 150% for actual weight guided by the severity of failure to thrive.

19.6   PROTEIN

Children with advanced CLD require protein intake of about 2–3 g/kg/day as sufficient to promote growth and endogenous protein synthesis [31]. Hyperammonemia may be observed and is due to liver insufficiency and portosystemic shunts related to portal hypertension. Cholestasis itself has an inhibitory effect on the urea cycle [32], causing, in turn, elevated plasma bicarbonate. Ammonia can still be partially detoxified by the glutamine synthesis pathway located in the perivenular zone of the liver lobule, a mechanism well maintained in the cirrhotic nodule [33]. Hyperammonemia in the absence of encephalopathy does not justify protein restriction. Ammonia levels may be reduced by the use of lactulose or sodium benzoate, but elevated levels of 120 mmol/L at least are acceptable without evident side effects [8]. Severe protein restriction lower than 2 g/kg/day should be avoided since it will lead to endogenous muscle protein consumption [27].

Systematic use of semielemental diet and protein hydrolysates are not justified, since there is no evidence of protein malabsorption in CLD, but intestinal mucosal atrophy is occasionally seen in severe malnutrition when semielemental diet can be used temporarily. It should be kept in mind that the poor palatability of semielemental diets might actually decrease the intake. Increased need for dietary branched-chain amino acids (BCAA) in CLD is mediated in part by increased leucine oxidation in the postabsorptive state [34]. Experimental and clinical evidence show that an increased intake of BCAAs may improve the body composition of cholestatic children. In an animal model of biliary obstruction, a formula enriched with BCAAs improved weight gain, protein mass, muscle mass, nitrogen balance, body composition, and bone mineral content with increased plasma BCAA, leading to the development of a feed enriched in BCAAs designed for cholestatic infants (Heparon Junior®, Nutricia, Bornem, Belgium). This product is not universally approved or available [5,35]. Additional clinical evidence shows a beneficial effect of a diet enriched in BCAAs in children with biliary atresia. Children receiving a semielemental formula enriched with BCAAs had an increase in total body potassium, mid upper-arm circumference, and subscapular skin-fold thickness, as compared with children receiving a standard semielemental formula. They also required fewer albumin infusions for management of ascites [5]. We suggest an ideal administration of protein as 3 g/kg day of whey proteins, being approximately 2.6 g/100 mL reconstituted formula, enriched in BCAA to 10%, in treating hyperammonemia if symptomatic rather than reducing protein intake.

Children with cholestatic liver disease should receive protein energy and electrolyte intake at least equivalent to that described in Table 19.2 according to tolerance.

TABLE 19.2
Nutritional Requirements in Cholestatic Infants

Nutritional Element	Daily Requirement	Products/Source	Means of Administration	Comments/ Monitoring
Total lipid/ MCT	30–50% of energy of which 30–70% MCT	Depending on product and level of malabsorption	As formula	
PUFA/LCP	Probably > 10% total energy	Rapeseed oil, egg yolk, walnut oil, fish oil, sunflower oil, soybean oil	Walnut oil added to feed/given separately	Products unpalatable Levels difficult to measure and interpret. Most centers lack access to clinical measurement.
Protein	3–4 g/kg (min 2 g/kg)	Whey protein	As formula	Avoid semielemental diet/hydrolysates if not necessary. Treat hyperammonemia instead of reducing protein intake.
BCAA	10% total AAs			
Energy	RDA for age or up to 150% of requirement for weight	2/3 as CHO and 1/3 as lipids approximately	As formula	
Carbohydrate		CHO polymer	As formula	Usually lactose free
Na/K	Minimum 2–3 mmol/kg		As formula	

Source: Baker A., Stevenson, R., Dhawan, A., Goncalves, I., Socha, P., and Sokal, E., *Pediatr Transplant*, 11, 825–834, 2007. With permission.

19.7 WATER AND ELECTROLYTES

Target total fluid should be normal for actual weight unless overload indicates restriction. Minimal sodium of 1 mmol/kg/day and low-normal potassium of 2 mmol/kg/day are usually appropriate. Do not correct the hyponatremia of liver failure with added sodium as fluid overload including ascites will probably result. Fluid restriction should be used instead. It may be impossible to achieve satisfactory energy intake in circumstances of necessary fluid restriction.

19.8 VITAMINS

Fat malabsorption is the primary cause of deficiency of fat-soluble vitamins (A, D, E, and K), but alterations in intermediary metabolism also contribute to decreased serum vitamin levels. It has been suggested that fat-soluble vitamin supplements should be given parenterally as soon as the serum bilirubin level exceeds 85 μmol/L [36], but high-dose oral formulations can be used with equal success and should be the standard recommendation unless insufficient availability is demonstrated. Recent progress in the use of a water-soluble form of vitamin E, D-α-tocopheryl polyethylene glycol-1000 succinate (TPGS-E), has enabled correction of vitamin E deficiency states [37,38] and has also allowed coadministration of other fat-soluble vitamins in patients with cholestasis [39].

Vitamin A deficiency causes dry skin, exophthalmia, and night blindness. Up to 40% of cholestatic children had subtle evidence of vitamin A deficiency [40].

Serum level is not an accurate indicator of vitamin A depletion. Vitamin A liver metabolism is usually preserved in cholestatic patients and although liver measurement is theoretically the best means to assess stores, it is not feasible in practice [41]. A useful ratio is plasma retinol/RBP molar ratio [calculated as serum retinol (μg/dL)/serum RBP (mg/dL) × 0.0734]. Vitamin A replete patients have levels between 0.8 and 2.0 [42]. Higher ratios can be associated with toxicity including liver fibrosis, hypercalcemia, pseudotumor cerebri, and painful bone lesions. Vitamin A toxicity is most effectively monitored from plasma levels of vitamin A esters.

Vitamin E deficiency is associated with progressive hypoflexia or areflexia, ataxia, peripheral neuropathy, and loss of vision. Oral TPGS-E supplementation in cholestatic children can quickly normalize serum vitamin E levels, but does not improve the increased lipid peroxidation and poor PUFA status [43]. Patients with Alagille syndrome and various types of progressive intrahepatic cholestasis are particularly at risk despite supplementation as recommended [44]. Vitamin E therapy monitoring uses vitamin E/total lipid ratio (normal > 0.8 mg/g, but with plasma vitamin E < 30 μg/mL). Toxicity is unusual and includes impaired neutrophil chemotaxis and vitamin K–dependent protein carboxylation.

Vitamin D deficiency is associated with hypocalcemia, hypophosphatemia, muscle hypotonia, and rickets. Among pediatric patients with cirrhosis lumbar bone mineral density was 22.4% less and bone mineral content 18.4% less than controls by dual x-ray absorption scanning [45]. Adequate supplements of 25-hydroxycholecalciferol (25-OH-D) and appropriate intake of calcium and phosphorus should be given. Sunlight exposure should be encouraged but not to excess. Serum levels of 25-OH-D exceeding 25 ng/mL must be achieved, whereas urinary calcium/creatinine ratio should be lower than 0.25. However, even with adequate levels of vitamin D, many infants with CLD remain osteopenic [46]. Hypercalcemia and pseudotumor cerebri are rare complications of excess.

Vitamin K was originally defined as a factor concerned with hemostasis, with deficiency resulting in hemorrhagic disease. Vitamin K deficiency leads to the synthesis of undercarboxylated proteins such as coagulation factors II, VII, IX, X, and bone proteins: matrix GLA protein, osteocalcin, and protein S. PIVKA II (protein induced in the absence of vitamin K) measured by enzyme-linked immunosorbent assay is available in specialist laboratories and is more sensitive than prothrombin time for monitoring vitamin K deficiency. PIVKA II > 3 ng/mL reflects vitamin K deficiency. Among cholestatic children, 54% had evidence of vitamin K deficiency despite supplementation, whereas those with noncholestatic liver disease had none

[47]. For managing vitamin K deficiency, success has been achieved by using a vitamin K compound micellar formulation solubilized in glycocholate and lecithin, KonaKion MM (Roche, Basel, Switzerland), which is safe and efficacious [48,49].

Water-soluble vitamins should also be supplemented due to the risk of altered hepatic metabolism. Chin et al. [6] documented low levels of minerals and trace elements in children with cholestasis. The suggested dose (but without evidence in CLD) is twice the recommended daily intake [recommended dietary allowance (RDA)] [50]. Selenium, zinc, calcium, and magnesium should be supplemented as guided by plasma levels. Iron may enhance oxidative stress, carcinogenesis, and fibrogenesis in patients with liver disease [51]. Iron deficiency is uncommon in CLD except with chronic blood loss. Serum iron and transferrin levels are not reliable indicators of deficiency. Thus, regular iron supplementation is not indicated. Children with cholestatic liver disease should receive vitamin supplementation equivalent to that described in Table 19.3.

19.9 AVAILABLE PRODUCTS

Available products are shown in Table 19.4. It may be possible to achieve improved growth with feed supplements, for example, maxijul glucose polymer or duocal CHO/lipid emulsion added to bottle feeds. Caprilon (SHS) is designed for oral feeding in cholestasis with MCT, but 17% of CHO is lactose. Specially designed liver feeds with up to 3.7 g/100 mL feed as protein, 32% BCAAs, 70% MCT, glucose polymer, and low sodium to permit preparation at higher concentration in fluid restriction are available (Generaid Plus, SHS). This product, although associated with good clinical response, is sufficiently unpalatable that nasogastric feeding is often required. It is not recommended by the Advisory Committee on Borderline Substances, a UK advisory committee advising on the prescription of products that are not drugs or medical devices for patients younger than 1 year old, but we have used it without problems in children as young as 6 months.

19.10 MEANS OF ADMINISTRATION

Many currently available commercial nutritional products are suitable for infants with CLD, but none are ideal for all situations. Additives are usually necessary in persistent failure to thrive although the practice of adding glucose polymers to increase energy alone is not recommended because this reduces the protein/energy ratio. The recommended ratio for catch-up growth is 9% [52]. Some centers use a modular feeding system with the various components combined for the needs and tolerance of the patient. Although this system works well for patients needing NGT feeding, it does not make for a palatable feed, and preparation is very demanding for the carers. Commercial preparations should form the first line of nutritional therapy with modular feeds used for special needs and refractory cases.

Anorexia is a common feature of severe liver disease as described above. It may be impossible to achieve energy requirements orally, especially with less palatable feeds. NGT feeding has been highly successful in overcoming these problems. Early use of nasogastric feeding is encouraged with gastrostomy feeding in selected cases

TABLE 19.3

Nutritional Requirements: Vitamins and Minerals

Nutritional Element	Daily Requirement	Products/Source	Means of Administration	Comments/Monitoring
Vitamin A	< 10 kg 5,000 IU > 10 kg 10,000 IU IM—50,000 IU	Ketovite liquid and tablets, Abidec	Oral	IM supplement only in severe refractory deficiency Serum retinol/RBP ≥ 0.8
Vitamin D	25-OH-D: 2–5 µg/kg IM, 30,000 IU 1–3 monthly	Ketovite liquid and tablets, Abidec has calciferol 400 IU/day, IM calciferol	Oral/IM	Supplementation with oral products containing calciferol may suffice. Refractory cases may require 25-OH-D or IM preps 25-OH-D serum levels > 20 ng/mL
Vitamin E	TPGS[a] 25 IU/kg IM 10 mg/kg (max 200 mg) every 3 weeks	TPGS from Eastman-Kodak or Orphan Europe. Others include Ketovite liquid and tablets, Abidec, Ephynal	Oral	Vitamin E/total lipids ≥ 0.6 mg/g Vitamin E < 30 µg/mL Look for reflexes!
Vitamin K	2 mg/day, weekly 5 mg: 5–10 kg, 10 mg > 10 kg IM, 5–10 mg every 2 weeks	KonaKion MM Micellar formulation or menadiol Phytomenadione	Oral, IM	Prothrombin time PIVKA II < 3 ng/mL
Water-soluble vitamins	Twice RDA	Children's multivitamins, Ketovite liquid and tablets	Oral	Supplement as needed
Minerals Calcium, selenium, zinc, phosphate	25–100 mg/kg 1–2 µg/kg 1 mg/kg 25–50 mg/kg		Oral	Supplement as needed

Source: Baker A., Stevenson, R., Dhawan, A., Goncalves, I., Socha, P., and Sokal, E., *Pediatr Transplant*, 11, 825–834, 2007. With permission.

[a] TPGS-Vitamin E prepared by esterifying D-α-tocopheryl acid succinate with polyethylene glycol 1000.

requiring long-term input but without severe portal hypertension. Bolus feeds are preferred in the first instance, being more physiological, but if they are associated with vomiting or if the target feed volume cannot be achieved for other reasons, continuous feeds administered by pump up to 20 hours per day often allow targets to be achieved. The period off feeds allows the gastric pH to fall to prevent bacterial

TABLE 19.4
Nutritional Products

Product/Company	Protein Source/Fat Source	Osmolality (mosm/kg per 100 mL Feed)	Pro (g) Fat (g) CHO (g) kcal	Indications
Caprilon/SHS	Whey protein, skimmed milk powder/MCT, 75% soybean oil	233	1.5 3.6 7 66	Fat malabsorption, pancreatic insufficiency, liver disease
Generaid Plus/SHS	Whey protein/MCT 35%/ Maize, coconut, palm kernel oil	up to 390	2.4 4.2 13.6 102	Fat malabsorption, pancreatic insufficiency, liver disease
Pepti-Junior/Cow and Gate	Whey hydrolysate supplementary amino acids MCT 50% maize, rapeseed, soybean oil	390	1.8 3.6 6.8 67	Whole protein or disaccharide intolerance, fat malabsorption
Pregestimil/Mead Johnson	Casein hydrolysate supplementary amino acids MCT 55% corn, soya, and safflower oils	330	1.89 3.8 6.9 68	Whole protein or disaccharide intolerance, fat malabsorption
Infatrini/Nutricia	Whey 60% casein 40% skimmed milk powder Vegetable oils, LCP—egg lipids, fish oils	310	2.6 5.4 10.3 100	Disease related malnutrition, growth failure in infants
Heparon Junior/ Nutricia	Casein hydrolysate 21%, BCAAs MCT 48.9%, soybean oil	357	2.0 3.6 11.6 68	Severe liver disease related malnutrition not galactosemia

Source: Baker A., Stevenson, R., Dhawan, A., Goncalves, I., Socha, P., and Sokal, E., *Pediatr Transplant,* 11, 825–834, 2007. With permission.

overgrowth. Overnight feeds of 8–10 hours giving half of the target intake may be a preferred strategy with the chance of maintaining some normal feeding behavior. Percutaneous endoscopic gastrostomy (PEG) may replace NGTs in long-term treatment, but there may be a problem of stomal variceal bleeding if portal hypertension is present.

Complications are seen in proportion to the severity of the underlying liver disease and malnutrition and duration of feeding. Fluid overload, especially with hyponatremia, is a particular problem. If fluid restriction is necessary, it may become impossible to meet nutritional targets. Infusions of human albumin solution 20% to maintain serum albumin above 35 g/L may help, but such a situation is evidence of very poor liver function and failure of nutritional care is an indication for liver transplantation. Vomiting is common and may respond to antireflux measures. Aspiration is rare. Gaseous bloating is common and frequent loose stools (five to eight times a day) is almost universal in infants.

Infants who are fed exclusively nasogastrically at about the age of 7 months may not develop normal feeding behavior and find all oral contact aversive. Once established, this situation can take months of hard work to correct. It is essential to maintain normal feeding behavior in some form alongside nasogastric or PEG feeding. Children should be encouraged to continue to take flavors and textures into their mouths appropriate to their age and begin to chew even if the nutritional contribution is negligible. Mealtimes should be respected. The opinion of a speech therapist with experience in this area may be very helpful.

19.11   REHABILITATION AFTER OLT

Most infants recover normal nutritional function and behavior rapidly after OLT [53–56]. Catch-up growth is most striking in those with worst previous malnutrition. Lactose and cow's milk protein intolerances are recognized complications. Feeding behavior may be severely deranged, requiring months of expert psychological and speech therapy input in some cases. This situation will require the sustained input of the nutritional care team including a speech therapist, psychologist, or local equivalent. All patients should undergo nutritional evaluation after transplant and rehabilitation if necessary.

19.12   PARENTERAL NUTRITION

PN is an accepted mode of delivery of calories and nutrients when the nasogastric route cannot be used because of risk of esophageal variceal hemorrhage, if the patient is intolerant to enteral nutrition because of diarrhea with osmotic disturbance, or if the patient fails to respond. The indications for PN are therefore diarrhea, vomiting (limiting the enteral caloric administration), or repeated episodes of GI hemorrhage. These indications are usually short term and also allow the limited simultaneous administration of enteral feeding. The use of PN in children with compensated liver disease, for example, cystic fibrosis, follows standard principles. Standard amino acid solutions are well tolerated. The role of BCAA-rich amino acid solutions remains unproven [57] and is limited by availability and cost. Lipids are well tolerated and help to optimize caloric intake. Special attention should be paid toward fluid, electrolyte (particularly sodium), and micronutrient (particularly manganese) balance. Normal IV trace element supplementation appears adequate even in severe cholestatic liver disease after the neonatal period.

The effect of prolonged PN on preexisting liver disease has not been studied in detail, but mild deterioration in biochemical parameters appears to be of little clinical significance. Abnormalities described in adults are mild elevations of liver enzymes with liver histology showing changes in steatosis and, in rare cases, cholestasis [58]. Guimber et al. [59] reported increase in Z scores in representing weight for age and weight for height, with no significant change in parameters of liver synthetic function in seven children with liver disease requiring PN. An increase in serum bilirubin was assumed to be a combined effect of the natural progression of underlying liver disease and line sepsis or PN. Simultaneous administration of enteral calories even in small volumes should be considered because prolonged PN is likely to adversely affect liver function and enteral feeding is protective. With the exception of those with concomitant intestinal failure, children with cholestatic liver disease should only receive PN when all possible means of enteral feeding have failed and in association with a nutritional care team. Prophylactic ursodeoxycholic acid has been shown to be of benefit in treating PNAC in adults and children [60,61] and may be indicated with PN.

19.13   CONCLUSIONS

Children with cholestatic liver disease require early and regular expert nutritional assessment including arm anthropometry. Early or prophylactic intervention is required with specialist feeds. Enteral nasogastric nutrition, if necessary, is preferred, with PN prescribed for patients in nutritional extremis or having primary GI disease. Energy intake is normal for age but increased by 40% or more for weight. Constituents are adapted to accommodate malabsorption and the metabolic derangement of liver disease. Feeding behavior should be maintained as close to normal as possible. Failure of intensive nutritional management is an indicator and an adverse prognostic marker for liver transplantation. Units caring for children with liver disease must have full multidisciplinary team resources and written protocols suitable for audit.

19.14   SUMMARY POINTS

- Neonatal cholestatic liver disease is uncommon.
- It is frequently accompanied by nutritional complications.
- Patients need regular nutritional review and care by a nutritional care team.
- Enteral feeding by NGT is the mainstay of treatment.
- Feeds tend to be unpalatable as they are supplemented with MCT and/or BCAAs.
- Fluid and electrolyte disturbances are a frequent obstruction to adequate or ideal intake.
- Fat-soluble vitamins must be supplemented and levels monitored.
- Problems related to feeding behavior are common after long-term nasogastric feeding.
- Many patients will ultimately proceed to liver transplantation, after which nutritional rehabilitation will be required.

ACKNOWLEDGMENTS

Contributions from Prof. A. Dhawan, Dr. I. Goncalves, Dr. P. Socha, and Prof. E. Sokal are acknowledged.

REFERENCES

1. Baker A., R. Stevenson, A. Dhawan, I. Goncalves, P. Socha, and E. Sokal. 2007. Guidelines for nutritional care for infants with cholestatic liver disease before liver transplantation. *Pediatr Transplant* 11:825–834.
2. Hurtado-López, E. F., A. Larrosa-Haro, E. M. Vásquez-Garibay, R. Macías-Rosales, R. Troyo-Sanromán, and M. C. Bojórquez-Ramos. 2007. Liver function test results predict nutritional status evaluated by arm anthropometric indicators. *J Pediatr Gastroenterol Nutr* 45:451–457.
3. Sokol, R. J., and C. Stall. 1990. Anthropometric evaluation of children with chronic liver disease. *Am J Clin Nutr* 52:203–208.
4. Cleghorn, G. J., and R. W. Shepherd. 2000. Value of total body potassium in assessing the nutritional status of children with end-stage liver disease. *Ann N Y Acad Sci* 904:400–405.
5. Moukarzel, A. A., I. Najm, J. Vargas, S. V. McDiarmid, R. W. Busuttil, and M. E. Ament. 1990. Effect of nutritional status on outcome of orthotopic liver transplantation in pediatric patients. *Transplant Proc* 22:1560–1563.
6. Chin, S. E., R. W. Shepherd, B. J. Thomas, G. J. Cleghorn, M. K. Patrick, J. A. Wilcox, T. H. Ong, S. V. Lynch, and R. Strong. 1992. The nature of malnutrition in children with end-stage liver disease awaiting orthotopic liver transplantation. *Am J Clin Nutr* 56:164–168.
7. Barshes, N. R., I. F. Chang, S. J. Karpen, B. A. Carter, and J. A. Goss. 2006. Impact of pretransplant growth retardation in pediatric liver transplantation. *J Pediatr Gastroenterol Nutr* 43:89–94.
8. Charlton, C. P., E. Buchanan, C. E. Holden, M. A. Preece, A. Green, I. W. Booth, and M. J. Tarlow. 1992. Intensive enteral feeding in advanced cirrhosis: Reversal of malnutrition without precipitation of hepatic encephalopathy. *Arch Dis Child* 67:603–607.
9. Baker, A., A. Dhawan, and N. Heaton. 1998. Who needs a liver transplant? (New disease specific indications). *Arch Dis Child* 79:460–464.
10. Thevenin, D. M., A. Baker, T. Kato, A. Tzakis, M. Fernandez, and M. Dowling. 2006. Neuodevelopmental outcomes for children transplanted under the age of 3 years. *Transplant Proc* 38:1692–1693.
11. Kalaitzakis, E., M. Simrén, R. Olsson, P. Henfridsson, I. Hugosson, M. Bengtsson, and E. Björnsson. 2006. Gastrointestinal symptoms in patients with liver cirrhosis: Associations with nutritional status and health-related quality of life. *Scand J Gastroenterol* 41:1464–1472.
12. Pierro, A., B. Koletzko, V. Carnielli, R. A. Superina, E. A. Roberts, R. M. Filler, J. Smith, and T. Heim. 1989. Resting energy expenditure is increased in infants and children with extrahepatic biliary atresia. *J Pediatr Surg* 24:534–538.
13. Heymsfield, S. B., M. Waki, and J. Reinus. 1990. Are patients with chronic liver disease hypermetabolic? *Hepatology* 11:502–505. Review.
14. Rovner, A. J., V. A. Stallings, D. A. Piccoli, A. E. Mulberg, and B. S. Zemel. 2006. Resting energy expenditure is not increased in prepubertal children with Alagille syndrome. *J Pediatr* 148:680–682.
15. Greer, R., M. Lehnert, P. Lewindon, G. J. Cleghorn, and R. W. Shepherd. 2003. Body composition and components of energy expenditure in children with end-stage liver disease. *J Pediatr Gastroenterol Nutr* 36:358–363.
16. Muller, M. J. 1998. Hepatic energy and substrate metabolism: A possible metabolic basis for early nutritional support in cirrhotic patients. *Nutrition* 14:30–38.
17. Holt, R. I., A. J. Baker, J. S. Jones, and J. P. Miell. 1998. The insulin-like growth factor and binding protein axis in children with end-stage liver disease before and after orthotopic liver transplantation. *Pediatr Transplant* 2:76–84.

18. Holt, R. I., J. P. Miell, J. S. Jones, G. Mieli-Vergani, and A. J. Baker. 2000. Nasogastric feeding enhances nutritional status in paediatric liver disease but does not alter circulating levels of IGF-I and IGF binding proteins. *Clin Endocrinol* 52:217–224.

19. Beath, S., I. Hooley, K. Willis, et al. 1993. Long chain triacylglycerol malabsorption and pancreatic function in children with protein energy malnutrition complicating severe liver disease. *Proc Nutr Soc* 52:252A.

20. Kaufman, S. S., N. D. Murray, R. P. Wood, B. W. Shaw, and J. A. Vanderhoof. 1987. Nutritional support for the infants with extrahepatic biliary atresia. *J Pediatr* 10:679–685.

21. Kaufmann, S. S., D. J. Scrivner, N. D. Murray, et al. 1992. Influence of Portagen and Pregestimil on essential fatty acid status in infantile liver disease. *Pediatrics* 89:151–154.

22. Bach, A., H. Schirardin, M. Bauer, and A. Weryha. 1977. Ketogenic response to medium-chain triglyceride load in the rat. *J Nutr* 107:1863–1870.

23. Pettei, M. J., S. Daftary, and J. J. Levine. 1991. Essential fatty acid deficiency associated with the use of a medium-chain-triglyceride infant formula in paediatric hepatobiliary disease. *Am J Clin Nutr* 53:1217–1221.

24. Beath, S. V., S. Johnson, K. D. Willis, D. A. Kelly, and I. W. Booth. 1996. Growth and luminal fat solubilisation in cholestatic infants on medium chain triglyceride (MCT). *J Pediatr Gastroenterol Nutr* 22:443.

25. Koletzko, B., C. Agostoni, S. E. Carlson, et al. 2001. Long chain polyunsaturated fatty acids (LC-PUFA) and perinatal development. *Acta Pediatr* 90:460–464.

26. Socha, P., B. Koletzko, P. Pawlowska, and J. Socha. 1997. Essential fatty acid status in children with cholestasis, in relation to serum bilirubin concentration. *J Pediatr* 131:700–706.

27. Socha, P., B. Koletzko, E. Świątkowska, J. Pawlowska, A. Stolarczyk, and J. Socha. 1998. Essential fatty acid metabolism in infants with cholestasis. *Acta Pediatr* 87:278–283.

28. Dupont, J., O. Amedee-Manesme, D. Pepin, and J. Chambaz. 1990. Eicosanoid synthesis in children with cholestatic disease. *J Inherit Metab Dis* 13:212–218.

29. Socha, P., B. Koletzko, I. Jankowska, A. Stolarczyk, J. Pawlowska, E. Świątkowska, H. Demmelmair, T. Kuryl, D. Korszyńska, and J. Socha. 2000. LCP-supplementation in infants with cholestasis. *J Pediatr Gastroenterol Nutr* 31 Suppl 2:S195 (abstract).

30. Lapillonne, A., C. Hakme, V. Mamoux, M. Chambon, V. Fournier, V. Chirouze, and A. Lachaux. 2000. Effects of liver transplantation on long-chain polyunsaturated fatty acid status in infants with biliary atresia. *J Pediatr Gastroenterol Nutr* 30:528–532.

31. Dewey, K. G., et al. 1996. Protein requirements in infants and children. *Eur J Clin Nutr* 50:S119–S150.

32. Powers-Lee, S. G., and L. Meister. 1988. Urea synthesis and ammonia metabolism. In *The Liver: Biology and Pathobiology*, ed. M. Arias, W. B. Jakoby, H. Popper, D. Schalter, and D. A. Shafritz, 317–330. New York: Raven Press.

33. Sokal, E. M., P. Trivedi, B. Portmann, and A. P. Mowat. 1990. Adaptive changes of metabolic zonation during the development of cirrhosis in growing rats. *Gastroenterology* 99:785–792.

34. Mager, D. R., L. J. Wykes, E. A. Roberts, R. O. Ball, and P. B. Pencharz. 2006. Mild-to-moderate chronic cholestatic liver disease increases leucine oxidation in children. *J Nutr* 136:965–970.

35. Sokal, E. M., M. C. Baudoux, E. Collette, V. Hausleithner, L. Lambotte, and J. P. Buts. 1996. Branched chain amino acids improve body composition and nitrogen balance in a rat model of extra-hepatic biliary atresia. *Pediatr Res* 40:66–71.

36. Sokal, E. M. 1993. Nutritional and medical care in chronic cholestasis. In *Management of Digestive and Liver Disorders in Infants and Children*, ed. J. P. Buts and E. M. Sokal, 537–542. Amsterdam: Elsevier.

37. Sokol, R. J., N. Butler-Simon, C. Conner, et al. 1993. Multicenter trial of D-α-tocopheryl polyethylene glycol-1000 succinate for treatment of vitamin E deficiency in children with chronic cholestasis. *Gastroenterology* 104:1727–1735.

38. Sokol, R. J. 1994. Fat-soluble vitamins and their importance in patients with cholestatic liver diseases. *Gastroenterol Clin North Am* 23:673–705.

39. Argao, E. A., and J. E. Heubi. 1993. Fat-soluble vitamin deficiency in infants and children. *Curr Opin Pediatr* 5:562–566.

40. Feranchak, A. P., J. Gralla, R. King, R. O. Ramirez, M. Corkill, M. R. Narkewicz, and R. J. Sokol. 2005. Comparison of indices of vitamin A status in children with chronic liver disease. *Hepatology* 42:782–792.

41. Amedée-Manesme, O., H. C. Furr, F. Alvarez, M. Hadchouel, D. Alagille, and J. A. Olson. 1985. Biochemical indicators of vitamin A depletion in children with cholestasis. *Hepatology* 5:1143–1148.

42. Hochman, J., and W. F. Balistreri. 1997. Neonatal cholestasis: Differential diagnosis, evaluation and management. In *Hepatobiliary, Pancreatic and Splenic Disease in Children*, ed. W. F. Balistreri, R. Ohi, T. Todani, and Y. Tsuchida. Amsterdam: Elsevier Science.

43. Socha, P., B. Koletzko, J. Pawlowska, K. Proszynska, and J. Socha. 1997. Treatment of cholestatic children with water-soluble vitamin E (alpha-tocopheryl polyethylene glycol succinate): Effects on serum vitamin E, lipid peroxides, and polyunsaturated fatty acids. *J Pediatr Gastroenterol Nutr* 24:189–193.

44. Davit-Spraul, A., C. Cosson, M. Couturier, M. Hadchouel, A. Legrand, F. Lemonnier, and P. Therond. 2001. Standard treatment of alpha-tocopherol in Alagille patients with severe cholestasis is insufficient. *Pediatr Res* 49:232–236.

45. Uslu, N., I. N. Saltik-Temizel, H. Demir, Y. Usta, H. Ozen, F. Gürakan, A. Yüce, and N. Koçak. 2006. Bone mineral density in children with cirrhosis. *J Gastroenterol* 41:873–877.

46. Argao, E. A., B. L. Specker, and J. E. Heubi. 1993. Bone mineral content in infants and children with chronic cholestatic liver disease. *Pediatrics* 91:1151–1154.

47. Mager, D. R., P. L. McGee, K. N. Furuya, and E. A. Roberts. 2006. Prevalence of vitamin K deficiency in children with mild to moderate chronic liver disease. *J Pediatr Gastroenterol Nutr* 42:71–76.

48. Mager, D. R., P. L. McGee, et al. 2000. Prevalence of vitamin K deficiency in children with chronic liver disease. *J Pediatr Gastroenterol Nutr* 31:193.

49. Amedée-Manesme, O., W. E. Lambert, D. Alagille, and A. P. De Leenheer. 1992. Pharmacokinetics and safety of a new solution of vitamin K_1 in children with cholestasis. *J Pediatr Gastroenterol Nutr* 14:160–165.

50. Ramaccioni, V., H. E. Soriano, et al. 2000. Nutritional aspects of chronic liver disease and liver transplantation in children. *J Pediatr Gastroenterol Nutr* 30:361–367.

51. Bonkovsky, H. L., B. F. Banner, et al. 1996. Iron in liver diseases other than haemochromatosis. *Semin Liver Dis* 16:65–82.

52. Plauth, M., M. Merli, A. Weimann, P. Ferenci, and M. J. Muller. 1997. ESPEN guidelines for nutrition in liver disease and transplantation. *Clin Nutr* 16:43–45.

53. Holt, R. I., E. Broide, C. R. Buchanan, J. P. Miell, A. J. Baker, A. P. Mowat, and G. Mieli-Vergani. 1997. Orthotopic liver transplantation reverses the adverse nutritional changes of end-stage liver disease in children. *Am J Clin Nutr* 65:534–542.

54. Pawlowska, J., H. Matusik, P. Socha, H. Ismail, J. Ryzko, E. Karczmarewicz, I. Jankowska, M. Teisseyre, and R. Lorenc. 2004. Beneficial effect of liver transplantation on bone mineral density in small infants with cholestasis. *Transplant Proc* 36:1479–1480.

55. Van Mourik, I. D., S. V. Beath, G. A. Brook, A. J. Cash, A. D. Mayer, J. A. Buckels, and D. A. Kelly. 2000. Long-term nutritional and neurodevelopmental outcome of liver transplantation in infants aged less than 12 months. *J Pediatr Gastroenterol Nutr* 30:269–275.

56. Ramaccioni, V., H. E. Soriano, R. Arumugam, and W. J. Klish. 2000. Nutritional aspects of chronic liver disease and liver transplantation in children. *J Pediatr Gastroenterol Nutr* 30:361–367.

57. Wolfe, B. M., B. K. Walker, D. B. Shaul, L. Wong, and B. H. Ruebner. 1998. Effect of total parenteral nutrition on hepatic histology. *Arch Surg* 123:1084–1090.

58. Balistreri, W. F. 1999. Liver disease in infancy and childhood. In *Schiff's Diseases of the Liver*, 8th edition, ed. E. R. Schiff, M. F. Sorrell, and W. C. Maddrey, 1357–1512. Philadelphia, PA: Lippincott Williams and Wilkins.

59. Guimber, D., L. Michaud, S. Ategbo, D. Turck, and F. Gottrand. 1999. Experience of parenteral nutrition for nutritional rescue in children with severe liver disease following failure of enteral nutrition. *Pediatr Transplant* 3:139–145.

60. Lindor, K., and J. Burnes. 1991. Ursodeoxycholic acid for the treatment of home parenteral nutrition associated cholestasis. *Gastroenterology* 101:250–253.

61. Spagnuolo, M. I., R. Iorio, J. E. Vagnete, L. Gramlich, et al. 1996. Ursodeoxycholic acid for treatment of cholestasis in children on long-term total parenteral nutrition: A pilot study. *Gastroenterology* 111:716–719.

20 Nutritional Considerations in Pediatric Liver Transplantation

Binita M. Kamath, Amanda Muir,
and Elizabeth B. Rand

CONTENTS

20.1   INTRODUCTION

General health, growth, and development in infancy, childhood, and adolescence are critically dependent on nutritional status. Chronic liver disease impacts nutritional status in a multifactorial manner by disrupting energy intake and expenditure, reducing absorption of macronutrients and micronutrients and altering metabolism. This chapter provides an overview of the nutritional consequences of chronic liver disease in pediatric patients with special attention to management of these issues leading up to and after liver transplantation. Nutritional therapy is perhaps the single most important treatment that can be provided for infants and children with chronic liver disease but requires attention to details of assessment as well as management of deficiencies.

20.2   NUTRITION AND LIVER TRANSPLANT EVALUATION

20.2.1   Assessment of Nutritional Status

Evaluation of nutritional status in children with chronic liver disease has three major goals: (1) identification of impairments in growth and development, (2) determination of specific needs/deficiencies in order to direct therapy, and (3) consideration of these factors with respect to the timing of liver transplantation. Precise assessment of nutritional status in children with chronic liver disease is difficult, however, because the assessment tools are directly altered by liver disease as well as any malnutrition.

Although weight is easy to measure, these children often have significant confounding variables, including organomegaly, fluid retention, and ascites, that make weight an unreliable estimate of body mass. Weight-for-height determination improves the utility of the assessment but is still compromised by the difficulties stated above. Body mass index is of limited use in pediatric chronic liver disease because of its emphasis on weight and the influence of pubertal status (Taylor et al., 2005). Anthropometric measurements such as mid-arm circumference and skin-fold thickness are a more accurate reflection of status, but require more time, special equipment, and trained personnel. Furthermore, anthropometrics generally are not useful for tracking short-term responses to interventions. Height z score has been shown to be the simplest and most accurate single measure to reflect nutritional status in liver disease, but this also has caveats. Height measurement may be inaccurate in young infants, and height compromise may be multifactorial in children with genetic disorders (e.g., Alagille syndrome). Head circumference is often preserved until late stages of malnutrition, but should be a standard part of evaluation (Taylor et al., 2005).

Serum protein levels have been used in nutritional assessment. Albumin, for example, with its serum half-life of 18–20 days, is generally depressed in long-standing malnutrition; however, hepatic insufficiency may cause further depression (and albumin or blood product administration may falsely elevate the level). Proteins with shorter serum half-life are most sensitive to acute changes but pose other problems. Transferrin, for example, which has a half-life of 8–9 days, is also synthesized in the liver. Prealbumin, with a half-life of 24–48 hours, is also an acute-phase reactant.

Retinol-binding protein is metabolized in the liver and, with a half-life of 12 hours, is most sensitive to acute changes; however, levels may be depressed in vitamin A or zinc deficiency, both of which are features of chronic liver disease (Taylor et al., 2005).

20.2.2 MACRONUTRIENTS IN PEDIATRIC LIVER DISEASE

20.2.2.1 Energy Requirements

Malnutrition is a common consequence of chronic liver disease in children, especially when the disease is cholestatic in nature and/or begins in infancy. Even in relatively well preserved noncholestatic adults with Child class A cirrhosis, malnutrition has been estimated to be as high as 25% of patients (Tsiaousi et al., 2008). In adults, dietary counseling of patients with Child A and B class cirrhosis alone resulted in improved nutritional parameters over a 3-month period (Manguso et al., 2005). Adults with ascites have been shown to have increased resting energy expenditure compared with those with cirrhosis, which is related perhaps to hyperdynamic circulation (Dolz et al., 1991; Taylor et al., 2003). Children have relatively greater nutritional needs to maintain normal growth and development, and the impact of deficiency is therefore greater. Various formulas for the calculation of resting energy expenditure in healthy children have been developed; however, these systems are not likely to be useful for children with chronic liver disease (Taylor et al., 2005). It has been estimated that infants and children with chronic liver disease require anywhere from 130 to 200 calories/kg/day to maintain growth (Guimber et al., 1999; Ramaccioni et al., 2000). Comprehensive examination showed that 21 infants with cholestatic liver diseases (predominantly biliary atresia) had a 27% increase in resting energy expenditure (ascribed largely to excess lipid oxidation during fasting and at rest) compared with 15 age-matched controls. Taken together, these findings support the use of high-calorie, high-protein, and carbohydrate diets with avoidance of fasting (Greer et al., 2003). Infants with cholestatic liver disease often exhibit delayed growth and are challenged by the combination of increased caloric requirements (baseline needs plus catch-up growth plus extra needs related to hospitalizations/surgery) with decreased delivery [anorexia, *nil per os* (NPO) status, poor absorption due to cholestasis]. Satisfaction of these needs may be difficult especially for infants and young children with anorexia and malabsorption, who will often require supplemental tube feedings (Francavilla et al., 2003; Guimber et al., 1999; Ramaccioni et al., 2000). In some cases, even supplemental tube feedings will be insufficient to meet caloric needs due to intolerance of feeding volumes or impaired utilization of calories. For this group with malnutrition resistant to enteral feeding, parenteral nutrition may be required and has been shown to be effective (Guimber et al., 1999).

20.2.2.2 Fat Requirements

Fat absorption is decreased in cholestasis causing decreased delivery of calories and also deficiency of individual fat-soluble micronutrients (discussed later in this chapter). Medium-chain triglycerides (MCTs) are an ideal source of fat calories in the cholestatic patient as absorption does not require micelle formation. MCT oil provides improved delivery of fat; however, it does not contain the essential fatty acids, and other fat-soluble micronutrients must be supplemented (Francavilla et al., 2003; Guimber et al., 1999; McDiarmid, 1996; Ramaccioni et al., 2000).

20.2.2.3 Protein Requirements

Protein needs are increased in children with liver disease due to their catabolic hypermetabolic state, in which ingested protein and lean body mass is sacrificed for gluconeogenesis. Although protein intake may be limited in adults with hyperammonemia and hepatic encephalopathy, protein intake should not be restricted in children with chronic liver disease.

20.2.2.4 Carbohydrate Requirements

Chronic liver disease results in impairment of hepatic storage and release of glucose. Failure of the liver to provide a source of glucose between feedings is a major cause of the catabolic state that favors protein breakdown for gluconeogenesis. In advanced disease, hypoglycemia may result; however, even in patients who maintain normal serum glucose, fasting should be avoided. Intravenous glucose containing solutions may be used during fasting for procedures; overnight feedings will also be helpful in this regard.

In summary, chronic liver disease results in an increase in overall caloric needs and specific increased requirements for each of the major macronutrients. Disorders with comorbidities affecting nutritional status pose additional difficulties; for example, Alagille syndrome and cystic fibrosis are diseases wherein chronic liver disease is complicated by pancreatic insufficiency causing an independent deleterious effect on nutritional status (Colombo et al., 2005; Rovner et al., 2002).

20.2.3 Micronutrients in Pediatric Liver Disease

A wide array of micronutrient disturbances have been demonstrated in pediatric liver disease, again with cholestasis a major factor in pathophysiology due to malabsorption.

20.2.3.1 Fat-Soluble Vitamins

Fat-soluble vitamin deficiencies have long been identified in cholestatic liver disease and attributed to failure of micellar solubilization (Table 20.1). The finding that markedly decreased intraluminal bile acid concentration correlated with depressed vitamin E absorption despite normal plasma transport and tissue uptake led to early recommendations to provide intramuscular vitamin E to profoundly cholestatic children (Sokol et al., 1983a, 1983b). Intramuscular administration was later replaced by oral D-α-tocopheryl succinate (TPGS) shown to be well absorbed despite cholestasis in pediatric patients (Sokol et al., 1987). TPGS has the additional advantage of improving the absorption of other lipid-soluble compounds (including the other fat-soluble vitamins) when coadministered. Like vitamin E, vitamin A is poorly absorbed in cholestasis, with deficiency reported in 43% of children studied (Feranchak et al., 2005; Ong et al., 1987). Supplementation is complicated by its potential hepatotoxicity and the difficulty in estimating body stores of vitamin A. Serum retinol levels are the most sensitive assay identifying 90% of deficient

TABLE 20.1

Recommended Doses of Vitamins and Minerals in Children with Chronic Liver Disease

Nutrient	Oral Dose
Vitamin A	5,000–15,000 IU/day
Vitamin D, 25-OH	4,000–12,000 IU/day
Vitamin E	25 IU/kg/day
Vitamin K	2.5–10 mg/day
Zinc	1 mg/kg/day

Note: Range of recommended fat-soluble vitamin and zinc doses.

patients (Feranchak et al., 2005). Although oral vitamin A is poorly absorbed in cholestasis, the absorption can be improved by coadministration with water-soluble TPGS described above (Feranchak et al., 2005). Similarly, vitamin K deficiency is common in children with cholestatic liver disease. Factors include poor absorption but also potential contributions from inhibition of vitamin K production in the liver and alterations in gut flora (due to antibiotics or Roux-en-Y loops) that reduce production or absorption of intestinal vitamin K. A comparison of children with mild-to-moderate cholestatic liver disease to those with noncholestatic liver disease and healthy children revealed striking vitamin K deficiency exclusive to the cholestatic children. Protein induced in vitamin K absence (PIVKA-II) was markedly elevated in the cholestatic group but not in noncholestatic or control children. Strikingly, 54% of cholestatic children taking vitamin K supplements were found to be deficient by this measure despite normal or near-normal clotting function, a reflection of the 50% reduction in prothrombin required before a rise in prothrombin time occurs (Mager et al., 2006a). As expected, vitamin K deficiency is compounded by pancreatic insufficiency; 100% of children with cystic fibrosis liver disease had elevated PIVKA-II levels (Rashid et al., 1999). Finally, vitamin D levels become depleted in pediatric liver disease, leading to calcium malabsorption and, ultimately, hepatic osteodystrophy. Adequate vitamin D levels are essential for calcium absorption from the gut, reabsorption in the renal tubule, and mineralization of bone. To obtain sufficient vitamin D, there must be adequate dietary intake, sufficient bile acids, and intact hepatocytes to metabolize vitamin D to 25-hydroxycholecalciferol (25-OH-D) as well as to make albumin and vitamin D–binding protein for transport to tissues (Bikle, 2007). Disruption of some or all of these pathways makes vitamin D supplementation before transplant routine practice.

Achieving adequate vitamin D supplementation to correct 25-OH-D levels, however, may not correlate with improved bone health. It has been shown that the bone mineral content of infants and children with chronic cholestasis may be as much as 3–5 standard deviations below the mean value for age (Bikle, 2007). However, only 29% of these patients have decreased serum 25-OH-D levels. Vitamin D supplementation should be administered at doses sufficient to normalize vitamin D levels and also parathyroid level and serum and urine calcium (Bikle, 2007).

20.2.3.2 Other Micronutrients

20.2.3.2.1 Branched-Chain Amino Acids

Supplementation of branched-chain amino acids (BCAAs) in children with chronic liver disease has been shown to increase growth and nitrogen balance, suggesting increased requirements for BCAA in this population. Chronic liver disease of a wide variety of liver disease (cholestatic and noncholestatic) has been characterized by altered amino acid patterns with lower concentrations of plasma BCAA (valine, leucine, and isoleucine) with corresponding increases in aromatic amino acids (phenylalanine and tyrosine). BCAA needs were estimated to be significantly higher in children with cholestatic liver disease as compared with norms using a stable isotope oxidation assay, and this elevation persisted (although at a lower level) in children after liver transplantation (Mager et al., 2006b, 2006c).

Mineral deficiency is observed in children with cholestatic or noncholestatic liver disease; other factors commonly noted are deficiencies in zinc, calcium, and magnesium, and those less well documented are deficiencies in manganese and selenium. Deficiency may be the result of poor intake and altered absorption, but hepatic synthetic compromise may also contribute insofar as serum albumin and other liver proteins are required for maintenance of serum levels. Deficiencies of minerals, in turn, exacerbate other deficiencies; for example, magnesium depletion is common among cholestatic patients and causes altered vitamin D metabolism by blunting parathyroid hormone response (Heubi et al., 1997).

20.2.3.2.2 Sodium Homeostasis

Cirrhosis is well known to alter sodium homeostasis in a complex manner. Patients with cirrhosis often experience massive whole-body sodium overload with or without retention of ascites, and this overload persists even in the face of decreased serum sodium levels. Discussion of the factors involved in this process is beyond the scope of this chapter; however, it is important to point out that iatrogenic (although not dietary) sodium intake must be closely monitored and restricted. Intravenous fluids and even flushes may deliver huge sodium loads, particularly in small infants who may also be receiving sodium in blood products and albumin infusions. Sodium content of antibiotics and other medications may be considerable and likewise deserves attention.

20.3 NUTRITION AND THE PERIOPERATIVE PERIOD

A period of not eating is inevitably mandated in the immediate perioperative period. In the majority of cases, when the operative course is smooth, this period only lasts 3–5 days. It is clear that surgical techniques will impact this duration. In infants in whom a new Roux-en-Y is fashioned, this period will be longer. In the frequent scenario of a child with biliary atresia who has undergone Kasai, a roux loop is already present, and therefore, the NPO period is not lengthened. The exception to this is in cases where surgical dissection is difficult after Kasai due to multiple adhesions and there may be vascular compromise of the roux—in this situation, the operating surgeon may mandate longer bowel rest. In general, since the NPO period is usually limited, interventions such as total parenteral nutrition are not necessary. It is clear that, if there are any particular complications lengthening the NPO period, such as a biliary leak or respiratory insufficiency requiring prolonged ventilation, then nutritional interventions become necessary. As always, enteral feeding is preferred over parenteral nutrition. In some centers, postpyloric enteral feeding tubes are placed intraoperatively in malnourished patients to facilitate early enteral feeding.

It is imperative to consider nutritional rehabilitation as soon as possible after surgery to begin the process of replenishing pretransplant deficits, as well as providing adequate calories to overcome the stress of abdominal surgery and hasten wound healing. Most children will eat well postoperatively, especially since underlying factors contributing to malaise and anorexia have been removed. Some children will require resumption of nasogastric feeds for a short period to maximize catch-up growth (van Mourik et al., 2000). In general, children eat better in their home surroundings rather than in the hospital setting, and it is important to consider a child's dietary intake in the postoperative period within this context, because it may reduce the need for unnecessary interventions.

20.4   NUTRITION AFTER LIVER TRANSPLANTATION

After liver transplantation, the underlying disease process is essentially cured in most cases, and one of the primary goals in the pediatric population is to realize the child's genetic growth potential. This ideal includes achieving age-appropriate weight and height parameters as well as the normal onset of puberty.

Growth impairment and pubertal delay are common in graft recipients who have had chronic liver disease for the reasons detailed above (Fine, 2002; Evans et al., 2005). Younger children (under the age of 1 year) are the most growth-impaired [Studies of Pediatric Liver Transplantation (SPLIT): year 2000 outcomes, 2001]. Current data suggest that although significant catch-up growth can be attained in many cases, it is often incomplete (Evans et al., 2005). Catch-up growth, a period of accelerated growth after transplant, occurs more rapidly for weight than for height. Data from the SPLIT database demonstrates that across age categories, weight normalizes by the end of the first posttransplant year (SPLIT: year 2000 outcomes, 2001). However, multiple studies reveal that catch-up linear growth is delayed until the second posttransplant year (Bartosh et al., 1999; McDiarmid et al., 1999; Saito et al., 2007). Catch-up growth continues for more than 5 years after liver transplant (Viner et al., 1999). However, height does not appear to entirely normalize and pediatric recipients of liver transplants consistently have some linear growth impairment when compared with the general population (SPLIT: year 2000 outcomes, 2001; McDiarmid et al., 1999; Viner et al., 1999; Saito et al., 2007).

20.4.1   FACTORS AFFECTING GROWTH POST–LIVER TRANSPLANTATION

Multiple factors may be correlated with or predict growth failure after liver transplantation and these have been substantiated by a multivariate analysis of growth impairment in 432 children from the SPLIT registry, as well as multiple other studies (Table 20.2) (Alonso, 2008; Bartosh et al., 1999; McDiarmid et al., 1999; Renz et

TABLE 20.2

Factors Affecting Post–Liver Transplant Growth in Children

Pretransplant factors
- Age at transplantation
- Degree of growth impairment at time of transplantation – height z score
- Primary hepatic diagnosis

Posttransplant factors
- Glucocorticoid exposure
- Graft function
- Posttransplant lymphoproliferative disorder
- Retransplantation

al., 2001). Age appears to be an important factor, with older children demonstrating more growth impairment. The height deficit that occurs after liver transplantation varies with age and is more pronounced in children who underwent transplantation at an older age in whom short stature is well established (Renz et al., 2001). Children younger than 2 years old who had undergone transplantation appear to achieve excellent catch-up growth and can achieve better final heights (McDiarmid et al., 1999; Viner et al., 1999; van Mourik et al., 2000; Renz et al., 2001). This age-related phenomenon may partly reflect the different diagnoses requiring transplantation in the different age groups. Clearly, most children younger than 2 years old undergoing liver transplantation have biliary atresia. In a study of biliary atresia patients alone, children demonstrated excellent catch-up growth with weight returning to normal within the first year after transplantation, but, as with other diagnoses, height remaining impaired even by the third posttransplantation year—of note, in this group there was no difference in catch-up growth in different age groups (younger or older than 2 years) (Saito et al., 2007; McDiarmid et al., 1999).

The primary liver disease is also an important factor in predicting growth after transplantation. In Alagille syndrome, the cause of growth failure is multifactorial and includes genetic, cardiac, pancreatic contributions, as well as cholestasis and liver disease. Therefore, after liver transplantation in Alagille syndrome, linear growth improves and becomes comparable to that of Alagille patients who had not undergone transplantation but remains below that which is expected of children who underwent transplantation for other indications (Quiros-Tejeira et al., 2000). In contrast, as mentioned above, a diagnosis of biliary atresia predicts better than expected catch-up growth.

Nutritional status at the time of transplantation is clearly important. As would be expected, children with higher z scores for height and weight at transplant are less likely to be growth-impaired after transplantation (McDiarmid et al., 1999). However, children with more growth retardation before transplantation, especially those younger than 2 years, demonstrate most catch-up growth (Bartosh et al., 1999; Viner et al., 1999). Overall, height, rather than weight, at the time of transplantation is the most important predictor of linear growth (Viner et al., 1999; Barshes et al., 2006).

Poor graft function and the need for a second transplant have been associated with poor height outcome (Viner et al., 1999). Graft type does not seem to impact posttransplant growth, with split graft and whole-size graft recipients having no significant differences in linear growth (Mejia et al., 2007).

Steroid exposure is a well-known cause of linear growth failure. SPLIT data suggest that children receiving steroids more than 18 months after transplant are more likely to be growth-impaired (Alonso, 2008). Although the degree of growth impairment does not appear to be dose-related, this concern has led to the development of protocols in which steroid administration is minimized and then eliminated between 6 and 18 months after transplantation.

20.4.2 INTERVENTIONS TO MAXIMIZE GROWTH AND NUTRITION AFTER LIVER TRANSPLANT

There are limited therapies available to maximize growth after liver transplant (Table 20.3). Aggressive nutritional monitoring and intervention is clearly important, as in the pretransplant period. In some children, continuation of pretransplant maneuvers such as enteral supplementation or tube feedings is required. However, most children eat well by mouth as liver function returns to normal, and they return to a state of overall well-being. This is demonstrated by the excellent catch-up weight that most children achieve. Complications necessitating prolonged or repeated hospitalizations clearly negatively impact return-to-normal eating patterns. A few children may require behavioral feeding therapy to assist with this.

It is important to pay special attention to electrolyte supplementation in the posttransplant period to maximize good nutrition. Calcineurin inhibitors are associated with wasting of magnesium, bicarbonate, and potassium, and these levels should be monitored and treated as required (Table 20.4). Hyperglycemia and diabetes mellitus are also known complications that may affect nutrition in the posttransplant period. Persistent hyperglycemia (hyperglycemia occurring more than 2 weeks after steroid induction and persisting for more 2 two weeks) was found in 17% of pediatric liver transplant recipients in one study (Romero et al., 2001). Insulin therapy (for longer than 4 months) was required in one-third of these children. This phenomenon is thought to be related to immunosuppressive agents. Frank diabetes mellitus has been reported to occur in 10% of pediatric long-term survivors of liver transplant, and it

TABLE 20.3
Strategies to Maximize Post–Liver Transplant Growth and Nutrition in Children

- Supplemental enteral feeds (by mouth or tube)
- Electrolyte supplementation
- Calcium and vitamin D supplementation
- Behavioral therapy for feeding difficulties
- Steroid minimization or avoidance
- Recombinant growth hormone treatment

TABLE 20.4

Immunosuppressants and Gastrointestinal and Nutritional-Related Side Effects

Medication	Gastrointestinal and Nutritional Side Effects
Cyclosporin A	Hyperglycemia, hypercholesterolemia, hyperkalemia, hypokalemia, hypomagnesemia
Prednisone	Water/sodium retention, increase in appetite and weight, hyperglycemia, impaired linear growth, osteoporosis, gastrointestinal ulcerations, pancreatitis
Azathioprine	Nausea, vomiting, altered taste, esophagitis, pancreatitis
Tacrolimus	Hyperkalemia, hypokalemia, hyperglycemia, hypomagnesemia, bicarbonate wasting
Mycophenolate mofetil	Nausea, vomiting, diarrhea, abdominal pain
Sirolimus	Nausea, diarrhea, mouth ulcers, hypercholesterolemia, hypertriglyceridemia

appears that the majority of these individuals were steroid-dependent (Avitzur et al., 2004). In the adult population, posttransplant diabetes is significantly more common (Driscoll et al., 2006).

Steroids are well known to impair linear growth; however, they still form an important part of the immunosuppressive regime at most centers. Steroid minimization is well accepted, and steroids are usually rapidly weaned in the first 6 months after liver transplantation. In a recent study comparing a steroid-free tacrolimus-basiliximab protocol to a conventional tacrolimus-steroid regimen, children demonstrated more rapid catch-up growth as well as successful attainment of normal height in the steroid-free treatment group (Gras et al., 2008).

Optimizing linear growth postpediatric liver transplant is challenging. Other than minimizing steroid exposure, the only other therapeutic option is growth hormone administration. Short- and long-term studies of recombinant growth hormone administration have shown improved linear growth (Puustinen et al., 2005; Rodeck et al., 2000). Treatment protocols require an extended period (> 1 year) of subcutaneous therapy, although minimal side effects have been reported. It has been shown that the improvement in linear growth peaks in the first year but is sustained above baseline for up to 5 years of treatment (Puustinen et al., 2005). Growth hormone administration seems a particularly appropriate option for height-impaired children in whom prolonged steroid exposure is necessary (such as with a primary diagnosis of autoimmune hepatitis).

20.4.3 BONE HEALTH AFTER LIVER TRANSPLANTATION

Cholestatic liver disease is known to impair bone mineral density. After liver transplantation, bone mineral density normalizes (Okajima et al., 2003; D'Antiga et al., 2004; Guthery et al., 2003). Children with prolonged or repeated steroid exposure or those with a primary diagnosis that affects bone, such as Alagille syndrome, remain

TABLE 20.5

Key Features of Pediatric Liver Transplantation

- Biliary atresia is the most frequent diagnosis requiring transplant.
- Growth impairment is a common indication for transplant.
- One-year patient survival rate is greater than 90%.
- Five-year patient survival rate is greater than 80%.
- Long-term complications after transplant commonly include posttransplant lymphoproliferative disorder and chronic renal failure.

vulnerable to impaired bone mineral density, and in these cases calcium and vitamin D supplementation is appropriate.

20.5 SUMMARY

Liver disease in children has a profound effect on nutritional status, which, in turn, impacts growth, development, progress of liver disease, and outcome of transplantation (Table 20.5). Nutritional disturbances may persist even after liver transplantation and may be exacerbated by medications or other treatments. Comprehensive medical management of pediatric liver disease and of liver transplant recipients includes careful nutritional assessment and individually tailored nutritional therapy.

20.6 SUMMARY POINTS

- Management of liver disease in children includes thorough nutritional assessment.
- Liver disease in children has profound impact on nutritional status.
- Altered nutritional status complicates the progress of liver disease in children.
- Both macronutrient and micronutrient balance may be affected by liver disease in children.
- Nutritional therapy is critical for optimal care of children with liver disease.
- Optimization of nutritional status has profound impact on the outcome of liver transplantation.
- Alterations in nutrition status may persist after transplant.
- After transplant, medications may continue to interfere with nutrition status and growth.

REFERENCES

Alonso, E. M. 2008. Growth and developmental considerations in pediatric liver transplantation. *Liver Transpl* 14:585–591.

Avitzur, Y., et al. 2004. Health status ten years after pediatric liver transplantation—looking beyond the graft. *Transplantation* 78:566–573.

Barshes, N. R., et al. 2006. Impact of pretransplant growth retardation in pediatric liver transplantation. *J Pediatr Gastroenterol Nutr* 43:89–94.

Bartosh, S. M., et al. 1999. Linear growth after pediatric liver transplantation. *J Pediatr*
135:624–631.

Bikle, D. D. 2007. Vitamin D insufficiency/deficiency in gastrointestinal disorders. *J Bone
Miner Res* 22:V50–V54.

Colombo, C., et al. 2005. Effects of liver transplantation on the nutritional status of patients
with cystic fibrosis. *Transpl Int* 18:246–255.

D'Antiga, L., et al. 2004. Long-term outcome of bone mineral density in children who underwent a successful liver transplantation. *Transplantation* 78:899–903.

Dolz, C., et al. 1991. Ascites increases the resting energy expenditure in liver cirrhosis.
Gastroenterology 100:738–744.

Driscoll, C. J., et al. 2006. Posttransplant diabetes mellitus in liver transplant recipients. *Prog
Transplant* 16:110–116.

Evans, I. V., et al. 2005. Post-transplantation growth among pediatric recipients of liver transplantation. *Pediatr Transplant* 9:480–485.

Feranchak, A. P., et al. 2005. Comparison of indices of vitamin A status in children with
chronic liver disease. *Hepatology* 42:782–792.

Fine, R. N. 2002. Growth following solid-organ transplantation. *Pediatr Transplant* 6:47–52.

Francavilla, R., et al. 2003. Hepatitis and cholestasis in infancy: Clinical and nutritional
aspects. *Acta Paediatr Suppl* 91:101–104.

Gras, J. M., et al. 2008. Steroid-free, tacrolimus-basiliximab immunosuppression in pediatric liver transplantation: Clinical and pharmacoeconomic study in 50 children. *Liver
Transpl* 14:469–477.

Greer, R., et al. 2003. Body composition and components of energy expenditure in children
with end-stage liver disease. *J Pediatr Gastroenterol Nutr* 36:358–363.

Guimber, D., et al. 1999. Experience of parenteral nutrition for nutritional rescue in children with severe liver disease following failure of enteral nutrition. *Pediatr Transplant*
3:139–145.

Guthery, S. L., et al. 2003. Bone mineral density in long-term survivors following pediatric
liver transplantation. *Liver Transpl* 9:365–370.

Heubi, J. E., et al. 1997. The role of magnesium in the pathogenesis of bone disease in childhood cholestatic liver disease: A preliminary report. *J Pediatr Gastroenterol Nutr*
25:301–306.

Mager, D. R., P. L. McGee, K. N. Furuya, and E. A. Roberts. 2006a. Prevalence of vitamin K deficiency in children with mild to moderate chronic liver disease. *J Pediatr
Gastroenterol Nutr* 42:71–76.

Mager, D. R., L. J. Wykes, E. A. Roberts, R. O. Ball, and P. B. Pencharz. 2006b. Branched-
chain amino acid needs in children with mild-to-moderate chronic cholestatic liver disease. *J Nutr* 136:133–139.

Mager, D. R., L. J. Wykes, E. A. Roberts, R. O. Ball, and P. B. Pencharz. 2006c. Effect of
orthotopic liver transplantation (OLT) on branched-chain amino acid requirement.
Pediatr Res 59:829–834.

Manguso, F., et al. 2005. Effects of an appropriate oral diet on the nutritional status of patients
with HCV-related liver cirrhosis: A prospective study. *Clin Nutr* 24:751–759.

McDiarmid, S. V. 1996. Risk factors and outcomes after pediatric liver transplantation. *Liver
Transpl Surg* 2:44–56.

McDiarmid, S. V., et al. 1999. Factors affecting growth after pediatric liver transplantation.
Transplantation 67:404–411.

Mejia, A., et al. 2007. Use of split-liver allografts does not impair pediatric recipient growth.
Liver Transpl 13:145–148.

Okajima, H., et al. 2003. Long-term effects of liver transplantation on bone mineral density in children with end-stage liver disease: A 2-year prospective study. *Liver Transpl* 9:360–364.

Ong, D. E., et al. 1987. Liver levels of vitamin A and cellular retinol-binding protein for patients with biliary atresia. *Hepatology* 7:253–256.

Puustinen, L., et al. 2005. Recombinant human growth hormone treatment after liver transplantation in childhood: The 5-year outcome. *Transplantation* 79:1241–1246.

Quiros-Tejeira, R. E., et al. 2000. Does liver transplantation affect growth pattern in Alagille syndrome? *Liver Transpl* 6:582–587.

Ramaccioni, V., et al. 2000. Nutritional aspects of chronic liver disease and liver transplantation in children. *J Pediatr Gastroenterol Nutr* 30:361–367.

Rashid, M., et al. 1999. Prevalence of vitamin K deficiency in cystic fibrosis. *Am J Clin Nutr* 70:378–382.

Renz, J. F., et al. 2001. Posttransplantation growth in pediatric liver recipients. *Liver Transpl* 7:1040–1055.

Rodeck, B., et al. 2000. Improvement of growth after growth hormone treatment in children who undergo liver transplantation. *J Pediatr Gastroenterol Nutr* 31:286–290.

Romero, R., et al. 2001. Persistent hyperglycemia in pediatric liver transplant recipients. *Transplant Proc* 33:3617–3618.

Rovner, A. J., et al. 2002. Rethinking growth failure in Alagille syndrome: The role of dietary intake and steatorrhea. *J Pediatr Gastroenterol Nutr* 35:495–502.

Saito, T., et al. 2007. Growth curves of pediatric patients with biliary atresia following living donor liver transplantation: Factors that influence post-transplantation growth. *Pediatr Transplant* 11:764–770.

Sokol, R. J., J. E. Heubi, and W. F. Balistreri. 1983a. Vitamin E deficiency in cholestatic liver disease. *J Pediatr* 103:663–664.

Sokol, R. J., J. E. Heubi, N. Butler-Simon, H. J. McClung, J. R. Lilly, and A. Silverman. 1987. Treatment of vitamin E deficiency during chronic childhood cholestasis with oral D-alpha-tocopheryl polyethylene glycol-1000 succinate. *Gastroenterology* 93:975–985.

Sokol, R. J., J. E. Heubi, S. Iannaccone, K. E. Bove, and W. F. Balistreri. 1983b. Mechanism causing vitamin E deficiency during chronic childhood cholestasis. *Gastroenterology* 85:1172–1182.

Studies of Pediatric Liver Transplantation (SPLIT): Year 2000 outcomes. 2001. *Transplantation* 72:463–476.

Taylor, R. M., et al. 2003. Can energy expenditure be predicted in critically ill children? *Pediatr Crit Care Med* 4:176–180.

Taylor, R. M., et al. 2005. Assessing nutritional status in children with chronic liver disease. *J Gastroenterol Hepatol* 20:1817–1824.

Tsiaousi, E. T., et al. 2008. Malnutrition in end stage liver disease: Recommendations and nutritional support. *J Gastroenterol Hepatol* 23:527–533.

van Mourik, I. D., et al. 2000. Long-term nutritional and neurodevelopmental outcome of liver transplantation in infants aged less than 12 months. *J Pediatr Gastroenterol Nutr* 30:269–275.

Viner, R. M., et al. 1999. Growth of long-term survivors of liver transplantation. *Arch Dis Child* 80:235–240.

21 Use of an Antioxidant Cocktail for Insulin Resistance Associated with Age and a High Sugar Diet: A Hepatic Mechanism

W. Wayne Lautt and Zhi Ming

CONTENTS

Aging is commonly associated with insulin resistance, characterized by a progressive impairment in glucose uptake and utilization primarily in skeletal muscle. Redistribution of body mass from muscle to fat and progressive hyperglycemia, hyperlipidemia, hyperinsulinemia, and hypertension (the "metabolic syndrome") often occur. Dysfunction of the central nervous system and the autonomic nervous system, including reduced parasympathetic and CNS cholinergic tone, are also

321

commonly seen with aging. We have recently suggested that the initiating metabolic defect that leads progressively to the metabolic syndrome, diabetes, and multiple organ failure is a postprandial defect in glucose sequestration that results in nutrient energy being shifted from normal storage as glycogen in skeletal muscle to production and storage of lipids and is typified by postprandial hyperglycemia, hyperinsulinemia, hyperlipidemia, and increased reactive oxidative stress.

In the normal healthy state, feeding results in a rapid meal-induced insulin sensitization (MIS). The mechanism of MIS has been demonstrated to result from insulin acting in the presence of feeding signals delivered to the liver resulting in the release of a hepatic insulin sensitizing substance (HISS), which acts selectively on skeletal muscle to stimulate glucose uptake. HISS action accounts for approximately 55% of the total glucose disposal response to a pulse of insulin in the fed state. MIS decreases with age and results in a progressive series of metabolic and tissue dysfunctions. Based on these concepts, the liver becomes the primary therapeutic target.

In this chapter, we focus on the MIS phenomenon and the impact of nutrition on both potentiating and attenuating the progressive development of absence of MIS (AMIS) and the consequent metabolic dysfunctions that normally occur with aging.

21.1   AGE AND PARASYMPATHETIC DYSFUNCTION

Aging is associated with a generalized reduction in parasympathetic nerve function demonstrated for the cardiovascular system (O'Brien et al., 1986; Ingall et al., 1990), eyes (Fitzgerald et al., 2005), gastrointestinal tract (Phillips and Powley, 2007), and urinary bladder (Schneider et al., 2005). Parasympathetic dysfunction can be identified before the development of diabetes (Lautt, 1980) and is later associated with the metabolic syndrome (Britton et al. 2007) and obesity (Skrapari et al., 2007; Von Kanel et al., 2007. Parasympathetic dysfunction in the liver results in blockade of HISS release and AMIS (for a review, see Lautt, 2004).

21.2   AGING AND OXIDATIVE STRESS

Increasing evidence suggests that reactive oxygen species are involved with, or even trigger, the process of aging (Biesalski, 2002). The free radical theory of aging was first proposed by Harman in 1956. According to this theory, endogenously produced free radicals continuously and progressively cause permanent tissue damage, finally leading to aging. Since the majority of free radicals are produced from the mitochondria, the current version of this theory is the mitochondrial free radical theory of aging. Oxidative damage to proteins has been found in association with age in a variety of tissues and cells including fibroblasts, brain, liver, heart, and skeletal muscles. (For a review, see Merker et al., 2001.)

21.3   POSTPRANDIAL HYPERGLYCEMIA, HYPERINSULINEMIA, HYPERLIPIDEMIA, AND OXIDATIVE STRESS

The majority of studies and diagnosis of metabolic diseases continue to focus on the fasted state. However, the importance of postprandial rather than fasting metabolic defects, as related to cardiovascular disease, is becoming increasingly recognized. Auto-oxidative glycosylation plays an important role in the pathophysiology associated with diabetes and aging (Wolff et al., 1989; Hunt et al., 1988). The relationship between glycosylated hemoglobin and plasma glucose in patients with type 2 diabetes was predicted by postprandial glycemic levels (Avignon et al., 1997). The strongest age- and sex-adjusted relative risk for all-cause and cardiovascular mortality was associated with 2-hour post-load plasma glucose levels (de Vegt et al., 1999). Increased mortality risk has been associated with 2-hour postload plasma glucose levels to a much greater extent than with fasting plasma glucose (Hanefeld et al., 1996; DECODE Study Group, 1999). Isolated postload hyperglycemia is a strong predictor of mortality (Simon et al., 1987; DECODE Study Group, 1999; Shaw et al., 1999; Vaccaro et al., 1999; Engelgau et al., 2000; Simon and Brandenberger, 2002).

It has been suggested that hyperglycemia-induced overproduction of superoxide by the mitochondrial electron transport chain accounts for the four main molecular mechanisms implicated in glucose-mediated vascular damage associated with blindness, renal failure, nerve damage, atherosclerosis, stroke, and hind limb amputation (Brownlee, 2001). Postprandial plasma glucose is an important determinant of both onset and development of nephropathy in patients with type 2 diabetes (Schchiri et al., 2000). Low-density lipoprotein oxidation increases after meals (Diwadkar et al., 1999) and directly relates to the degree of hyperglycemia (Ceriello et al., 1999). Acute hyperglycemia is associated with an acute increase in clotting factor VII (Ceriello et al., 1998) and enhanced thrombin activity that is proportional to the level of hyperglycemia (Ceriello et al., 1996). The synthesis of fibrinogen, which is a strong risk factor for cardiovascular disease in both diabetic and nondiabetic subjects, increases during food intake in diabetic patients (Ceriello, 1997).

Acute hyperglycemia also stimulates increased expression of proadhesive proteins including intercellular adhesion molecule 1 (Ceriello, 2003). Dunn and Grant (2005) reviewed the relationship between the hypercoagulable prothrombic state occurring in type 2 diabetes and cardiovascular disease risk. In a review of the importance of postprandial hyperglycemia on the development of cardiovascular disease, Haffner (1998) suggested that atherosclerotic changes start to develop in the prediabetic state when postprandial blood glucose levels are only moderately elevated above normal levels. He suggested, however, that increased insulin resistance and hyperinsulinemia may be responsible for the atherosclerotic changes and that hyperglycemia may be a marker but not a cause of these changes. The role of postprandial hyperglycemia, hyperlipidemia, hyperinsulinemia, and oxidative stress on cardiovascular disease has recently been reviewed (Lautt, 2007). A negative influence of postprandial hypertriglyceridemia on endothelial function is seen in diabetic subjects (Bae et al., 2001; Anderson et al., 2001). Postprandial hypertriglyceridemia is a recognized independent predictor of cardiovascular pathology (Anderson et al., 2001). Ingelsson et al. (2005) suggested that obesity may be a coincidental predictor of cardiovascular dysfunction and is simply a marker of insulin resistance, which is compensated for by hyperinsulinemia, and suggested that hyperinsulinemia was a cardiovascular risk factor through several possible mechanisms.

Ceriello, recognizing the strong relationship between processing a meal and the production of oxidative stress, concluded that "paradoxically, the vast majority of the studies on cardiovascular disease risk factors have been conducted by measuring them in strictly fasting conditions. This simply means that most of the data available to date may not reflect the real situation" (Ceriello, 2000). Meal consumption in healthy subjects acutely reduces antioxidant defenses (Ceriello et al., 1998) and produces oxidative stress that is linked to the pathogenesis of cardiovascular disease (Griendling and Alexander, 1997) and hypertension (Nakazono et al., 1991).

21.4 ANTIOXIDANTS

The effects of antioxidants or free radical scavengers have been widely tested for the prevention and treatment of acute and chronic diseases. However, the efficacy of antioxidant treatment in clinical trials has been generally unimpressive. We have suggested that the major reason is that, although the production of the free radicals with various chemical properties is widely spread out throughout the different tissue and cellular components, the chemical property of an individual antioxidant can only allow it to scavenge the free radicals located in a specific cellular component, for example, the lipid or aqueous phase. The efficacy of an antioxidant substance is also dependent on the redox state of the cell. In situations where an imbalanced redox state preexisted, antioxidant treatment may be ineffective or even detrimental.

We have recently demonstrated a unique synergistic interaction among three antioxidants selected to specifically target different cellular components. The combination of S-adenosylmethionine and vitamins E and C has been shown to protect against liver damage and the development of HISS-dependent insulin resistance (HDIR) that occurs as a result of acute exposure to the hepatotoxic thioacetamide (Ming et al., 2006). All three compounds play an important and different but interacting, role in scavenging free radicals. The water-soluble property of vitamin C makes it the first-order antioxidant to protect cell components from free radical–induced damage by quenching various water-soluble radicals, for example, superoxide anion. Vitamin E is a lipid-soluble molecule and can transfer its phenolic hydrogen to a peroxyl free radical of a peroxidized polyunsaturated fatty acid, thereby breaking the radical chain reaction, thus preventing the lipid peroxidation in cellular and subcellular membrane phospholipids, especially those of mitochondria and microsomes. S-Adenosylmethionine is a natural, nontoxic regulator of glutathione (GSH). GSH is the main intracellular defense against free radicals. GSH stores are significantly depleted in liver injury induced by oxidative stress. Administration of S-adenosylmethionine represents an effective means of restoring intracellular GSH stores especially in mitochondria, thus improving the cellular ability to scavenge free radicals (Lieber, 1999). The unique synergistic activity of this antioxidant cocktail, referred to as Samec for convenience, was shown by the demonstration that the combination of vitamins C and E did not confer protection of serum alanine aminotransferase or aspartate aminotransferase levels 24 hours after exposure to thioacetamide. Similarly, S-adenosylmethionine presented alone did not confer protection, whereas the combination cocktail conferred very significant protection. Similarly, the activity of HISS was virtually eliminated by the acute hepatotoxin and was protected only by the combined cocktail (Ming et al., 2006).

21.5 MEAL-INDUCED INSULIN SENSITIZATION

MIS is a readily quantified phenomenon that has been only recently identified (Lautt, 1999; Lautt et al., 2001; Sadri et al., 2006). Despite the potential significance of this observation, it has apparently not been studied by anyone other than our group. MIS is seen as a dramatic increase in the glucose disposal response to insulin immediately after a meal. The phenomenon of MIS is defined from the observation that the dynamic response to insulin determined after a 24-hour fast is doubled when tested 100 minutes after administration of a mixed meal in rats (Sadri et al., 2006) and humans (Patarrao et al., 2008). The process of MIS is a result of the action of HISS, which is released from the liver in response to a pulse of insulin and acts selectively to stimulate glucose uptake in skeletal muscle (Xie and Lautt, 1996). Although the chemical identity of HISS remains unknown, its action can be quantified (see Lautt, 2003) and a homeostatic role has been suggested (see Lautt, 2004).

For MIS to be quantified, an index of insulin sensitivity must be used that can be carried out in both the fed and fasted states. The acute dynamic response to insulin used to demonstrate MIS has been shown using changes in arterial-venous glucose gradients (glucose extraction) across various organs, the use of the insulin tolerance test, and a rapid insulin sensitivity test (RIST).

RIST is a rapidly sampled transient euglycemic clamp in response to a bolus administration of insulin. The operating procedure for the RIST has been described (Lautt et al., 1998) and methods for differentiating and quantifying HISS-dependent and HISS-independent insulin actions have been reviewed (Lautt, 2003). The RIST index is the amount of glucose required to be infused to maintain a euglycemic baseline after a bolus administration of insulin.

MIS can be quantified using two different approaches as shown in Figure 21.1 (from Sadri et al., 2006). A RIST index is determined first after a 24-hour fast where HISS release is minimal or absent (Lautt et al., 2001). The phenomenon of MIS is then demonstrated by carrying out the RIST approximately 100 min after administration of a mixed meal and after a new euglycemic baseline has been established. In Figure 21.1, the study was carried out in conscious rats where the meal was administered as a mixed liquid test meal directly into the stomach through an implanted catheter. A similar degree of MIS can be demonstrated in conscious animals that have voluntarily consumed a meal of normal rat chow (Latour and Lautt, 2002). The difference in RIST index between the 24-hour fasted and fed states is attributed to HISS action on skeletal muscle.

The second method to quantify MIS is to determine the RIST index in the recently fed state and then again after HISS release has been blocked by any of several means known to interfere with the feeding signals (Lautt et al., 2001). In Figure 21.1, the MIS phenomenon is completely blocked by intravenous administration of atropine, which acts on muscarinic receptors in the liver to block HISS release. From this figure, it can be seen that quantification of the MIS phenomenon is similar using either method. The most straightforward method technically is to allow feeding in the conscious state and then to carry out the tests under anesthesia before and after atropine to differentiate the HISS component.

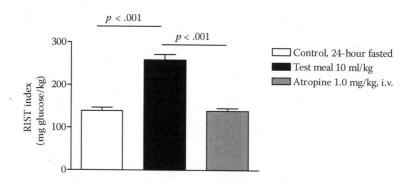

FIGURE 21.1 Quantification of meal-induced insulin sensitization (MIS). The rapid insulin sensitivity test (RIST) index was determined after a 24-hour fast (control), following administration of a liquid test meal and then after atropine (to block HISS release). MIS can be quantified either from the difference in response to insulin comparing 24-hour-fasted to fed responses, or from comparing fed responses to post-atropine responses. Both methods have advantages and disadvantages depending on the question. (From Sadri, P., Reid, M. A. G., Afonso, R. A., et al., *Br J Nutr*, 95, 288–295, 2006. With permission.)

HISS release from the liver is dependent on receiving three simultaneous signals. Two permissive "feeding signals" are required to be delivered to the liver. The first signal is an elevation of hepatic GSH levels that increase by approximately 30% after a meal (Tateishi et al., 1974; Guarino et al., 2003) and the second signal is delivered by the hepatic parasympathetic nerves, which release acetylcholine to act on muscarinic receptors, resulting in activation of nitric oxide synthase and generation of nitric oxide. In the presence of these two feeding signals, a pulse of insulin results in the release of a pulse of HISS. Figure 21.2 shows the dynamic RIST curves obtained in fed anesthetized rats before and after HISS release has been blocked by inhibition of hepatic muscarinic receptors using atropine, blockade of hepatic nitric oxide synthase using N^G-monomethyl-L-arginine (L-NMMA) or by surgical denervation of the liver (Lautt et al., 2001). The pulsatile nature of HISS action is evident.

21.6 ABSENCE OF MEAL-INDUCED INSULIN SENSITIZATION

Blockade of HISS release prevents both the development of MIS in response to a meal and blocks MIS once it has been developed (Sadri et al., 2006). HISS-dependent insulin action accounts for 55% of the response to a pulse of insulin in the fed rat (Lautt et al., 2001), 45% in fed mice (Latour and Chan, 2002), and 67% in fed humans (Patarrao et al., 2008). HISS action decreases progressively with the duration of fasting to become insignificant after a 24-hour fast. In the absence of HISS release, a state of HISS-dependent insulin resistance (HDIR) is said to exist. Although HDIR is appropriate in the fasted state in order to reduce the hypoglycemic impact of insulin, HDIR in the fed state results in AMIS. We have suggested that AMIS represents the earliest metabolic deficiency that leads to a definable and predictable series of consequences including "syndrome X" and diabetes.

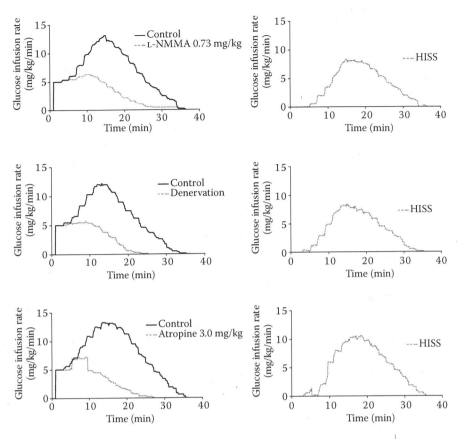

FIGURE 21.2 Dynamic insulin action demonstrating the HISS-dependent and HISS-independent components. The mean ($n = 8$–18) dynamic RIST response to a bolus of 50 mU/kg insulin showing the rate of glucose infusion required to maintain a euglycemic baseline in fed rats (control) and after HISS release was blocked by inhibition of hepatic nitric oxide synthase (L-NMMA), surgical denervation of the liver, and blockade of hepatic muscarinic receptors (atropine). The difference between the two curves on the left panel is shown as HISS action in the right panels. (From Lautt, W. W., Macedo, M. P., Sadri, P., Takayama, S., Ramos, F. D., and Legare, D. J., *Am J Physiol Gastrointest Liver Physiol*, 281, G29–G36, 2001. With permission.)

The normal response to a meal results in a considerably amplified response to insulin secondary to HISS acting on skeletal muscle (Xie and Lautt, 1996; Moore et al., 2002) leading to nutrient storage primarily as glycogen in skeletal muscle. When HDIR results in AMIS, the postprandial condition is typified by hyperglycemia, compensatory hyperinsulinemia, and resultant hyperlipidemia. All of these conditions are associated with increased free radical production, which has been suggested to account for virtually all of the complications associated with the "metabolic syndrome." We have suggested that HDIR and the resultant AMIS could account for the cardiovascular and other risks associated with insulin resistance, obesity, and diabetes (Lautt, 2007; Lautt et al., 2008; Ming et al., 2008). Because AMIS results

TABLE 21.1

Key Features of the Absence of Meal-Induced Insulin Sensitization (AMIS) Syndrome: Basic "Take-Home" Messages

1. The ability of insulin to remove glucose from blood is approximately doubled immediately after meal.
2. This meal-induced insulin sensitization results in glucose being stored in muscle.
3. AMIS, through a defined mechanism regulated by the liver, results in nutrients being stored as fat and in the response to a meal resulting in metabolic disturbances including increased free radical stress.
4. Metabolic disturbances associated with AMIS result in a wide range of progressive dysfunctions including obesity, impaired heart function, impaired blood vessel responses associated with high blood pressure, dysfunctions of the eye and kidney, and generation of foot ulcers. AMIS can be triggered by a wide range of stressors including inappropriate diet through high sugar intake.
5. AMIS and the related symptoms can be attenuated by incorporation of an antioxidant either through mixed foods or a unique pharmaceutical antioxidant cocktail.

in a mechanistic-based, predictable, and manipulatable progression of dysfunctions, we suggest it could be referred to as an AMIS syndrome (Table 21.1).

21.6.1 AMIS, AGE, AND SUCROSE

Aging is associated with a decrease in lean body mass and a relative increase in fat mass (Barbieri et al., 2001). Insulin resistance associated with aging is closely related to fat accumulation (Kohrt et al., 1993). The insulin resistance seen with aging in rats is completely accountable for by a decrease in HISS action with the HISS-independent component of insulin action, detectable after atropine administration, being undiminished (Macedo et al., 2002).

We have recently demonstrated that a diet high in sucrose provided either as an additional supplement through drinking of water or through an isocaloric replacement for starch in solid rat chow results in insulin resistance that is accountable for by HDIR with the HISS-independent component remaining unaltered (Ribeiro et al., 2005).

21.7 HDIR ASSOCIATED WITH AGE ACCELERATED BY SUCROSE SUPPLEMENT AND ATTENUATED BY SAMEC

HDIR and resultant AMIS associated with normal aging can be positively and negatively impacted by nutrition (Lautt et al., 2008; Ming et al., 2009). A low-dose sucrose supplement was used to accelerate HDIR during the aging process up to 1 year. In addition, the antioxidant cocktail, Samec, consisting of S-adenosylmethione, vitamin C, and vitamin E formulated into the chow, demonstrated a strong protective effect for HDIR and AMIS associated with aging and with the sucrose diet. The objective was to test the AMIS syndrome hypothesis, which proposes that HDIR is an initiating metabolic defect that leads progressively to dysfunctions associated with syndrome X or the metabolic syndrome, obesity, and type 2 diabetes.

The RIST index in 9-week-old rats dramatically decreased from 175 ± 7 to 100 ± 6 by 6 months of age and further to 79 ± 4 mg/kg by 12 months with the HISS-dependent component accounting for virtually all of the decrease. HISS action accounted for $52 \pm 2\%$ of the response to insulin in young (9 weeks) animals, but decreased to $30 \pm 3\%$ at 6 months and $17 \pm 3\%$ by 1 year (Figure 21.3). The antioxidant cocktail attenuated the decrease in the HISS component, which remained at $44 \pm 2\%$ and $41 \pm 2\%$ at 6 and 12 months of age, respectively.

Figure 21.4 shows the detrimental effect of the low-dose sucrose supplement and the protective effect of the antioxidant on HISS action when administered concomitantly with the sucrose supplement. The effects on the HISS-independent component of insulin action were quantitatively minor and the impact on the RIST index could be accounted for almost entirely by changes in the HISS component of insulin action.

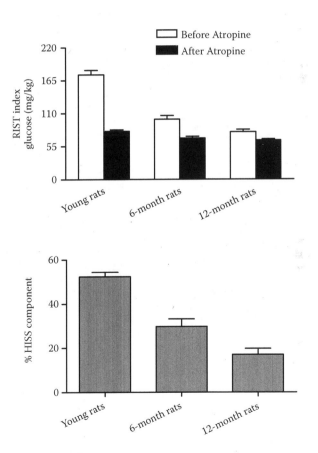

FIGURE 21.3 Effect of age on insulin action. Age results in reduced dynamic response to insulin attributable to HISS action with the HISS-independent (post-atropine) component of insulin action being modestly affected. (From Lautt, W. W., Ming, Z., Macedo, M. P., and Legare, D. J., *Exp Gerontol*, 43, 790–800, 2008. With permission.)

The hypothesis that HISS action inversely relates to adiposity is critically tested by the data shown in Figure 21.5, where HISS action and adiposity (whole body based on electrical impedance and confirmed by measurement of regional fat depots from perinephric, perienteric, and epididymal masses) are shown. These data are pooled for several groups including normal aged and sucrose and antioxidant combinations at each age. Considering the diversity of long-term interventions, the correlation is remarkable. Adiposity was predicted by determining the HISS component of insulin action.

HISS action correlated with other components associated with the metabolic syndrome. Fasting glucose, insulin, triglyceride, and total cholesterol levels and postprandial insulin and glucose correlated significantly with HISS action. The antioxidant supplement afforded protection against development of AMIS with age and completely prevented the negative effect of sucrose on development of AMIS. Correlation analysis showed that HISS action could be manipulated over a sufficiently wide range to demonstrate significant and strong correlation with parameters associated with the metabolic syndrome, diabetes, and obesity (Lautt et al., 2008; Ming et al., 2009).

Initial predictions of the AMIS syndrome have been demonstrated. Whereas the connection among absence of HISS action, adiposity, hyperglycemia, hyperlipidemia, and hyperinsulinemia have been demonstrated, specific tissue and organ dys-

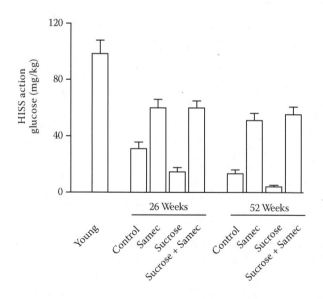

FIGURE 21.4 Interaction of age, sucrose, and antioxidants on HISS action. HISS-dependent insulin action assessed from the RIST index decreases with age and is made worse by a low dose (5%) sucrose supplement. The antioxidant cocktail (Samec) attenuated the decline in HISS action resulting from age and completely prevented the impact of sucrose. (Calculated from the data of Lautt, W. W., Ming, Z., Macedo, M. P., and Legare, D. J., *Exp Gerontol*, 43, 790–800, 2008.)

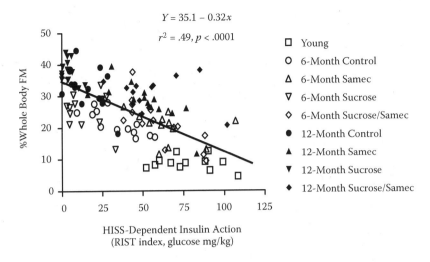

$$Y = 35.1 - 0.32x$$
$$r^2 = .49, p < .0001$$

□ Young
○ 6-Month Control
△ 6-Month Samec
▽ 6-Month Sucrose
◇ 6-Month Sucrose/Samec
● 12-Month Control
▲ 12-Month Samec
▼ 12-Month Sucrose
◆ 12-Month Sucrose/Samec

HISS-Dependent Insulin Action
(RIST index, glucose mg/kg)

FIGURE 21.5 Manipulation of HISS action results in changes in adiposity. Adiposity can be predicted from HISS action shown by pooled data from normal aging (9, 26, and 52 weeks), age plus sucrose, age plus antioxidant (Samec), and age plus sucrose plus antioxidant (Samec). Whole-body fat mass was estimated from bioelectrical impedance, but the relationship is similar for adiposity determined from regional adiposity based on weighed fat mass from perinephric, perienteric, and epididymal fat pads. As HISS action decreases, adiposity increases. (Calculated from the data of Lautt, W. W., Ming, Z., Macedo, M. P., and Legare, D. J., *Exp Gerontol*, 43, 790–800, 2008.)

functions have not yet been reported. The AMIS hypothesis defines a central role of the liver in regulating nutrient partitioning to fat or glycogen.

21.8   IMPLICATIONS AND APPLICATIONS

These studies suggest that some of the major impairments that are associated with aging can be attributed to HDIR, and HDIR can be positively and negatively affected by nutrition. The historical and epidemiological relationship between sugar consumption and the characteristics that we suggest can be considered as the AMIS syndrome implies that a major contributor to the current epidemic of metabolic syndrome, adiposity, and diabetes is preventable by reduction of intake of sugars. The importance of an antioxidant balance is also amply demonstrated in these studies. Epidemiological studies demonstrate that diets high in antioxidants have health benefits, whereas individual dietary supplements have generally provided minimal advantage and, because of the imbalance imposed by a high dose of a single compound, can result in toxicities. Even a modest sucrose supplement approximately doubled the rate of development of HDIR with aging, and an antioxidant cocktail conferred complete protection against the sucrose impact and also significantly attenuated age-related HDIR and a cluster of dysfunctions predicted by the AMIS syndrome. The impact of other lifestyle interventions, such as exercise, on HDIR and resultant AMIS has not been examined.

21.9 SUMMARY POINTS

- Increased postprandial skeletal muscle responses to insulin are determined by the liver through release of a HISS.
- In the normal state, feeding leads to doubling the whole-body response to insulin.
- MIS results from insulin releasing HISS from the liver to act selectively on skeletal muscle.
- Lack of HISS results in AMIS.
- Insulin resistance associated with age is attributable to lack of HISS and resultant AMIS.
- The AMIS syndrome accounts for postprandial hyperglycemia, hyperinsulinemia, hyperlipidemia, and increased reactive oxygen generation.
- HISS release and MIS are affected by nutrition, inhibited by sucrose, and potentiated by antioxidants.
- As HISS action changes, adiposity changes as do other components of the AMIS syndrome including postprandial insulin and glucose, and fasting insulin, triglycerides, cholesterol, and blood pressure.
- Resistance to the direct effect of insulin develops slower and later than resistance to HISS.
- Therapeutic targeting of the liver restores HISS release and reverses AMIS.

ACKNOWLEDGMENTS

The authors acknowledge the assistance of Karen Sanders and the long-term conceptual input of Dallas Legare and Paula Macedo and her group in Lisbon. Research upon which this chapter is based was funded by the Canadian Institutes for Health Research and the Canadian Diabetes Association.

REFERENCES

Anderson, R. A., M. L. Evans, G. R. Ellis, et al. 2001. The relationship between post-prandial lipaemia, endothelial function and oxidative stress in healthy individuals and patients with type 2 diabetes. *Atherosclerosis* 154:475–483.

Avignon, A., A. Radauceanu, and L. Monnier. 1997. Nonfasting plasma glucose is a better marker of diabetic control than fasting plasma glucose in type 2 diabetes. *Diabetes Care* 20:1822–1826.

Bae, J. H., E. Bassenge, K. B. Kim, et al. 2001. Postprandial hypertriglyceridemia impairs endothelial function by enhanced oxidant stress. *Atherosclerosis* 155:517–523.

Barbieri, M., M. R. Rizzo, D. Manzella, and G. Paolisso. 2001. Age-related insulin resistance: Is it an obligatory finding? The lesson from healthy centenarians. *Diabetes Metab Res Rev* 17:19–26.

Biesalski, H. K. 2002. Free radical theory of aging. *Curr Opin Clin Metab Care* 5:5–10.

Britton, A., M. Shipley, M. Malik, K. Hnatkova, H. Hemingway, and M. Marmot. 2007. Changes in heart rate and heart rate variability over time in middle-aged men and women in the general population (from the Whitehall II Cohort Study). *Am J Cardiol* 100:524–527.

Brownlee, M. 2001. Biochemistry and molecular cell biology of diabetic complications. *Nature* 414:813–819.

Ceriello, A. 1997. Fibrinogen and diabetes mellitus. Is it time for intervention trials? *Diabetologia* 40:731–734.

Ceriello, A. 2000. The post-prandial state and cardiovascular disease: Relevance to diabetes mellitus. *Diabetes Metab Res Rev* 16:125–132.

Ceriello, A. 2003. The possible role of postprandial hyperglycaemia in the pathogenesis of diabetic complications. *Diabetologia* 46:M9–M16.

Ceriello, A., N. Bortolotti, E. Motz, et al. 1998. Meal-generated oxidative stress in type 2 diabetic patients. *Diabetes Care* 21:1529–1533.

Ceriello, A., N. Bortolotti, E. Motz, et al. 1999. Meal-induced oxidative stress and low-density lipoprotein (LDL) oxidation in diabetes: The possible role of hyperglycemia. *Metabolism* 48:1503–1508.

Ceriello, A., C. Taboga, L. Tonutti, et al. 1996. Post-meal coagulation activation in diabetes mellitus: The effect of acarbose. *Diabetologia* 39:469–473.

DECODE Study Group, on behalf of the European Diabetes Epidemiology Group. 1999. Glucose tolerance and mortality comparison of WHO and American Diabetes Association diagnostic criteria. *Lancet* 354:617–621.

De Vegt, F., J. M. Dekker, H. G. Ruhe, et al. 1999. Hyperglycaemia is associated with all-cause and cardiovascular mortality in the Hoorn population: The Hoorn study. *Diabetologia* 42:926–931.

Diwadkar, V. A., J. W. Anderson, S. R. Bridges, et al. 1999. Postprandial low density lipoproteins in type 2 diabetes are oxidized more extensively than fasting diabetes and control samples. *Proc Soc Exp Biol Med* 222:178–184.

Dunn, E. J., and P. J. Grant. 2005. Type 2 diabetes: An atherothrombotic syndrome. *Curr Mol Med* 5:323–332.

Engelgau, M. M., K. M. V. Narayan, and W. H. Herman. 2000. Screening for type 2 diabetes. *Diabetes Care* 23:1563–1580.

Fitzgerald, M. E., E. Tolley, B. Jackson, et al. 2005. Anatomical and functional evidence for progressive age-related decline in parasympathetic control of choroidal blood flow in pigeons. *Exp Eye Res* 81:478–491.

Griendling, K. K., and R. W. Alexander. 1997. Oxidative stress and cardiovascular disease. *Circulation* 96:3264–3265.

Guarino, M. P., R. A. Afonso, N. Raimundo, J. F. Raposo, and M. P. Macedo. 2003. Hepatic glutathione and nitric oxide are critical for hepatic insulin-sensitizing substance action. *Am J Physiol Gastrointest Liver Physiol* 284:G588–G594.

Haffner, S. M. 1998. The importance of hyperglycemia in the nonfasting state to the development of cardiovascular disease. *Endocrine Rev* 19:583–592.

Hanefeld, M., S. Fischer, U. Julius, et al. 1996. Risk factors for myocardial infarction and death in newly detected NIDDM: The Diabetes Intervention Study, 11-year follow-up. *Diabetologia* 39:1577–1583.

Harman, D. 1956. Aging: A theory based on free radical and radiation chemistry. *J Gerontol* 11:298–300.

Hunt, J. V., R. T. Dean, and S. P. Wolff. 1988. Hydroxyl radical production and autoxidative glycosylation. Glucose autoxidation as the cause of protein damage in the experimental glycation model of diabetes mellitus and ageing. *Biochem J* 256:205–212.

Ingall, T. J., J. G. McLeod, and P. C. O'Brien. 1990. The effect of ageing on autonomic nervous system function. *Aust NZ J Med* 20:570–577.

Ingelsson, E., J. Sundstrom, J. Arnlow, et al. 2005. Insulin resistance and risk of congestive heart failure. *JAMA* 294:334–341.

Kohrt, W. M., J. P. Kirwan, M. A. Staten, et al. 1993. Insulin resistance in aging is related to abdominal obesity. *Diabetes* 42:273–281.

Latour, M. G., and C. C. Chan. 2002. A rapid insulin sensitivity test (RIST) in the anesthetized mice (Abstract). *Diabetes* 51(Suppl 2):A422.

Latour, M. G., and W. W. Lautt. 2002. Insulin sensitivity regulated by feeding in the conscious unrestrained rat. *Can J Physiol Pharmacol* 80:8–12.

Lautt, W. W. 1980. Hepatic parasympathetic neuropathy as a cause of maturity-onset diabetes? *Gen Pharmacol* 11:343–345.

Lautt, W. W. 1999. The HISS story overview: A novel hepatic neurohumoral regulation of peripheral insulin sensitivity in health and diabetes. *Can J Physiol Pharmacol* 77:553–562.

Lautt, W. W. 2003. Practice and principles of pharmacodynamic determination of HISS-dependent and HISS-independent insulin action: Methods to quantitate mechanisms of insulin resistance. *Med Res Rev* 23:1–14.

Lautt, W. W. 2004. A new paradigm for diabetes and obesity: The hepatic insulin sensitizing substance (HISS) hypothesis. *J Pharmacol Sci* 95:9–17.

Lautt, W. W. 2007. Postprandial insulin resistance as an early predictive cardiovascular risk factor. *Ther Clin Risk Manag* 3:761–770.

Lautt, W. W., M. P. Macedo, P. Sadri, S. Takayama, F. D. Ramos, and D. J. Legare. 2001. Hepatic parasympathetic (HISS) control of insulin sensitivity determined by feeding and fasting. *Am J Physiol Gastrointest Liver Physiol* 281:G29–G36.

Lautt, W. W., Z. Ming, M. P. Macedo, and D. J. Legare. 2008. HISS-dependent insulin resistance (HDIR) in aged rats is associated with adiposity, progresses to syndrome X, and is attenuated by a unique antioxidant cocktail. *Exp Gerontol* doi:10.1016/j.exger.2008.04.013.

Lautt, W. W., X. Wang, P. Sadri, D. J. Legare, and M. P. Macedo. 1998. Rapid insulin sensitivity test (RIST). *Can J Physiol Pharmacol* 76:1080–1086.

Lieber, C. S. 1999. Role of *S*-adenosyl-L-methionine in the treatment of liver diseases. *Hepatology* 30:1155–1159.

Macedo, M. P., R. A. Afonso, and R. T. Ribeiro. 2002. Aged Wistar rats show a hepatic insulin sensitizing substance (HISS)–dependent insulin resistance. *Proc West Pharmacol Soc* 45:245.

Merker, K., A. Stolzing, and T. Grune. 2001. Proteolysis, caloric restriction and aging. *Mech Ageing Dev* 122:595–615.

Ming, Z., Y.-J. Fan, X. Yang, and W. W. Lautt. 2006. Synergistic protection by *S*-adenosylmethionine with vitamins C and E on liver injury induced by thioacetamide in rats. *Free Radic Biol Med* 40:617–624.

Ming, Z., D. J. Legare, and W. W. Lautt. 2009. Is HISS-dependent insulin resistance (HDIR) the precursor to the metabolic syndrome, type 2 diabetes, and obesity? *Can J Physiol Pharmacol* (submitted).

Moore, M. C., S. Satake, B. Baranowski, P. S. Hsieh, D. W. Neal, and A. D. Cherrington. 2002. Effect of hepatic denervation on peripheral insulin sensitivity in conscious dogs. *Am J Physiol Endocrinol Metab* 282:E286–E296.

Nakazono, K., N. Watanabe, K. Matsuno, et al. 1991. Does superoxide underlie the pathogenesis of hypertension? *Proc Natl Acad Sci U S A* 88:10045–10048.

O'Brien, I. A. D., P. O'Hare, and R. J. M. Corrall. 1986. Heart rate variability in healthy subjects: Effect of age and the derivation of normal ranges for tests of autonomic function. *Br Heart J* 55:348–354.

Patarrao, R. S., W. W. Lautt, M. P. Guarino, et al. 2008. Meal-induced insulin sensitization (MIS) and parasympathetic regulation of MIS in humans. *Can J Physiol Pharmacol* 86:880–888.

Phillips, R. J., and T. L. Powley. 2007. Innervation of the gastrointestinal tract: Patterns of aging. *Auton Neurosci* 136:1–19.

Ribeiro, R. T., W. W. Lautt, D. J. Legare, and M. P. Macedo. 2005. Insulin resistance induced by sucrose-feeding is due to an impairment of the hepatic parasympathetic nerves. *Diabetologia* 48:976–983.

Sadri, P., M. A. G. Reid, R. A. Afonso, et al. 2006. Meal-induced insulin sensitization in conscious and anesthetized rat models comparing liquid mixed meal with glucose and sucrose. *Br J Nutr* 95:288–295.

Schchiri, M., H. Kishikawa, Y. Ohkubo, et al. 2000. Long-term results of the Kumamoto Study on optimal diabetes control in type 2 diabetic patients. *Diabetes Care* 23:B21–B29.

Schneider, T., P. Hein, M. B. Michel-Reher, and M. C. Michel. 2005. Effects of ageing on muscarinic receptor subtypes and function in rat urinary bladder. *Naunyn Schmiedebergs Arch Pharmacol* 372:71–78.

Shaw, J. E., A. M. Hodge, M. de Courten, et al. 1999. Isolated post-challenge hyperglycemia confirmed as a risk factor for mortality. *Diabetologia* 42:1050–1054.

Simon, C., and G. Brandenberger. 2002. Ultradian oscillations of insulin secretion in humans. *Diabetes* 51:S258–S261.

Simon, C., M. Follenius, and G. Brandenberger. 1987. Postprandial oscillations of plasma glucose insulin and C-peptide in man. *Diabetologia* 30:769–773.

Skrapari, I., N. Tentolouris, D. Perrea, C. Bakoyiannis, A. Papazafiropoulou, and N. Katsilambros. 2007. Baroreflex sensitivity in obesity: Relationship with cardiac autonomic nervous system activity. *Obesity* 15:1685–1693.

Tateishi, N., T. Higashi, S. Shinya, A. Naruse, and Y. Sakamoto. 1974. Studies on the regulation of glutathione level in rat liver. *J Biochem* 75:93–103.

Vaccaro, O., G. Ruffa, G. Imperatore, et al. 1999. Risk of diabetes in the new diagnostic category of impaired fasting glucose. *Diabetes Care* 22:1490–1493.

Von Kanel, R., R. A. Nelesen, M. G. Ziegler, B. T. Mausbach, P. J. Mills, and J. E. Dimsdale. 2007. Relation of autonomic activity to plasminogen activator inhibitor–1 plasma concentration and the role of body mass index. *Blood Coagul Fibrinolysis* 18:353–359.

Wolff, S. P., Z. A. Bascal, and J. V. Hunt. 1989. "Autoxidative glycosylation": Free radicals and glycation theory. *Prog Clin Biol Res* 304:259–275.

Xie, H., and W. W. Lautt. 1996. Insulin resistance of skeletal muscle produced by hepatic parasympathetic interruption. *Am J Physiol* 270:E858–E863.

22 Nutrition in End-Stage Liver Disease

Jens Kondrup

CONTENTS

22.1 INTRODUCTION

Indication for diet therapy is given by the randomized controlled trials showing a beneficial effect on clinical outcome. According to the guidelines issued by the European Society of Clinical Nutrition and Metabolism (ESPEN), there is indication for nutrition support, such as enteral feeding, when patients with cirrhosis cannot meet their nutritional requirements from normal food (Plauth et al., 2006). This is a level A recommendation based on the results of randomized trials and an earlier thorough analysis of randomized trials, which indicated that a decrease in mortality

TABLE 22.1

Features of End-Stage Liver Disease

Failing liver function leads to	Fatigue. The liver supports all other organs in the body by modifying the nutrients absorbed to the requirements of other organs, by storing glycogen to later starvation periods, by synthesizing a large number of plasma proteins with essential functions, by producing hormones (e.g., insulin-like growth factor 1) and metabolic intermediates (e.g., for synthesis of creatine, glutathione, and vitamin D).
	The liver also plays a vital role in elimination of drugs and other potentially toxic substances that enter the body.
	Failure of all these functions probably contributes to the fatigue.
	Bleeding episodes due to failing production of coagulation factors in the liver
	Malnutrition (see this chapter)
Portal hypertension leads to	Ascites, which is plasma fluid trapped in the peritoneum of the abdomen because of the high pressure in the portal vein.
	Varices are distended veins in the esophagus through which the blood bypasses the portal vein to return to the heart. These veins may rupture causing fatal bleeding episodes.
	Encephalopathy is a particular mental disturbance characterized by fluctuations in orientation and memory. It is believed to be mainly caused by metabolites from nutrients and intestinal (bacterial) products that bypass the usual elimination by the liver.

Note: Most features are due to the failing liver function and shrinkage of the liver, which causes blood from the intestines (splanchnic area) to bypass the liver and portal hypertension.

is likely when nutrition support is given to patients with low energy and protein intake due to complications of the disease (Kondrup and Müller, 1997) (Table 22.1).

22.2 CARBOHYDRATE-LIPIDS ENERGY

22.2.1 GLUCOSE METABOLISM

Many patients with cirrhosis have glucose intolerance or frank diabetes. A frequency of 20–30% has been reported (Gentile et al., 1993). Glucose intolerance does not seem to be related to clinical or biochemical indices of the disease nor to the etiology of the disease (Lecube et al., 2004; Müller et al., 1994b). On the other hand, glucose intolerance has been found to be related to the prognosis of patients with cirrhosis, also in a multivariate analysis (Nishida et al., 2006). Glucose intolerance seems to be due to several factors: a decrease in meal-induced insulin secretion (Marchesini et al., 1985), a higher meal-induced systemic appearance of glucose (Kruszynska et al., 1993), and a decreased peripheral glucose utilization (Proietto et al., 1980). The decreased peripheral utilization is reflected in decreased glucose membrane transport and decreased nonoxidative glucose disposal, that is, glycogen synthesis (Selberg et al., 1993). Insulin-induced glucose oxidation (4–5 g/kg/day) is not decreased (Petrides et al., 1994). Total glucose turnover reaches a maximum of 5–6 g glucose/kg/day (Selberg et al., 1993).

22.2.1.1 Practical Applications

Glucose should not be given in doses larger than 5–6 g glucose/kg/day. Blood glucose should be monitored closely.

22.2.2 Lipid Metabolism

Intestinal fat absorption may be reduced in patients with cirrhosis, especially in patients with cholestatic syndromes (Kestell and Lee, 1993). Without clinically obvious cholestasis, fecal energy content, or fecal fat, is usually not increased (Cabre et al., 2005; Nielsen et al. 1995).

Patients with cirrhosis have an elevated rate of fat oxidation after an overnight fast, similar to that seen in healthy volunteers after a 3-day fast. This is associated with a decrease in glucose oxidation. This increase in fat oxidation was explained as a more rapid switch to a prolonged fasting pattern because of low hepatic glycogen stores (Owen et al., 1981). In agreement with this, the rate of fat oxidation normalizes after 1 month's refeeding (Campillo et al., 1995). The rate of ketogenesis was also decreased, despite increased levels of plasma free fatty acids, probably secondary to the decreased liver function (Owen et al., 1981). When infusing a long-chain triglyceride (LCT) emulsion intravenously, fat oxidation, plasma free fatty acids, and plasma triglycerides were the same in patients with cirrhosis as in controls, whereas the increase in ketone bodies was less in the patients. This indicates that whole-body removal of exogenously administered LCT is unaltered in cirrhosis and supports the notion that hepatic ketogenesis is reduced (Müller et al., 1992).

A study of oral fat intake (Cabre et al., 2005) showed that patients with cirrhosis, as compared with healthy controls, accumulate less fat in chylomicrons and very low density lipoprotein postprandially and exhibit a more rapid rise in plasma free fatty acids. These changes were more pronounced in patients with ascites (portal hypertension). The results were interpreted as indicating that fatty acids derived from fat in food are absorbed via the portal route to a higher degree in patients with cirrhosis. Lipid oxidation saturates at a fat intake of about 1 g/kg/day and the surplus of lipids is metabolized by storage as triglyceride (Müller et al., 1992).

22.2.2.1 Practical Applications

Lipids should not be given in doses larger than 1 g/kg/day. Larger doses lead to storage as triglyceride.

22.2.3 Energy

Most studies on energy expenditure in cirrhosis found a normal mean resting energy expenditure (REE) in groups of patients, as compared with predictions of REE by standard equations, such as the Harris-Benedict equation (Müller et al., 1994a). The Harris-Benedict equation gives reliable results in groups of patients when applying actual body weight, and also in patients with ascites (Dolz et al., 1991; Müller et al.,

1994a). Measurements of REE before and after removal of several liters of ascites by paracentesis both agreed with the Harris-Benedict equation when applying the actual body weights before and after paracentesis (Dolz et al., 1991). This result suggests that ascites is not simply a volume of water, but a fluid compartment with its own energy requirements.

However, there is a larger variance in measured REE among patients with cirrhosis, as compared with healthy individuals, since more than 50% of the patients are outside the ±10% prediction range. Both hypermetabolism and hypometabolism exist (Müller et al., 1994a). In one large study of 473 patients, the average REE was found to be normal, as compared with values predicted by the Harris-Benedict equation, but 34% of the patients had an REE of > 120% of the expected value. In these hypermetabolic patients, total body potassium was lower, suggesting an association between increased REE and malnutrition, at least in some patients (Müller et al., 1999). The Harris-Benedict equation can therefore be used as a first clinical approximation, but to identify the high number of outliers, it is recommended to use indirect calorimetry.

Both exercise-induced increase in oxygen uptake (Riggio et al., 2003) and diet-induced energy expenditure (Müller et al., 1993) are within normal range in patients with cirrhosis.

REE was compared between well-nourished and malnourished cirrhotic patients, and it was observed that REE was lower in absolute terms in malnourished patients, that energy expenditure associated with physical activity was equal in the two groups, and that both groups were in energy balance (Riggio et al., 2003). Only 2 of 50 cirrhotic patients were hypermetabolic in that study. This study concluded that the state of malnutrition is not associated with a negative energy balance, confirming a similar previous study in malnourished cirrhotic patients (Nielsen et al. 1993). In both studies (Nielsen et al., 1993; Riggio et al., 2003), REE and dietary intake were decreased in proportion to body size, and both REE and dietary intake were lower than those observed in the healthy population. In addition, energy expenditure associated with physical activity, as calculated from a 24-hour activity factor, is lower in patients with cirrhosis when compared with the healthy population (Nielsen et al., 1993). Therefore, hypermetabolism may contribute to the development of malnutrition, but when the state of malnutrition is reached, it appears that a new steady state usually is reached, that is, that REE, mainly determined by lean body mass, is adequate for the new condition and that total energy expenditure is adequate for the low physical activity. The cause may be that energy intake is limited because of anorexia and the patients adapt by loss of lean body mass and decreased physical activity (see Section 22.5).

In controlled studies showing an improvement of clinical outcome, an average of about 40 kcal/kg/day was given (Kondrup and Müller, 1997). In a 6-week refeeding study involving an ordinary diet in patients with cirrhosis, a mean time averaged intake of about 40 kcal/kg/day allowed for synthesis of lean body mass and fat mass at rates similar to those of malnourished individuals without organ disease (Kondrup and Nielsen 1996; Nielsen et al., 1995). At the end of the refeeding study, energy intake was about 45 kcal/kg/day, and therefore, in a nutrition plan aiming at repletion, energy intake should be 40–50 kcal/kg/day. The enteral guideline from the ESPEN recommends an energy intake of 35–40 kcal/kg/day (Plauth et al., 2006).

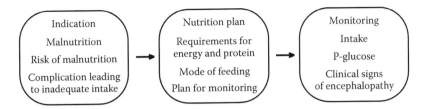

FIGURE 22.1 Structured process for nutritional support in end-stage liver disease. The structured process of nutritional support includes identifying the patients who will benefit clinically, working out a nutrition plan, and the monitoring scheme. See text for further details. (After Kondrup, J., Allison, S. P., Elia, M., Vellas, B., and Plauth, M., *Clin Nutr* 22, 415–421, 2003.)

22.2.3.1 Practical Applications

Energy requirements for maintenance of body weight in patients with cirrhosis can be estimated by the Harris-Benedict equation, allowing for physical activity, for example, by the use of a 24-hour activity factor.

In malnourished patients needing nutritional support because of inadequate intake, for example, due to intercurrent complications, 35–40 kcal/kg/day should be administered. Actual body weight including ascites is used for this calculation (Figure 22.1).

In clinically stable malnourished patients for whom the aim is repletion, 40–50 kcal/kg/day should be administered.

There are no specific guidelines for the energy distribution of the macronutrients. For the healthy population, 30 energy% fat and 55 energy% carbohydrate is recommended. With 40 kcal/kg/day, this would equal to about 1.3 g/kg fat and 5.4 g/kg carbohydrate per day, not far from the limits given above.

22.3 AMINO ACID AND PROTEIN METABOLISM

In the fasting state, the plasma amino acid composition in patients with cirrhosis is characterized by an increase in aromatic amino acids and a decrease in branched-chain amino acids (BCAAs) (Clemmesen et al., 2000; Rosen et al., 1978). Increase in aromatic amino acids may be due to a reduced hepatic capacity for their elimination, and decrease in BCAAs may reflect their increased use for removal of ammonia (Hayashi et al., 1981).

Protein requirement is increased in clinically stable patients with cirrhosis, to an average requirement of about 0.8 g/kg/day. With the customary addition of 2 standard deviations, this gives a recommended intake of about 1.2 g/kg/day (Kondrup and Nielsen, 1996; Nielsen et al., 1995; Swart et al., 1989a). Much research has been carried out to explain the increased requirement. Protein requirement can be increased due to (1) decreased absorption/increased intestinal protein loss, (2) decreased synthesis of body protein, (3) increased degradation of body protein, or (4) increased hepatic urea production with increased urinary nitrogen excretion.

Protein is generally not malabsorbed in patients with cirrhosis (Kondrup et al., 1997; Mueller et al., 1983). However, in patients given lactulose, fecal mass and nitrogen increase, probably due to bacterial proliferation, leading to apparent malabsorption (Mueller et al., 1983). Accordingly, cirrhotic patients given a high-fiber vegetable diet have an increased fecal bacterial nitrogen excretion (Weber et al., 1985). In the studies mentioned above, which demonstrated increased protein requirements, there was no increase in fecal nitrogen excretion.

Investigations with stable isotopes suggested that a single meal does not increase whole-body protein synthesis in patients with cirrhosis, as compared with the increase seen in healthy volunteers. This defect was suggested to be due to the insulin insensitivity also observed in that study (Tessari et al., 2002).

Other studies with stable isotopes indicated that there is an increased rate of endogenous protein degradation both in the fasting state (Swart et al., 1988) and in the diurnal fasting and fed states (Kondrup et al., 1997). The increase in breakdown of body protein in the latter study was associated with a rise in the level of plasma amino acids, suggesting that the primary event is increased protein breakdown, leading to increased plasma levels of amino acids and secondarily to increased urea formation and urinary nitrogen loss. The increased degradation of protein in the fasting state (Swart et al., 1988) may be due to low glycogen reserves, prompting an early switch to gluconeogenesis from amino acids derived from body protein stores (Owen et al., 1981). Preliminary data suggest that the increased protein breakdown in the diurnal fasting and fed states (Kondrup et al., 1997) may be due to a relative lack of BCAAs, for example, caused by increased consumption for removal of ammonia (Hayashi et al., 1981; Kondrup, 2000).

Taken together, these studies suggest that the increased protein requirement is attributable to both a defect in meal-induced protein synthesis due to insulin insensitivity and increased protein degradation during feeding as well as fasting due to low energy stores and altered metabolism of BCAAs.

Stable malnourished patients with cirrhosis are in nitrogen balance at a protein intake (per person) that is lower than that of the healthy population, suggesting that they have reached a steady state with decreased lean body mass with the low intake (Nielsen et al., 1995). In the 6-week refeeding study mentioned above, the mean time averaged protein intake was 1.5 g/kg/day (Nielsen et al., 1995), and at the end of the refeeding period, protein intake was 1.8 g/kg/day, and therefore, in a nutrition plan aiming at repletion, protein intake should be 1.5–1.8 g/kg/day (Table 22.2).

TABLE 22.2

Macronutrient Recommendations for Weight Maintenance or Repletion in Patients with Cirrhosis

	Maintenance	Repletion
Carbohydrate (g/kg/day)	5.0	6.0
Lipids (g/kg/day)	1.0	1.5
Protein (g/kg/day)	1.2	1.5–1.8
Energy (kcal/kg/day)	35	45

In situations when acute exacerbations further decrease the intake (e.g., due to infections, tense ascites, bleeding, or encephalopathic episodes), the possible increase in REE and further increase in protein requirement will, of course, rapidly aggravate the nutritional status.

The guidelines from ESPEN recommend a protein intake of 1.2–1.5 g/kg/day (Plauth et al., 2006).

22.3.1 PROTEIN INTOLERANCE

It was commonly believed that hepatic encephalopathy (HE) develops after excess protein intake. The frequency of protein intolerance relative to other causes of HE, such as fluid and electrolyte disturbances, or infections, has, however, never been documented in series of patients with HE. It is likely that protein intolerance does exist as rare cases at spontaneous protein intake (Horst et al., 1984), but it is a mistake to believe that protein restriction should be a routine part of the treatment (see further below). In the literature analysis mentioned above (Kondrup and Müller, 1997), there was no indication that an adequate dietary intake, including protein, aggravated existing HE.

The ESPEN guideline (Plauth et al., 2006) states that in malnourished patients who have an inadequate dietary intake and are at risk for fatal complications, low-grade HE (grades I–II) should not be considered a contraindication to nutrition support, including an adequate protein supply. This is supported by an intervention trial of tube feeding (Cordoba et al., 2004) in which malnourished encephalopathic patients in stages 1–4, median stage 2, were randomized to a gradual increase in protein intake or to an adequate protein intake, 1.2 g/kg/day, from day 1. All patients received standard therapy for HE (lactulose followed by neomycin). Outcome of HE and mortality was identical in both groups. The adequate protein group had a positive nitrogen balance from day 2, and plasma ammonia at the end of the study was similar in both groups. This study clearly shows that no harm is done when treating malnourished encephalopathic patients with adequate amounts of protein. This new approach with adequate protein feeding in HE has received considerable support (Mullen and Dasarathy, 2004; Shawcross and Jalan, 2005) and replaces earlier protein restriction and iatrogenic malnutrition in patients who, in fact, have increased protein requirements.

Nevertheless, protein intolerance may develop in a few patients during refeeding with a high protein diet (Nielsen et al., 1995). It is recommended to follow the patients closely with respect to clinical signs of HE and by simple HE tests such as number connection test or a test of continuous reaction time (Nielsen et al., 1995). If symptoms of HE appear, it is recommended to ascertain that the patient has not become obstipated, to reduce protein intake for a couple of days only, or to use a supplement with BCAAs.

22.3.2 BRANCHED CHAIN AMINO ACIDS

BCAAs are investigated as nutritional supplement to improve nutritional status and clinical outcome and/or to ameliorate HE.

For recent reviews of the nutritional effects, see Bianchi et al. (2005). A recent multicenter 1-year trial among 174 not-malnourished and not-encephalopathic cirrhotic patients (Marchesini et al., 2003) showed that BCAA reduced the rate of death, the further severe progression of liver disease, and the rate of hospital admission, as well as improved appetite rating and quality of life. Another recent study lasting for 2 years among 646 patients, included because of hypoalbuminemia and/or the presence of ascites, peripheral edema, or HE, showed that BCAA improved event-free survival (death by any cause, development of liver cancer, rupture of esophageal varices, or progress of hepatic failure) and quality of life (Muto et al., 2005). It therefore appears from recent large studies that BCAA is able to improve clinical outcome. The mechanism may be that one of the BCAAs, leucine, appears to have a special anabolic role as a coregulator of the rate of protein breakdown and, in experimental animals, also of the rate of protein synthesis (Garlick, 2005).

BCAAs have also been investigated as a treatment of HE, in order to reduce brain uptake of tryptophan (Bianchi et al., 2005). In a meta-analysis of studies using BCAA for treatment of HE, BCAA was significantly effective when all studies were included. However, when low-quality studies (unknown randomization method, unknown blinding) were excluded, only a few studies remained in the analysis, and the effect on HE was not statistically significant (Als-Nielsen et al., 2003).

One of the first studies to use BCAA was carried out in patients who were protein-intolerant, that is, tolerating less than 40 g of protein. They were randomized to increase their protein intake to 70 g, either in the form of casein or with a BCAA supplement (Horst et al., 1984). When HE worsened, it was considered a treatment failure and the patient was withdrawn from the study. Seven out of 12 patients in the casein group experienced worsening HE, but only 1 out of 14 in the BCAA group had worsening HE. This study combines the two potential uses of BCAA: (1) as nutritional treatment and (2) as prevention of HE in malnourished patients who cannot be refed because of protein intolerance.

22.3.3 PRACTICAL APPLICATIONS

It is recommended to administer 1.2 g/kg protein per day to patients with cirrhosis because of their increased protein requirements. Actual body weight including ascites is used for this calculation. With 40 kcal/kg/day, this will equal 12 energy%, not far from the level of intake in the healthy population. The development of HE in rare cases should be discovered by clinical observation and/or an objective measurement such as a test of continuous reaction time. In protein-intolerant patients, it is recommended to give a supplement of BCAA. The use of BCAA as an anabolic agent is gaining support from recent controlled intervention trials.

22.4 VITAMINS AND MINERALS

Patients with liver cirrhosis often have low plasma levels of vitamins and minerals, but the specific functional or clinical implications of these abnormalities are not known in detail. Thiamine deficiency is known to be common in alcoholic cirrhosis and found equally frequently in hepatitis C virus–related cirrhosis (Levy et al., 2002).

It was therefore recommended that all patients with cirrhosis should receive thiamine. Deficiency of fat-soluble vitamins is observed in patients with steatorrhea due to cholestasis and bile salt deficiency, and in alcohol abusers (Plauth et al., 1997).

Magnesium depletion is common in end-stage liver disease (Koivisto et al., 2002). Zinc deficiency is also common and seems to be caused by decreased absorption as well as a diuretic-induced increase in urinary excretion (Yoshida et al., 2001). Supplementation with zinc improves glucose tolerance (Marchesini et al., 1998).

22.4.1 PRACTICAL APPLICATIONS

To cover any possible deficiency it is advised to prescribe a standard vitamin/mineral tablet (Plauth et al., 1997).

22.5 ANOREXIA

Many studies have shown that patients with cirrhosis have a low dietary intake and also that the low dietary intake is associated with impaired clinical outcome (Campillo et al., 2003). Liver disease may impair food intake, for example, by reduced clearance of satiation mediators such as cholecystokinin or by splanchnic production of cytokines, which impair hypothalamic appetite stimulation (Davidson et al., 1999). In addition, the mechanical effect of ascites and intestinal edema may play a role.

As mentioned above, the dietary intake of malnourished patients with cirrhosis matches their energy expenditure and protein requirements (Nielsen et al., 1993; Riggio et al., 2003), that is, they do not show spontaneous compensatory excess intake to ensure weight gain. Young healthy individuals increase their intake in excess of their expenditure after an experimental weight loss, resulting in weight gain (Roberts et al., 1994), whereas elderly did not increase their intake and did not regain weight. The biochemical basis of this abnormality in the elderly may be inadequate secretion of ghrelin (Schneider et al., 2008). In malnourished patients with cirrhosis, there is an increased level of ghrelin, but perhaps not sufficient to increase food intake enough to ensure weight gain (Kalaitzakis et al., 2007). Few studies have tested ways of improving appetite and intake. A supplement with BCAA did improve appetite ratings in patients with cirrhosis (Marchesini et al., 2003).

22.6 MEAL PATTERN

After an overnight fast, splanchnic metabolism in patients with cirrhosis was similar to that in healthy volunteers after a 3-day fast. In particular, gluconeogenesis from peripherally derived amino acids was substantially increased (Owen et al., 1981). Nitrogen balance can be improved by splitting the daily protein intake between four and six meals rather than the usual three meals (Swart et al., 1989b) or by administering a late evening oral dose of glucose (Zillikens et al., 1993).

22.6.1 PRACTICAL APPLICATIONS

It is important to reduce the length of the evening and nighttime periods of starvation in patients with cirrhosis.

22.7   SUMMARY POINTS

- Patients with cirrhosis often exhibit inadequate dietary intake.
- Controlled trials show improved clinical outcome, including increased survival, with nutritional support.
- In malnourished patients needing nutritional support because of inadequate intake, for example, due to intercurrent complications, 35–40 kcal/kg/day should be administered.
- In clinically stable malnourished patients for whom the aim is repletion, 40–50 kcal/kg/day should be administered.
- Because of insulin insensitivity, glucose should not be given in doses larger than 5–6 g glucose/kg/day.
- Because of increased protein requirements, protein should be given in doses of 1.2–1.8 g/kg protein per day.
- Actual body weight including ascites is used for these calculations.
- The development of HE in rare cases should be discovered by clinical observation and/or an objective measurement such as a test of continuous reaction time.
- A standard vitamin/mineral tablet should be prescribed.
- The length of starvation during the evening and nighttime should be reduced in patients with cirrhosis.

REFERENCES

Als-Nielsen, B., R. L. Koretz, L. L. Kjaergard, and C. Gluud. 2003. Branched-chain amino acids for hepatic encephalopathy. *Cochrane Database Syst Rev* CD001939.

Bianchi, G., R. Marzocchi, F. Agostini, and G. Marchesini. 2005. Update on branched-chain amino acid supplementation in liver diseases. *Curr Opin Gastroenterol* 21:197–200.

Cabre, E., J. M. Hernandez-Perez, L. Fluvia, C. Pastor, A. Corominas, and M. A. Gassull. 2005. Absorption and transport of dietary long-chain fatty acids in cirrhosis: A stable-isotope-tracing study. *Am J Clin Nutr* 81:692–701.

Campillo, B., P. Bories, M. Leluan, B. Pornin, M. Devanlay, and P. Fouet. 1995. Short-term changes in energy metabolism after 1 month of a regular oral diet in severely malnourished cirrhotic patients. *Metabolism* 44:765–770.

Campillo, B., J. P. Richardet, E. Scherman, and P. N. Bories. 2003. Evaluation of nutritional practice in hospitalized cirrhotic patients: Results of a prospective study. *Nutrition* 19:515–521.

Clemmesen, J. O., J. Kondrup, and P. Ott. 2000. Splanchnic and leg exchange of amino acids and ammonia in acute liver failure. *Gastroenterology* 118:1131–1139.

Cordoba, J., J. Lopez-Hellin, M. Planas, P. Sabin, F. Sanpedro, F. Castro, R. Esteban, and J. Guardia. 2004. Normal protein diet for episodic hepatic encephalopathy: Results of a randomized study. *J Hepatol* 41:38–43.

Davidson, H. I., R. Richardson, D. Sutherland, and O. J. Garden. 1999. Macronutrient preference, dietary intake, and substrate oxidation among stable cirrhotic patients. *Hepatology* 29:1380–1386.

Dolz, C., J. Raurich, J. Ibanez, A. Obrador, P. Marsè, and J. Gayà. 1991 Ascites increases the resting energy expenditure in liver cirrhosis. *Gastroenterology* 100:738–744.

Garlick, P. J. 2005. The role of leucine in the regulation of protein metabolism. *J Nutr* 135:1553S–1556S.

Gentile, S., C. Loguercio, R. Marmo, L. Carbone, and C. Del Vecchio Blanco. 1993. Incidence of altered glucose tolerance in liver cirrhosis. *Diabetes Res Clin Pract* 22:37–44.

Hayashi, M., H. Ohnishi, Y. Kawade, Y. Muto, and Y. Takahashi. 1981. Augmented utilization of branched-chain amino acids by skeletal muscle in decompensated liver cirrhosis in special relation to ammonia detoxication. *Gastroenterol Jpn* 16:64–70.

Horst, D., N. D. Grace, H. O. Conn, E. Schiff, S. Schenker, A. Viteri, D. Law, and C. E. Atterbury. 1984. Comparison of dietary protein with an oral, branched chain-enriched amino acid supplement in chronic portal-systemic encephalopathy: A randomized controlled trial. *Hepatology* 4:279–287.

Kalaitzakis, E., I. Bosaeus, L. Ohman, and E. Bjornsson. 2007. Altered postprandial glucose, insulin, leptin, and ghrelin in liver cirrhosis: Correlations with energy intake and resting energy expenditure. *Am J Clin Nutr* 85:808–815.

Kestell, M. F., and S. Lee. 1993 Clinical nutrition in acute and chronic liver disease. *Sem Gastrointest Dis* 4:116–126.

Koivisto, M., P. Valta, K. Hockerstedt, and L. Lindgren. 2002. Magnesium depletion in chronic terminal liver cirrhosis. *Clin Transplant* 16:325–328.

Kondrup, J. 2000. Metabolic basis of increased protein requirement in patients with liver cirrhosis (abstract). *Clin Nutr* 19:40.

Kondrup, J., S. P. Allison, M. Elia, B. Vellas, and M. Plauth. 2003. ESPEN Guidelines for Nutrition Screening 2002. *Clin Nutr* 22:415–421.

Kondrup, J., and M. J. Müller. 1997. Energy and protein requirements of patients with chronic liver disease. *J Hepatol* 27:239–247.

Kondrup, J., and K. Nielsen. 1996. Protein requirement and protein utilization in patients with liver cirrhosis. *Z Gastroenterol* 34:26–31.

Kondrup, J., K. Nielsen, and A. Juul. 1997. Effect of long-term refeeding on protein metabolism in patients with cirrhosis of the liver. *Br J Nutr* 77:197–212.

Kruszynska, Y. T., A. Meyer-Alber, F. Darakhshan, P. D. Home, and N. McIntyre. 1993. Metabolic handling of orally administered glucose in cirrhosis. *J Clin Invest* 91: 1057–1066.

Lecube, A., C. Hernandez, J. Genesca, J. I. Esteban, R. Jardi, and R. Simo. 2004. High prevalence of glucose abnormalities in patients with hepatitis C virus infection: A multivariate analysis considering the liver injury. *Diabetes Care* 27:1171–1175.

Levy, S., C. Herve, E. Delacoux, and S. Erlinger. 2002. Thiamine deficiency in hepatitis C virus and alcohol-related liver diseases. *Dig Dis Sci* 47:543–548.

Marchesini, G., G. Bianchi, M. Merli, P. Amodio, C. Panella, C. Loguercio, F. Rossi Fanelli, R. Abbiati, and Italian BCAA Study Group. 2003. Nutritional supplementation with branched-chain amino acids in advanced cirrhosis: A double-blind, randomized trial. *Gastroenterology* 124:1792–1801.

Marchesini, G., E. Bugianesi, M. Ronchi, R. Flamia, K. Thomaseth, and G. Pacini. 1998. Zinc supplementation improves glucose disposal in patients with cirrhosis. *Metabolism* 47:792–798.

Marchesini, G., A. Melli, G. A. Checchia, L. Mattioli, M. Capelli, S. Cassarani, M. Zoli, and E. Pisi. 1985. Pancreatic beta-cell function in cirrhotic patients with and without overt diabetes. C-peptide response to glucagon and to meal. *Metabolism* 34:695–701.

Mueller, K. J., L. O. Crosby, J. L. Oberlander, and J. L. Mullen. 1983. Estimation of fecal nitrogen in patients with liver disease. *J Parenter Enteral Nutr* 7:266–269.

Mullen, K. D., and S. Dasarathy. 2004. Protein restriction in hepatic encephalopathy: Necessary evil or illogical dogma? *J Hepatol* 41:147–148.

Müller, M., J. Böttcher, and O. Selberg. 1993 Energy expenditure and substrate metabolism in liver cirrhosis. *Int J Obes Relat Metab Disord* 17:S102–S106.

Müller, M. J., K. H. W. Böker, and O. Selberg. 1994a. Review: Are patients with liver cirrhosis hypermetabolic? *Clin Nutr* 13:131–144.

Müller, M. J., J. Böttcher, O. Selberg, S. Weselmann, K. H. Böker, M. Schwarze, A. von zur Mühlen, and M. P. Manns. 1999. Hypermetabolism in clinically stable patients with liver cirrhosis. *Am J Clin Nutr* 69:1194–1201.

Müller, M. J., M. Pirlich, H. J. Balks, and O. Selberg. 1994b. Glucose intolerance in liver cirrhosis: Role of hepatic and non-hepatic influences. *Eur J Clin Chem Clin Biochem* 32:749–758.

Müller, M. J., A. Rieger, O. Willmann, H. U. Lautz, H. J. Balks, A. Von Zur Muhlen, H. Canzler, and F. W. Schmidt. 1992. Metabolic responses to lipid infusions in patients with liver cirrhosis. *Clin Nutr* 11:193–206.

Muto, Y., S. Sato, A. Watanabe, H. Moriwaki, K. Suzuki, A. Kato, M. Kato, T. Nakamura, K. Higuchi, S. Nishiguchi, and H. Kumada. 2005. Effects of oral branched-chain amino acid granules on event-free survival in patients with liver cirrhosis. *Clin Gastroenterol Hepatol* 3:705–713.

Nielsen, K., J. Kondrup, L. Martinsen, H. Dossing, B. Larsson, B. Stilling, and M. G. Jensen. 1995. Long-term oral refeeding of patients with cirrhosis of the liver. *Br J Nutr* 74:557–567.

Nielsen, K., J. Kondrup, L. Martinsen, B. Stilling, and B. Wikman. 1993. Nutritional assessment and adequacy of dietary intake in hospitalized patients with alcoholic liver cirrhosis. *Br J Nutr* 69:665–679.

Nishida, T., S. Tsuji, M. Tsujii, S. Arimitsu, Y. Haruna, E. Imano, M. Suzuki, T. Kanda, S. Kawano, N. Hiramatsu, N. Hayashi, and M. Hori. 2006. Oral glucose tolerance test predicts prognosis of patients with liver cirrhosis. *Am J Gastroenterol* 101:70–75.

Owen, O. E., F. A. Reichle, M. A. Mozzoli, T. Kreulen, M. S. Patel, I. B. Elfenbein, M. Golsorkhi, K. H. Chang, N. S. Rao, H. S. Sue, and G. Boden. 1981. Hepatic, gut, and renal substrate flux rates in patients with hepatic cirrhosis. *J Clin Invest* 68:240–252.

Petrides, A. S., C. Vogt, D. Schulze Berge, D. Matthews, and G. Strohmeyer. 1994. Pathogenesis of glucose intolerance and diabetes mellitus in cirrhosis. *Hepatology* 19:616–627.

Plauth, M., E. Cabre, O. Riggio, M. Assis-Camilo, M. Pirlich, J. Kondrup, P. Ferenci, E. Holm, S. Vom Dahl, M. J. Muller, and W. Nolte. 2006. ESPEN Guidelines on Enteral Nutrition: Liver disease. *Clin Nutr* 25:285–294.

Plauth, M., M. Merli, J. Kondrup, A. Weimann, P. Ferenci, and M. J. Muller. 1997. ESPEN guidelines for nutrition in liver disease and transplantation. *Clin Nutr* 16:43–55.

Proietto, J., F. P. Alford, and F. J. Dudley. 1980. The mechanism of the carbohydrate intolerance of cirrhosis. *J Clin Endocrinol Metab* 51:1030–1036.

Riggio, O., S. Angeloni, L. Ciuffa, G. Nicolini, A. F. Attili, C. Albanese, and M. Merli. 2003. Malnutrition is not related to alterations in energy balance in patients with stable liver cirrhosis. *Clin Nutr* 22:553–559.

Roberts, S. B., P. Fuss, M. B. Heyman, W. J. Evans, R. Tsay, H. Rasmussen, M. Fiatarone, J. Cortiella, G. E. Dallal, and V. R. Young. 1994. Control of food intake in older men. *JAMA* 272:1601–1606.

Rosen, H. M., P. B. Soeters, J. H. James, J. Hodgman, and J. Fisher. 1978. Influences of exogenous intake and nitrogen balance on plasma and brain aromatic amino acid concentration. *Metabolism* 27:393–404.

Schneider, S. M., R. Al-Jaouni, C. Caruba, J. Giudicelli, K. Arab, F. Suavet, P. Ferrari, I. Mothe-Satney, E. Van Obberghen, and X. Hebuterne. 2008. Effects of age, malnutrition and refeeding on the expression and secretion of ghrelin. *Clin Nutr* 27:724–731.

Selberg, O., W. Burchert, J. v.d. Hoff, G. J. Meyer, H. Hundeshagen, E. Radoch, H. J. Balks, and M. J. Muller. 1993. Insulin resistance in liver cirrhosis. Positron-emission tomography scan analysis of skeletal muscle glucose metabolism. *J Clin Invest* 91:1897–1902.

Shawcross, D., and R. Jalan. 2005. Dispelling myths in the treatment of hepatic encephalopathy. *Lancet* 365:431–433.

Swart, G. R., J. W. O. van den Berg, J. K. van Vuure, T. Tietveld, D. L. Wattimena, and M. Frenkel. 1989a. Minimum protein requirements in liver cirrhosis determined by nitrogen balance measurements at three levels of protein intake. *Clin Nutr* 8:329–336.

Swart, G. R., J. W. O. van den Berg, J. L. D. Wattimena, T. Rietveld, J. K. Van Vuure, and M. Frenkel. 1988. Elevated protein requirement in cirrhosis of the liver investigated by whole body protein turnover studies. *Clin Sci* 75:101–107.

Swart, G. R., M. C. Zillikens, J. K. van Vuure, and J. W. van den Berg. 1989b. Effect of a late evening meal on nitrogen balance in patients with cirrhosis of the liver. *Br Med J* 299:1202–1203.

Tessari, P., R. Barazzoni, E. Kiwanuka, G. Davanzo, G. De Pergola, R. Orlando, M. Vettore, and M. Zanetti. 2002. Impairment of albumin and whole body postprandial protein synthesis in compensated liver cirrhosis. *Am J Physiol Endocrinol Metab* 282:E304–E311.

Weber, F. L., Jr., D. Minco, K. M. Fresard, and J. G. Banwell. 1985. Effects of vegetable diets on nitrogen metabolism in cirrhotic subjects. *Gastroenterology* 89:538–544.

Yoshida, Y., T. Higashi, K. Nouso, H. Nakatsukasa, S. I. Nakamura, A. Watanabe, and T. Tsuji. 2001. Effects of zinc deficiency/zinc supplementation on ammonia metabolism in patients with decompensated liver cirrhosis. *Acta Med Okayama* 55:349–355.

Zillikens, M. C., J. W. van den Berg, J. L. Wattimena, T. Rietveld, and G. R. Swart. 1993. Nocturnal oral glucose supplementation. The effects on protein metabolism in cirrhotic patients and in healthy controls. *J Hepatol* 17:377–383.

23 Nutrition in Adult Liver Transplantation

Teodoro Grau and Juan Carlos Montejo

CONTENTS

23.1 INTRODUCTION

Orthotopic liver transplantation (OLT) is a life-saving procedure for selected patients with end-stage liver disease (ESLD) and acute failure. In Spain, 8269 patients underwent OLT in the period 2000–2007, more than 700 of them in our unit. The main indications for OLT were cirrhosis of any etiology (59%), hepatic neoplasm (21%), chronic rejection in previous OLT (6%), and fulminant hepatic failure (3%) (Figure 23.1) [1]. The nutritional and metabolic derangements of candidates to OLT occurred before the surgical procedure, and malnutrition is common in patients with advanced liver disease. As far as the disease progresses, protein and caloric malnutrition is an established feature that increases the postoperative morbidity of these patients [2,3]. The interval between listing and transplantation, usually many months, provides a therapeutic window to institute nutritional management before the surgical procedure. Once it is performed, the liver transplantation recipient has a metabolic stress response similar to other major surgical procedures. The risk of nosocomial

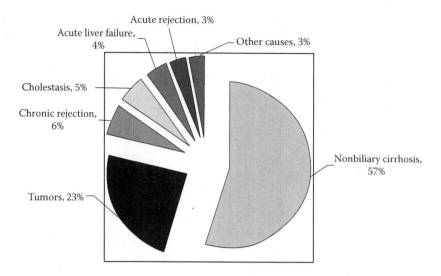

FIGURE 23.1 Primary diagnosis of patients waiting for orthotopic liver transplantation (OLT) in Spain, 2007. The main indication for OLT was cirrhosis and the next one was tumors. Note that rejection was the third reason for transplantation.

infections related to immunosuppression or the secondary effects of these drugs enhance the need for establishing a nutritional program after transplantation. We can distinguish three different periods: (1) pretransplantation nutrition assessment and nutritional intervention; (2) acute postsurgical situation, where nutritional support is needed; and (3) follow-up period after recovery from the procedure when nutritional counseling and prevention of complications relating to immunosuppression are the recommended mode of the nutritional support.

23.2 NUTRITIONAL ASSESSMENT AND INTERVENTION IN PATIENTS ELIGIBLE FOR LIVER TRANSPLANTATION

Protein energy malnutrition (PEM) is common in patients with ESLD and is highly prevalent in all forms of chronic liver disease, regardless of etiology, and increases the risk of death. Malnutrition correlates with the degree of liver dysfunction and the etiology of the disease. The incidence of malnutrition is higher in patients with alcoholic liver disease compared with those with nonalcoholic cirrhosis, and patients with acute liver failure have better nutritional status than patients with ESLD [4]. Between 20% and 50% of patients undergoing liver transplantation have moderate degrees of malnutrition, and 3–25% of them show severe malnutrition, depending on the different selection criteria for transplantation [5]. Patients with cirrhosis who are malnourished have higher rates of encephalopathy, infection, variceal bleeding or refractory ascites, and death [6]. Indeed, malnutrition has significant implications for liver transplantation because it has been shown that patients with poor nutritional status before transplantation have increased complications postoperatively, particularly infections and variceal bleeding, shorter graft survival, and higher mortality rates [7].

In patients with advanced liver disease, major causes of malnutrition include anorexia, disease-related complications, and main nutrient-related metabolic changes (Table 23.1). The primary etiology of malnutrition in ESLD is poor oral intake due to different factors. Dietary restrictions are commonly recommended to these patients, and oral intake is discouraged. Mechanical compression secondary to massive ascites promotes early satiety, and frequently, these patients show high levels of leptin and proinflammatory cytokines that have an anorexic effect [8]. Moreover, the presence of low grades of encephalopathy, muscular weakness, and fatigue discourage oral intake. Patients with cholestatic disease usually present more caloric depletion and deficiency in fat-soluble vitamins secondary to malabsorption. Other metabolic disturbances can contribute to malnutrition in patients with ESLD. These patients show metabolic derangements including increased energy expenditure, insulin resistance, and low respiratory quotient, indicating reduced glucose and increased lipid oxidation that may also contribute to nutritional depletion in the early stages of the disease [9].

TABLE 23.1
Etiology of Malnutrition in Patients Waiting for Orthotopic Liver Transplantation

Decreased oral intake
   Dietary restrictions
   Mechanical compression secondary to ascites
   Encephalopathy
   Upper gastrointestinal bleeding
   Muscular weakness and fatigue
Metabolic derangements
   Increased energy expenditure
   Decreased protein synthesis
   Insulin resistance
   Increased lipid oxidation
Malabsortion
   Cholestasis
   Portal hypertension enteropathy
   Pancreatic insufficiency
Drugs
   Steroids
   Lactulose
   Neomycin
Recurrent infections

Note: Key factors involved in the development of malnutrition in patients with end-stage liver disease. Recurrent infections increase the risk of malnutrition because patients increase their metabolism rate and can decrease caloric intake.

Up to 30% of these patients develop overt diabetes mellitus and insulin resistance and become catabolic during overnight fasting, and exacerbated muscle catabolism is also observed [10]. Lipid metabolism alters if malabsorption occurs and the liver functions deteriorate. Moreover, essential fatty acids deficiency has been associated with severity of the liver disease and malnutrition [11]. Increased protein catabolism is a hallmark in these patients and, as far as the disease progresses, protein deficiency worsens. There is an imbalance between branched-chain amino acids (BCAAs) and aromatic amino acids, which is difficult to control at the final stages of the disease without protein restriction, but with an increased risk of protein malnutrition.

23.2.1 NUTRITIONAL ASSESSMENT

The presence of malnutrition in cirrhosis is obvious in patients with an advanced stage of the disease who are markedly cachectic. However, because PEM may occur early in the course of the disease, the diagnosis of malnutrition should be established by a combination of different methods: medical history, anthropometric measurements, biochemical parameters, and body composition. Unfortunately, most of the clinical parameters used are modified by the disease itself and there is no gold standard for the nutritional assessment of patients with ESLD [12]. However, such technical limitations do not justify the omission of nutritional assessment in patients eligible for liver transplantation. Following the recommendations of the European Society for Clinical Nutrition and Metabolism's (ESPEN) Guidelines for Nutrition Screening, it is our practice to perform nutritional screening tests for the initial assessment of a patient's nutritional status, even when they are not specifically indicated for advanced chronic liver disease [13]. Subjective global assessment (SGA) combines different parameters such as weight loss, changes in dietary intake, and changes in the physical examination, and is easy to perform [14]. Moreover, when it is used in combination with other anthropometric measures, SGA has a reasonable specificity and is a reliable tool in evaluating the nutritional status of liver transplantation patients [15]. The use of anthropometric measurements such as body weight, triceps skin-fold thickness, and mid-arm muscle circumference in patients has been discouraging because most patients with edema ascites have rendered these tests unreliable. Most useful is the assessment of muscle function using the handgrip strength and respiratory muscle strength taken serially. Handgrip strength is highly sensitive and can overestimate the degree of malnutrition but is a good predictor of complications in ESLD patients before transplantation and seems to be better than SGA in assessing the outcome of patients with cirrhosis [16]. Other study has shown that the combined criteria of handgrip strength of less than 30 kg and mid-arm muscle circumference of less than 23 cm have a sensitivity of 94% and a negative predictive value of 97% in identifying patients with depleted body cell mass [7].

Most of the laboratory tests used for nutritional assessment are commonly altered in patients with ESLD. Anemia, hypoalbuminemia, high bilirubin, low lymphocyte count, thrombocytopenia, or prolonged prothrombin time is more of an indication of the severity of the liver disease rather than the degree of malnutrition. In any case, iron, zinc, and vitamin deficiency should be ruled out. Most interesting is the assessment of body mass composition (BMC) to estimate the nutritional status.

Dual-energy x-ray absorptiometry provides an accurate measurement of total body bone mineral, fat, and fat-free soft tissue mass. Although use of this method has been reported in some patients with cirrhosis, usually used in combination with other methods, its accuracy in patients with water and salt imbalance remains to be established [7]. Bioelectrical impedance analysis is another method to estimate BMC. It measures the difference between the electrical conduction through fat tissue and water. The accuracy of a bioimpedance analysis depends on the applicability of the regression equation relating current resistance through the body to body composition parameters and can be inaccurate when patients retain water, particularly ascites. Despite this, some groups advocate its usefulness in the assessment of patients with advanced liver disease [18].

23.2.2 PRETRANSPLANT NUTRITIONAL SUPPORT

Patients manifesting malnutrition at the time when they are to be included in the transplantation list and patients at risk should receive a nutritional intervention. The aim of nutritional support is to preserve lean body mass, immune function, and liver metabolism; prevent further nutritional depletion; and improve outcome after OLT. First, patients well nourished or with mild degree of malnutrition must receive nutritional counseling alone or in combination with oral nutritional supplements if they are unable to achieve their energy requirements. Caloric restriction is not indicated unless the patient is stable and suffers from obesity due to inactivity and continued oral intake. Stable patients should have normal protein intake in the range 1.2–1.5 g/kg/day. Until recently, it remained unclear whether a formula enriched in BCAAs is superior to a standard whole protein formula; even in patients with a mild degree of encephalopathy, long-term nutritional supplementation with oral BCAA granulate as oral supplement seems to be useful in slowing down the progression of hepatic failure and prolonging event-free survival [19–20]. In addition, vitamins and other supplements should be administered to patients waiting for OLT.

The decision to start specialized nutritional support is based on clinical judgment and objective nutritional parameters. Patients with moderate to severe malnutrition, as assessed by the SGA method, and unable to achieve their caloric requirements should receive artificial nutrition immediately. The primary endpoint of nutritional support in these patients is to improve protein-caloric malnutrition and correct nutritional deficiencies. Nevertheless, OLT should not be delayed to allow additional nutritional replacement. Energy requirements in these patients considerably vary according their clinical status and the method of assessment.

The ESPEN guidelines recommend 35–40 kcal/kg/day for patients with liver cirrhosis [21], but it seems to be excessive when compared with measurements performed with indirect calorimetry studies or estimates of resting energy expenditure using the Harris-Benedict equation. Our approach is to give no more than 20–25 kcal/kg/day to avoid overfeeding and complications relating to hyperglycemia such as infectious complications. Providing substrates significantly exceeding the energy expenditure with the goal of achieving an unattainable anabolic state will be more harmful than beneficial. Protein requirements are in the range of 1–1.5 g/kg/day based on different guidelines [22]. In addition, patients with a mild degree of encephalopathy can tolerate up to 1.2 g/kg/day without any significant deterioration, and protein restrictions do not affect the outcome [23]. Patients with ESLD have diminished glycogen stores and are at risk for developing hypoglycemia, and they usually have an exacerbated lipid oxidation; we recommend that the 60–70% of nonprotein calories should be given as carbohydrates.

Artificial nutrition should be started when oral intake, with or without supplements, is suboptimal. The enteral route is the preferred choice because it is more physiological and cost-effective and the risk of infectious complications is lower. Soft feeding tubes are usually well tolerated, easy to place, and do not increase the risk of bleeding in the presence of esophageal varices. If the patient cannot tolerate gastric feeding, the tube can be placed in the jejunum, but the use of a percutaneous gastrostomy or jejunostomy is not recommended because there is an increased risk of ascites leakage and peritonitis. Total parenteral nutrition (TPN) should be used only when enteral nutrition fails or if the patient has gastrointestinal dysfunction. The clinician should be aware of the infectious complications as well as fluid and electrolyte shifts when using TPN in these patients. We use TPN only in selected cases when ESLD is complicated with spontaneous peritonitis or severe encephalopathy or when enteral nutrition is not tolerated (Table 23.2).

Unfortunately, most of the recommendations regarding nutritional support among liver transplant candidates are based on expert suggestions rather than prospective, randomized clinical trials. Patients with acute liver failure as well as other critically ill individuals need nutritional support. In patients with ESLD, available studies suggest an improvement of nutritional variables and a trend of decreased mortality; however, sample sizes of most of these studies are small. Furthermore, most of the studies have been conducted in patients with ESLD, particularly in patients with alcoholic cirrhosis, and may not accurately represent the typical patient waiting for a liver transplant. The only randomized trial that addressed this question in this group

---

TABLE 23.2
Recommendations for Pretransplant Nutritional Support

Nutrients	Recommendations
Energy requirements	$1.0-1.2 \times REE$ 20–25 kcal/kg/day
Proteins	1–1.5 g/kg/day Consider the use of BCAAs
Carbohydrates/fat ratio	60:40
Vitamins	Consider additional supplements if with alcohol addiction, malabsorption, or drugs
Other metabolic issues	Correct phosphorus, copper, and manganese deficiencies

Note: Nutritional protocol recommended for patients waiting for orthotopic liver transplant that are malnourished. REE, resting energy expenditure; BCAAs, branched-chain amino acids.

of patients did not show any prognostic benefit after the transplantation, probably because the sample size was too small to detect significant differences [24].

23.3 NUTRITIONAL SUPPORT AFTER LIVER TRANSPLANTATION

Liver transplantation is a major surgical procedure usually performed in patients with poor nutritional status before transplant who will receive high dose of steroids and immunosuppressive drugs. Although this procedure allows resolution of some of the metabolic derangements of patients with ESLD, nutritional support and monitoring should be maintained for a long period. Surgical stress is the cornerstone of metabolic derangements in the first days after transplantation but is rapidly modified by the effect of immunosuppressive drugs. Another misunderstood factor is the metabolic and nutritional status of the donor liver. Once the patient reassumes oral intake, the nutritional team should be aware of the nutritional derangements secondary to the immunosuppressive drugs, and the aim is the prevention of several metabolic complications.

23.3.1 EARLY NUTRITIONAL SUPPORT AFTER LIVER TRANSPLANTATION

Most of the recommendations regarding nutritional support after liver transplantation are extrapolated from studies conducted on surgical patients, and reports stemming from the experience are few. For undernourished patients, or if it is anticipated that oral intake will be inadequate for more than 7 days, artificial nutrition should be given. Most patients undergoing a liver transplant can reassume oral intake in the first 5 days after surgery, and nutritional support should be provided only to malnourished patients with complications or delayed oral intake after organ transplant [25].

23.3.1.1 Acute Energy and Nutritional Requirements after Liver Transplant

Usually, patients are not hypermetabolic unless sepsis develops, and resting energy expenditure measured by indirect calorimetry varies from 20% to 30% more than the predicted value. Hence, in our practice, we provide 30–35 kcal/kg/day, in agreement with other recommendations [25]. Protein requirements are affected by surgical stress, surgical losses, use of steroids, and previous nutritional status. Untreated patients can show nitrogen urinary losses higher than 200 g in the first week after transplantation. For these patients, 1.5–2 g/kg/day is the usual amount of delivered proteins to avoid exaggerated catabolism. The new liver should be able to manage the increased plasmatic pool of amino acids for gluconeogenesis and acute phase proteins synthesis, and protein metabolism is closely linked to an adequate hepatic function. If graft failure occurs, amino acid metabolism is impaired and nutritional support fails to improve protein catabolism. Furthermore, peripheral oxidation of aromatic amino acids promotes the development of encephalopathy. Graft function can be assessed using sophisticated methods such as branched-chain/aromatic amino acid ratio in plasma, but in clinical practice, liver function is assessed using conventional tests such as hepatic enzymes and coagulation tests. A mixture of carbohydrates and fat should be used to provide energy in a ratio of 70:30 of the nonprotein calories. A limiting factor for the use of glucose is the hyperglycemia secondary

TABLE 23.3

Recommendations of Nutritional Support after Liver Transplantation

Intervention	Recommendations
Time and route of feeding	Artificial nutrition should start in the first 24 hours
	Use the enteral route through nasojejunal tube
	Start oral feedings as soon as possible
	Limit the use of TPN
Energy requirements	1.3–1.5 × REE
	25–30 kcal/kg/day
Proteins	1.2–1.5 g/kg/day
	Consider the use of arginine and other pharmaconutrients
Carbohydrates/fat ratio	60:40 to 50:50
	Tight glycemic control
Vitamin and electrolytes	Standard amounts of vitamins
	Consider fluid restriction

Note: Nutritional protocol recommended for all patients receiving an orthotopic liver transplant. TPN, total parenteral nutrition; REE, resting energy expenditure.

to the use of steroids that may necessitate increasing the amount of fat up to 50% of the caloric intake (Table 23.3).

23.3.1.2 The Donor Liver

There are no specific recommendations published with regard to optimal organ donor nutritional support. To avoid preservation and reperfusion injury as much as possible, the donor should maintain normothermia, cardiac function, and pulmonary gas exchange. Nutritional status of the donor also seems to influence the degree of liver dysfunction and primary failure of the graft [26]. Livers obtained from patients with prolonged intensive care unit (ICU) length of stay deteriorated more frequently as compared with patients with shorter stay. Depletion of nucleotides and glycogen stores seems to be one of the main reasons, and it has been confirmed by studies that show lesser reperfusion injury when glucose and insulin were infused in the portal vein of donor's liver during organ preservation [27]. Another issue is the presence of some degree of hepatic steatosis in the donor liver. Usually, livers with more than 30% of steatosis are rejected, but grafts with some degree of fat infiltration are prone to develop graft failure more frequently. There are no specific interventions to treat donors to avoid these phenomena, and there is no standard protocol to nourish donors before organ harvest.

23.3.1.3 Nutritional Support after Liver Transplant

Most patients reassume oral diet in the first 5 days after the procedure. Patients are extubated in the first 24 hours and proceed to liquid diets within a day or two. The primary goal of nutritional support in this period is to give adequate substrates to promote recovery from surgical stress and correct nutritional deficiencies. The use of TPN has been restricted because of the higher risk of infection and is used only when enteral nutrition is impossible. TPN was used initially when it was demonstrated to be better than conventional fluid repletion in terms of nitrogen balance, duration of mechanical ventilation, and ICU length of stay. Nevertheless, enteral nutrition is the method of choice to feed these patients. It has been demonstrated that enteral nutrition is well tolerated and has similar nutritional effect to TPN [28]. Enteral nutrition given early after the procedure decreases length of stay and reduces the number of viral infections when compared with conventional fluid therapy [29]. A European survey has shown that most centers use early enteral nutrition in the first hours after the procedure [30]. Nasojejunal tubes or jejunostomies are the preferred route to administer feeding whose only limitation is the type of surgery. The surgeon can place nasojejunal tubes or surgical tubes to overcome the stomach before finishing the surgical procedure. This approach is useful because gastric palsy is the main reason of tube feeding intolerance. Biliary anastomosis on a Roux-en-Y jejunal loop makes this approach difficult and could delay the use of enteral nutrition for several days. Recent reports have extensively reviewed the use of enteral nutrition in liver transplant, and there is no doubt about its efficacy and superiority over TPN [25]. The latter should be used in patients with a very complicated course that do not tolerate enteral feeding. Our practice is to place a nasojejunal tube intraoperatively and to start with feedings when the patient is rewarmed and hemodynamically stable, usually in the first 12 hours after the procedure. We use full-strength polymeric iso-osmolal diets starting at 25 mL/h, and infusion rate is increased in the next 24–48 hours until the caloric goal is achieved. Once the patient is extubated, liquid supplements and oral diet are initiated and enteral nutrition is maintained until the patients reassume more than 50% of the caloric requirements by the oral route. We use TPN when enteral nutrition is not feasible, following the recommendations published elsewhere for patients who underwent major surgical procedures [31,32]. We avoid the simultaneous use of TPN and enteral nutrition to avoid overfeeding. It is our practice to start TPN early, in the first 24 hours, with 20 kcal/kg/day and 1 g/kg/day of proteins, and increase the infused volume daily until energy requirements are achieved in 3–5 days.

Some substrates deserve special interest as pharmaconutrients. Studies on surgical patients have demonstrated that arginine, fish oil, and nucleotides are beneficial in reducing postoperative infectious complications and length of hospital stay, in both malnourished and well-nourished patients [33]. One study conducted on liver transplant recipients has shown that this type of diet improves nutritional status and decreases the number of infectious complications [34]. Nevertheless, European recommendations do not support the use of these diets routinely. Probiotics and fiber added to enteral nutrition have been also studied and seem to have beneficial effects on the outcome but have not been recommended until now [35]. In our practice, we routinely use diets containing arginine, omega-3 fatty acids, and nucleotides, but we do not use fiber and probiotics.

Hyperglycemia is prevalent in the posttransplant population and theoretically may influence infection rates. Surgical patients admitted in the ICU show better outcomes when a tight glucose is achieved by insulin perfusion drips [36]. Liver transplant patients who develop an infectious complication during ICU stay show higher insulin resistance and increased insulin needs compared with other surgical patients. Despite the lack of data, we have implemented an ICU glucose control protocol with a target level of glycemia, 6.6 and 8.25 mmol/L (Table 23.3).

23.3.2 LONG-TERM MONITORING AND NUTRITIONAL SUPPORT

Once the liver transplant patients reassume oral feeding and leave the hospital, the main purpose of nutritional support is prevention. Oral intake should be maximized with the addition of supplements or by increasing the number of small meals to avoid satiety or vomiting. Complications such as acute rejection, intestinal complications, or infections can disturb oral intake, and sometimes enteral nutrition should be reassumed. Several metabolic complications such as diabetes mellitus, hyperlipidemia, obesity, metabolic syndrome, and osteoporosis are common after OLT, and increase morbidity and mortality [37]. Immunosuppressive drugs are responsible not only for infectious complications but also for several metabolic and nutritional derangements. Steroids, tracolimus, sirolimus, and cyclosporine produce hyperglycemia and hyperlipidemia (Table 23.4). Up to 30% of patients develop new-onset diabetes and this increases with the age of the liver transplant recipient and in patients with chronic hepatitis C [38]. These patients should be followed up closely in order to achieve tight glycemic control and prevent diabetes mellitus–related complications.

Hyperlipidemia and an accelerated form of arteriosclerosis have been also described in patients receiving a liver transplant. Of these patients, 43% will develop hypercholesterolemia and 38% will develop hypertriglyceridemia within 18 months after the procedure. They have an increased risk for the development of coronary disease when compared with their preoperative cardiovascular risk [39]. Patients should receive dietary advice and hypolipidemic drugs such as statins. This group of drugs is not free of adverse effects and can increase the risk of malabsorption, fat-soluble vitamins, and hepatic dysfunction and should be closely monitored. One important consequence of hyperlipidemia is the development of obesity and metabolic syndrome. The greatest weight gain appears in the first 6 months and affects between 60% and 70% of patients. These patients usually have a history of diabetes mellitus, hyperlipidemia, hypertension, or arteriosclerosis, but the effect of steroids and other immunosuppressive drugs should not be minimized. Patients should be aware of the increased cardiovascular risk of obesity and hyperlipidemia and the need to modify their nutritional practice because there are identifiable and treatable [40].

Osteoporosis and low bone mineral density following liver transplantation are frequently seen. Patients show a wide range of bone loss (between 1.5% and 24%), and it is frequently observed within the first 6 months after transplantation. Some risk factors exist even before the transplant, such as physical inactivity, lean body mass losses, and liver disease by itself [41]. Immunosuppressive drugs accelerate this process in the immediate period after the transplant, and the highest incidence of fractures appears in the first year in 20–30% of patients [42]. Alendronate has been recently tested in an uncontrolled study in order to prevent bone loss in liver transplant patients [43].

TABLE 23.4
Metabolic and Nutritional Derangements of Immunosuppressive Drugs

Drug	Mechanism of Action	Adverse Effects
Azathioprine	Purine synthesis inhibitor	• Nausea • Vomiting • Diarrhea • Taste changes • Pancreatitis
Cyclosporine	Inhibits lymphokine production and interleukin release, and reduces function of effector T cells	• Hyperglycemia • Hyperlipidemia • Renal toxicity • CNS toxicity • Hepatic toxicity • Hypomagnesemia • Vitamin D deficiency
Steroids	Decrease immune response, modify carbohydrate metabolism, and increase protein metabolism	• Hyperglycemia • Hyperlipidemia • Increased metabolic rate • Overweight • Osteoporosis • Pancreatitis
Daclizumab	Monoclonal antibody to the IL-2 receptor of T cells that blocks T lymphocyte activation	• Nausea • Vomiting
Mofetil micofenolate	Inhibits purine synthesis and lymphocyte T and B production	• Nausea • Vomiting • Diarrhea • Gastrointestinal hemorrhage
Sirolimus	Inhibits lymphocytes T and B proliferation	• Nausea • Vomiting • Diarrhea • Hyperlipidemia
Antilymphocytic serum	Decreases total lymphocyte count	• Nausea • Vomiting • Diarrhea • Abdominal pain
Tacrolimus	Inhibits lymphocytes T and B proliferation, and IL-2 synthesis	• Nausea • Vomiting • Diarrhea • Hyperglycemia • Hypomagnesemia • CNS toxicity

Note: Summary of the adverse effects of immunosuppressive drugs used to prevent rejection after liver transplantation. CNS, central nervous system; IL-2, interleukin 2.

23.4   SUMMARY POINTS

- A significant number of patients with ESLD who are candidates for OLT suffer from malnutrition at the moment of their inclusion in the waiting list.
- Nutritional assessment and a nutritional plan is a standard of care for these patients.
- SGA and handgrip strength, alone or in combination, are useful tools for clinical assessment of nutritional status.
- Patients with moderate to severe malnutrition should be nourished artificially in the interval between listing and transplantation.
- In the first days after the procedure, patients should be fed artificially until they achieve their energy requirements by the oral route.
- The route of choice for artificial feeding must be the enteral one. TPN should be reserved for complicated cases. Overfeeding should be avoided.
- The nutritional team should be aware of the adverse effects of immunosuppressive drugs. Nutritional counseling and dietary intervention are necessary to prevent overweight and metabolic syndrome.

REFERENCES

1. ONT: Spanish Transplantation Organization. Statistics 2007. Madrid, Spain. http://www.ont.es//estadistica (accessed May 25, 2008).
2. Pikul, J., M. D. Sharpe, R. Lowndes, and C. N. Ghent. 1994. Degree of preoperative malnutrition is predictive of postoperative morbidity in liver transplant recipients. *Transplantation* 57:469–472.
3. Alberino, F., A. Gatta, P. Amodio, et al. 2000. Nutrition and survival in patients with liver cirrhosis. *Nutrition* 17:445–450.
4. Cabre, E., and M. A. Gassull. 2000. Nutritional and metabolic issues in cirrhosis and liver transplantation. *Curr Opin Clin Nutr Metab Care* 3:345–354.
5. Sanchez, A. J., and J. Aranda-Michel. 2006. Nutrition for the liver transplant patient. *Liver Transpl* 12:1310–1316.
6. Moller, S., F. Bendtsen, E. Christensen, and J. H. Henriksen. 1994. Prognostic variables in patients with cirrhosis and oesophageal varices without previous bleeding. *J Hepatol* 21:940–946.
7. Figueiredo, F., E. R. Dickson, T. Pasha, et al. 2000. Impact of nutritional status on outcomes after liver transplantation. *Transplantation* 70:1347–1352.
8. Ockenga, J., S. C. Bischoff, H. L. Tillmann, et al. 2000. Elevated bound leptin correlates with energy expenditure in cirrhotics. *Gastroenterology* 119:1656–1662.
9. Scolapio, J. S., J. Bowen, G. Stoner, and V. Tarrosa. 2000. Substrate oxidation in patients with cirrhosis: Comparison with other nutritional markers. *JPEN J Parenter Enteral Nutr* 24:150–153.
10. Nishida, T., S. Tsuji, M. Tsuji, et al. 2006. Oral glucose tolerance test predicts prognosis of patients with liver cirrhosis. *Am J Gastroenterol* 101:70–75.
11. Cabre, E., A. Abad-Lacruz, M. C. Nunez, et al. 1993. The relationship of plasma polyunsaturated fatty acid deficiency with survival in advanced liver cirrhosis: Multivariate analysis. *Am J Gastroenterol* 88:718–722.
12. De Luis, D. A., O. Izaola, M. C. Velicia, et al. 2006. Impact of dietary intake and nutritional status on outcomes after liver transplantation. *Rev Esp Enferm Dig* 98:6–13.

13. Kondrup, J., S. Allison, M. Elia, B. Vellas, and M. Plauth. 2003. ESPEN Guidelines for Nutrition Screening 2002. *Clin Nutr* 22:415–421.
14. Detsky, A. S., J. R. McLaughlin, J. P. Baker, et al. 1987. What is subjective global assessment of nutritional status? *JPEN J Parenter Enteral Nutr* 11:8–13.
15. Stephenson, G. R., E. W. Moretti, H. El-Moalem, P. A. Clavien, and J. E. Tuttle-Newhall. 2001. Malnutrition in liver transplant patients: Preoperative subjective global assessment is predictive of outcome after liver transplantation. *Transplantation* 72:666–670.
16. Alvares-da-Silva, M. R., and T. Reverbel da Silveira. 2005. Comparison between handgrip strength, subjective global assessment, and prognostic nutritional index in assessing malnutrition and predicting clinical outcome in cirrhotic outpatients. *Nutrition* 21:113–117.
17. Kyle, U. G., L. Genton, G. Mentha, et al. 2001. Reliable bioelectrical impedance analysis estimate of fat-free mass in liver, lung and heart transplantation. *JPEN J Perenter Enteral Nutr* 25:45–51.
18. Als-Nielsen, B., R. L. Koretz, L. L. Kjaergard, and C. Gluud. 2003. Branched-chain amino acids for hepatic encephalopathy. *Cochrane Database Syst Rev* (2):CD001939.
19. Muto, Y., S. Sato, A. Watanabe, et al., for the LOTUS group. 2005. Effects of oral branched chain amino acid granules on event-free survival in patients with liver cirrhosis. *Clin Gastroenterol Hepatol* 3:705–713.
20. Plauth, M., E. Cabré, O. Riggio, et al. 2006. ESPEN Guidelines on Enteral Nutrition: Liver disease. *Clin Nutr* 25:285–294.
21. Plauth, M., M. Merli, J. Kondrup, P. Ferenci, A. Weimann, and M. J. Muller. 1997. ESPEN guidelines for nutrition in liver disease and transplantation. *Clin Nutr* 16:43–55.
22. Jiménez Jiménez, F. J., J. C. Montejo González, and R. Nuñez Ruiz. 2005. Spanish Society of Intensive Care Recommendations. Artificial nutrition in liver failure. *Nutr Hosp* 20:22–24.
23. Cordoba, J., J. Lopez-Hellın, M. Planas, et al. 2004. Normal protein for episodic hepatic encephalopathy: Results of a randomized trial. *J Hepatol* 41:38–43.
24. Le Cornu, K. A., F. J. McKiernan, S. A. Kapadia, and J. M. Neuberger. 2000. A prospective randomized study of preoperative nutritional supplementation in patients awaiting elective orthotopic liver transplantation. *Transplantation* 69:1364–1369.
25. ASPEN Board of Directors and The Clinical Guidelines Task Force. Guidelines for the Use of Parenteral and Enteral Nutrition in Adult and Pediatric Patients. 2002. Solid organ transplant. *JPEN J Parent Ent Nutr* 26 (Suppl 1):74–76.
26. Clavien, P. A., P. R. C. Harvey, and S. M. Strasberg. 1992. Preservation and reperfusion injuries in liver allografts. *Transplantation* 53:957–958.
27. Cywes, R., P. D. Greig, J. R. Sanabria, et al. 1992. Effect of intraportal glucose infusion on hepatic glycogen content and degradation, and outcome in liver transplantation. *Ann Surg* 1216:235–246.
28. Wicks, C., S. Somasundaram, I. Bjarnason, et al. 1994. Comparison of enteral feeding and total parenteral nutrition after liver transplantation. *Lancet* 344:837–840.
29. Hasse, J. M., L. S. Blue, G. U. Liepa, et al. 1995. Early enteral nutrition support in patients undergoing liver transplantation. *JPEN J Parenter Enteral Nutr* 19:437–443.
30. Weimann, A., E. R. Kuse, W. O. Bechstein, J. M. Neuberger, M. Plauth, and R. Pichlmayr. 1998. Perioperative parenteral and enteral nutrition for patients undergoing orthotopic liver transplantation. Results of a questionnaire from 16 European transplant units. *Transpl Int* 11 (Suppl 1):S289–S291.
31. Heyland, D. K., R. Dhaliwal, J. W. Drover, L. Gramlich, P. Dodek, and the Canadian Critical Care Clinical Practice Guidelines Committee. 2003. Canadian clinical practice guidelines for nutrition support in mechanically ventilated, critically ill adult patients. *JPEN J Parenter Enteral Nutr* 27:355–373.

32. Ortiz Leyba, C., J. C. Montejo Gonzalez, F. J. Jiménez Jimenez, and the Spanish Society of Intensive Care Recommendations. 2005. Recommendations for nutritional assessment and specialized nutritional support of critically ill patients. *Nutr Hosp* 20:1–4.
33. Montejo, J. C., A. Zarazaga, J. Lopez-Martinez, et al., and the Spanish Society of Intensive Care Medicine and Coronary Units. 2003. Immunonutrition in the intensive care unit. A systematic review and consensus statement. *Clin Nutr* 22:221–233.
34. Plank, L. D., J. L. McCall, E. J. Gane, et al. 2005. Pre- and postoperative immunonutrition in patients undergoing liver transplantation: A pilot study of safety and efficacy. *Clin Nutr* 24:288–296.
35. Rayes, N., D. Seehofer, T. Theruvath, et al. 2005. Supply of pre- and probiotics reduces bacterial infection rates after liver transplantation: A randomized, double-blind trial. *Am J Transplant* 5:125–130.
36. Van den Berghe, G., P. Wouters, F. Weekers, et al. 2001. Intensive insulin therapy in the critically ill patients. *N Engl J Med* 345:1359–1367.
37. Stegall, M. D., G. Everson, G. Schroter, B. Bilir, F. Karrer, and I. Kam. 1995. Metabolic complications after liver transplantation. Diabetes, hypercholesterolemia, hypertension, and obesity. *Transplantation* 60:1057–1060.
38. Mirabella, S., A. Brunati, A. Ricchiuti, A. Pierini, A. Franchello, and M. Salizzoni. 2005. New-onset diabetes after liver transplantation. *Transplant Proc* 37:2636–2637.
39. Munoz, S. J., R. O. Deems, M. J. Moritz, P. Martin, B. E. Jarrell, and W. C. Maddrey. 1991. Hyperlipidemia and obesity after orthotopic liver transplantation. *Transplant Proc* 23:1480–1483.
40. Baum, C. L. 2001. Weight gain and cardiovascular risk after organ transplantation. *JPEN J Parenter Enteral Nutr* 25:114–119.
41. Sanchez, A. J., and J. Aranda-Michel. 2006. Liver disease and osteoporosis. *Nutr Clin Pract* 21:273–278.
42. Leslie, W. D., C. N. Bernstein, M. S. Leboff, and the American Gastroenterological Association Clinical Practice Committee. 2003. AGA technical review on osteoporosis in hepatic disorders. *Gastroenterology* 25:941–966.
43. Millonig, G., I. W. Graziadci, D. Eichler, K. P. Pfeiffer, et al. 2005. Alendronate in combination with calcium and vitamin D prevents bone loss after orthotopic liver transplantation: A prospective single-center study. *Liver Transpl* 11:960–966.

Index